Understanding and Treating
Anxiety in Autism

by the same authors

Understanding and Treating Self-Injurious Behavior in Autism
A Multi-Disciplinary Perspective
Edited by Stephen M. Edelson and Jane Botsford Johnson
Foreword by Temple Grandin
ISBN 978 1 84905 741 7
eISBN 978 1 78450 189 1

Infantile Autism
The Syndrome and Its Implications for a Neural Theory
of Behavior by Bernard Rimland, Ph.D.
50th Anniversary updated edition
Edited by Stephen M. Edelson
Forewords by Temple Grandin, Ph.D. and Margaret L. Bauman, M.D.
ISBN 978 1 84905 789 9
eISBN 978 1 78450 057 3

Siblings
The Autism Spectrum Through Our Eyes
Jane Johnson and Anne Van Rensselaer
ISBN 978 1 84905 829 2
eISBN 978 0 85700 281 5

Families of Adults with Autism
Stories and Advice for the Next Generation
Edited by Jane Johnson and Anne Van Rensselaer
ISBN 978 1 84310 885 6
eISBN 978 1 84642 766 4

UNDERSTANDING AND TREATING ANXIETY IN AUTISM

A MULTI-DISCIPLINARY APPROACH

EDITED BY STEPHEN M. EDELSON AND JANE BOTSFORD JOHNSON

FOREWORD BY DR. DAVID G. AMARAL

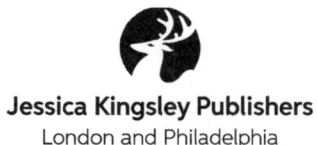

Jessica Kingsley Publishers
London and Philadelphia

First published in Great Britain in 2021 by Jessica Kingsley Publishers
An Hachette Company

2

Copyright © Jessica Kingsley Publishers 2021

Figure 6.1 reproduced from Miller *et al.* 2007 by permission of
the American Occupational Therapy Association.
Figure 6.2 reproduced from Autism, 2nd Edition by Sue Fletcher-Watson and
Francesca Happé, published by Routledge. © 2019 Sue Fletcher-Watson and
Francesca Happé. Reproduced by arrangement with Taylor & Francis Books UK.
Figures 9.1–9.4 reproduced by permission of the Groden Center.

Front cover background artwork by Starkow.

A CIP catalogue record for this title is available from the
British Library and the Library of Congress

ISBN 978 1 78775 152 1
eISBN 978 1 78775 153 8

Printed and bound in Great Britain by CPI Group

Jessica Kingsley Publishers' policy is to use papers that are natural, renewable and recyclable
products and made from wood grown in sustainable forests. The logging and manufacturing
processes are expected to conform to the environmental regulations of the country of origin.

Jessica Kingsley Publishers
73 Collier Street
London N1 9BE, UK

www.jkp.com

CONTENTS

Foreword

David G. Amaral, Ph.D., U.C. Davis Distinguished Professor, Department of Psychiatry and Behavioral Sciences, U.C. Davis MIND Institute

Even from the first formal description of its symptoms, anxiety has been a prominent component of autism. In his seminal article describing the characteristics of autism, Kanner (1943) mentions the fears of several of his first 11 patients. He writes about Case 8, "Alfred," who "frets when the bread is put in the oven to be made into toast, and is afraid it will get burned and be hurt. He is upset when the sun sets. He is upset because the moon does not always appear in the sky at night." While the appreciation that people with autism also suffer from anxiety came early, clinicians and researchers have struggled ever since to differentiate anxiety from the core features of autism. Kanner described "Donald," who was willing to play on a slide at the playground when alone but was "horrorstruck" when other children were present. His avoidance of children may have reflected social disinterest or awkwardness, which is consistent with the core features of autism or, as Kanner actually suggested, a fear of being in the presence of other children, which is more consistent with anxiety. To make things more complicated, his fear may have been related to worrying about what people thought of him (which is consistent with social anxiety disorder) or could have been a concern about anticipating and interpreting social interaction (which could be viewed as symptoms of autism). These difficulties in determining when an autistic individual also has anxiety have led to studies suggesting that anywhere between 11 and 84 percent of children with autism may experience clinically significant anxiety (Kerns and Kendall, 2012). It has also been unclear how IQ is associated with anxiety in autism. Some studies have suggested that higher IQ is associated with greater anxiety symptoms, but this finding has not been universal. Some have suggested that clinically significant anxiety may be equally prevalent in autistic children with and without intellectual impairment when varied forms of anxiety are considered.

The vast majority of studies of anxiety in autism have relied on parent report measures of anxiety rather than semi-structured interviews. The ability of these brief assays to differentiate between autism and anxiety symptoms and capture distinct presentations of anxiety in autism may be limited, given that most measures were developed and validated for children without autism. We have recently been fortunate to collaborate with Dr. Connor Kerns, a clinical psychologist, currently at the University of British Columbia, who is an expert on anxiety in autism. She has developed the Autism Spectrum Addendum (Kerns *et al.*, 2017), which is a series of prompts and guidelines that are woven into the Anxiety Disorders Interview Schedule–IV–Parent Interview (ADIS-P) protocol, to tailor the instrument for children with autism. The ADIS-P is a semi-structured interview conducted with parents to assess the presence of childhood anxiety disorders with strong inter-rater and test-retest reliability. We have used this instrument to evaluate a large population of children who are about 11 years old at the U.C. Davis MIND Institute (Kerns *et al.*, 2020). We found that 69 percent of the children with autism had clinically significant anxiety in comparison to 8 percent of a comparison group of typically developing children. We also broke down anxiety into DSM-type, such as generalized anxiety disorder or social phobia, and "distinct anxiety," which includes idiosyncratic fears (e.g., fears of toilets, specific sounds, glasses, beards) and other social fears (which include social fears related to social confusion rather than fear of negative evaluation). We found that the rates of both DSM-anxiety disorders and distinct anxiety were not significantly different for children with or without intellectual impairment. However, the vast majority of DSM anxiety disorders in children with intellectual disability were specific phobias, while DSM anxiety disorders (other than phobia) were significantly less common in children with (8%) versus without (36%) intellectual impairment. Thus, autistic individuals with intellectual disability also have concerning symptoms of anxiety, but they appear to be qualitatively different from those of individuals without cognitive disability. A take-home message from this study is that accurate assessment is critical to ensure that all children suffering from anxiety problems are identified and given access to appropriate interventions.

The prominence of anxiety in the behavioral challenges associated with autism also has implications for an understanding of the neurobiology of the disorder. Fear and anxiety have been major areas of fundamental neuroscience research for well over half a century (LeDoux and Pine, 2016). Several brain regions have been implicated in the mediation of fear and anxiety: chief among them is a small, almond-shaped structure in the temporal lobe of the brain called the amygdala. Thirty years ago, Brothers suggested that the amygdala also plays a prominent role in guiding social behavior (Brothers, Ring, and Kling, 1990). Given that early postmortem studies by Kemper and Bauman (1993) indicated that the amygdala demonstrated pathology, Baron-Cohen suggested that dysfunction of the amygdala might be the neurobiological substrate of the altered behaviors of autism (Baron-Cohen *et al.*, 2000). Based on our basic research studies of the amygdala, we proposed the contrary hypothesis that the amygdala does not play a primary role in the social alterations of autism but likely is important as a substrate for co-occurring anxiety (Amaral, Bauman, and Schumann, 2003; Amaral and Corbett, 2003). Researchers are still debating the relative merits of these hypotheses. There is no doubt, however, that the structure, connectivity, and function of the amygdala is altered in some individuals with autism (Avino *et al.*, 2018; Nordahl *et al.*, 2012), and research is ongoing to determine whether alterations in the structure and function of the amygdala can predict who on the autism spectrum will also be at risk for anxiety disorders. The principle that emerges is that many but not all individuals with autism have significant anxiety, nor do all individuals have identifiable alterations in amygdala structure and function.

The current book is an important contribution to the autism community. As with its predecessor, which focused on self-injurious behavior, Edelson and Johnson have identified a highly common co-occurring condition in autism and brought together authors who describe steps that are being taken now to alleviate anxiety in autistic people. In 1998, when the U.C. Davis MIND Institute was established, the parent founders gave us the mission of "curing" autism. In the intervening 20 years, I believe that the world of autism researchers and clinicians has come to appreciate that this may be the wrong goal. Educated by the neurodiversity movement, we have learned that autism per se is not the enemy, but rather the debilitating conditions associated with it such as anxiety, epilepsy, gastrointestinal problems, and sleep disorders. The benefit of this perspective is that while we do not have effective treatments directed at the core features of autism, there are many excellent interventions for conditions such as anxiety. This book provides summaries of both behavioral approaches, such as cognitive behavior therapy, and pharmaceutical strategies, such as selective serotonin reuptake inhibitors. Of course, much research needs to be done to determine if having autism necessitates modifications of these therapies from what is done with typically developing individuals. But this is refining strategy rather than starting from scratch. Unfortunately, for reasons that are complex, individuals with autism appear to have more medical problems than typically developing individuals (Croen *et al.*, 2015), which also shortens their average lifespan (Hirvikoski *et al.*, 2016). By bringing awareness of how common anxiety is in autism to the greater autism community, Edelson and Johnson are doing a tremendous service. It goes without saying that accurate diagnosis and effective treatment of anxiety in autistic individuals will not solve all of their problems—but it will certainly improve the quality of their lives. This may also have the added benefit of allowing them to be more open to interventions that are directed at other core and co-occurring conditions.

References

Amaral, D. G., Bauman, M. D., and Schumann, C. M. (2003). The amygdala and autism: implications from non-human primate studies. *Genes, Brain and Behavior, 2*(5), 295–302.

Amaral, D. G., and Corbett, B. A. (2003). The amygdala, autism and anxiety. *Novartis Foundation Symposium, 251*, 177–187; discussion 187–197, 281–297.

Avino, T. A., Barger, N., Vargas, M. V., *et al.* (2018). Neuron numbers increase in the human amygdala from birth to adulthood, but not in autism. *Proceedings of the National Academy of Sciences USA, 115*(14), 3710–3715.

Baron-Cohen, S., Ring, H. A., Bullmore, E. T., Wheelwright, S., Ashwin, C., and Williams, S. C. (2000). The amygdala theory of autism. *Neuroscience & Biobehavioral Reviews, 24*(3), 355–364.

Brothers, L., Ring, B., and Kling, A. (1990). Response of neurons in the macaque amygdala to complex social stimuli. *Behavioural Brain Research, 41*(3), 199–213.

Croen, L. A., Zerbo, O., Qian, Y., *et al.* (2015). The health status of adults on the autism spectrum. *Autism, 19*(7), 814–823.

Hirvikoski, T., Mittendorfer-Rutz, E., Boman, M., Larsson, H., Lichtenstein, P., and Bolte, S. (2016). Premature mortality in autism spectrum disorder. *British Journal of Psychiatry, 208*(3), 232–238.

Kanner, L. (1943). Autistic disturbances of affective contact. *Nervous Child, 2* 217–250.

Kemper, T. L., and Bauman, M. L. (1993). The contribution of neuropathologic studies to the understanding of autism. *Neurologic Clinics, 11*(1), 175–187.

Kerns, C. M., and Kendall, P. C. (2012). The presentation and classification of anxiety in autism spectrum disorder. *Clinical Psychology: Science and Practice, 19*(4), 323–347.

Kerns, C. M., Renno, P., Kendall, P. C., Wood, J. J., and Storch, E. A. (2017). Anxiety Disorders Interview Schedule-Autism Addendum: Reliability and validity in children with autism spectrum disorder. *Journal of Clinical Child & Adolescent Psychology, 46*(1), 88–100.

Kerns, C. M., Winder-Patel, B., Iosif, A. M., *et al*. (2020). Clinically significant anxiety in children with autism spectrum disorder and varied intellectual functioning. *Journal of Clinical Child & Adolescent Psychology*, 1–16, doi: 10.1080/15374416.2019.1703712.

LeDoux, J. E., and Pine, D. S. (2016). Using neuroscience to help understand fear and anxiety: A two-system framework. *American Journal of Psychiatry, 173*(11), 1083–1093.

Nordahl, C. W., Scholz, R., Yang, X., *et al*. (2012). Increased rate of amygdala growth in children aged 2 to 4 years with autism spectrum disorders: a longitudinal study. *Archives of General Psychiatry, 69*(1), 53–61.

Introduction

Lauren J. Moskowitz, Ph.D., St. John's University, New York, and
Stephen M. Edelson, Ph.D., Autism Research Institute, California

Many people on the autism spectrum suffer from anxiety, significantly reducing their quality of life. Understanding the biology that underlies anxiety, as well as its relationship to observable behaviors in individuals with autism spectrum disorders (ASD), will allow clinicians to better recognize and treat this complex and challenging condition.

This book is a practical resource for clinicians and researchers as well as for those with ASD and their parents. The chapters provide a detailed description of the published research and also offer an overview of treatment interventions involving neurology, medicine, nutrition, cognition, and behavior.

History of Anxiety in ASD

Although anxiety is not part of the diagnostic criteria for ASD, it is increasingly being recognized that it is one of the most common presenting problems for individuals with ASD (White *et al.*, 2009). In fact, in the earliest description of children with autism, Kanner (1943) noted that several of these children exhibited significant fear (e.g., fear of vacuum cleaners) and anxiety; for example, Alfred displayed a "good deal of 'worrying': he frets when the bread is put in the oven to be made into toast, and is afraid it will get burnt and be hurt. He is upset when the sun sets" (p.233). Kanner believed that the restricted and repetitive behaviors that are characteristic of autism were driven by the "anxiously obsessive desire for the maintenance of sameness" (ibid., p.245). For example, he described how Susan T. "noticed some cracks in the office ceiling and walls. She kept asking anxiously and repeatedly who had cracked the ceiling and could not be calmed by any answer given her. She was obviously unhappy and every time she was in the office, she kept exclaiming: 'Who cracked the ceiling?' 'How did it crack itself?'" (Kanner, 1951).

Why Might Individuals with ASD be Predisposed to Anxiety?

Fear and anxiety are more prevalent in youth with ASD than in typically developing youth and those with other developmental disabilities. It is likely that there are many characteristics inherent to autism—such as the need to maintain sameness and sensory sensitivities, as well as difficulties in communication, social interaction, forming or sustaining friendships, and understanding other people's actions and intentions—that predispose individuals with ASD to be more anxious than those without ASD, or that can predispose them to stressful experiences that lead to anxiety. For example, it is hard for individuals with ASD to pick up on social cues and "read" other people, and this could make the world a more unpredictable and scary place (Rodgers, 2018). Those with ASD could also experience increased anxiety when their behaviors are in conflict with social expectations or demands or when their behaviors cause punishing reactions from others (Wood and Gadow, 2010).

Why is Anxiety Often Overlooked in ASD?

Recent research suggests that approximately 40 percent of youth with ASD meet criteria for at least one anxiety disorder (van Steensel, Bogels, and Perrin, 2011), with as many as 84 percent experiencing some degree of impairing anxiety (White *et al.*, 2009). There is much less research on anxiety in adults with ASD, but a recent systematic review estimated the current and lifetime prevalence was 27 and 42 percent, respectively (Hollocks *et al.*, 2019). Both of these percentages are likely an underestimate, given that anxiety is often overlooked in this population. Despite longstanding clinical accounts of anxiety in children with ASD (e.g., Kanner, 1943, 1951), historically, applied assessment and treatment research focused almost exclusively on behaviors without acknowledging the role of affect and cognitions in the lives of these individuals. Thus, affective states such as fear, anxiety, or sadness were rarely discussed or acknowledged. This is in large part due to the difficulty of assessing or measuring anxiety in people with ASD, given that they often lack the ability to self-report or communicate their thoughts and emotions and may express these thoughts or emotions in idiosyncratic ways.

Communication Deficits

One reason anxiety is so difficult to assess is due to the inherent communication impairments in ASD. "Anxiety" is a multi-component construct that involves *feelings* or affective states (e.g., subjective fear and panic experienced), *cognitions* (thoughts, beliefs, and images, such as worry and dread), *behavioral* escape or avoidance of the feared situation (and nonverbal behaviors such as crying, whining, and visible muscle tension), and associated *physiological arousal* (Barlow, 2000; Wolpe, 1958). Unlike behaviors, the thoughts, subjective emotional/affective state, and physiological arousal that are part of the construct of anxiety often cannot be directly observed. This makes it difficult to assess or identify anxiety, particularly in those who also have intellectual disability (ID) and/ or minimal verbal ability. This is because anxiety in typically developing (TD) individuals is usually assessed through self-reports on thoughts, feelings, and behaviors ("self-report"), and/or asking parents, teachers, staff, or other caregivers to report on the individual's thoughts, feelings, and behaviors ("other-informant report"). Given that people with ASD often cannot report or articulate their emotional states, traditional assessment of anxiety using paper-and-pencil self-reports or verbal self-reports (interviews) is often difficult or impossible (Hagopian and Jennett, 2008). After all, communication in ASD is universally impaired to some degree; approximately 30 percent of children with ASD are functionally nonverbal (Tager-Flusberg and Kasari, 2013), and even those who have verbal language tend not to signal their emotional states to others (Rogers, 1998) and often have difficulty describing their mental states, mental experiences, and daily life experiences (Leyfer *et al.*, 2006).

For example, in an interview with Mark Rimland, a 63-year-old man with ASD, he did not describe himself as being *afraid* of elevators, bridges, or cafés, but he did acknowledge that he *avoids* them. When asked why he avoids elevators, he explained, "Slow elevators make me not sure that it's going to open. I have trouble believing that the door is going to open when it gets there. It feels more safer to ride in the fast elevators, it feels more like it's working." In response to probing about his feared outcome if the elevator did not open, he said, "I hope that I won't die of starvation." Similarly, Mark also stated that, "It's hard for me to walk across bridges." When asked about his feared outcome, similar to the elevator, his fear seemed to be about physical harm befalling him; he responded, "If I walk too far, I might get dizzy and fall." He also described his avoidance of cafés: "When I hear lots of talking and I don't know what people are talking about, I'm worried that they're saying I'm not a good person and I'm going to jail." Once he thought a person at a café said something negative about him, so he avoided that café for a couple of months, but he did eventually go back. He described rituals he engages in to reduce his anxiety in these situations, although once again he did not use the term "anxiety." He stated, "I sing inside my head over and over, 'Hello my name is Mark Rimland, hello my name is Mark Rimland' while walking across the bridge. It seems to be a help with being able to make it over the bridge, but it still seems very hard to make it across." When asked why or how repeating that phrase seemed to help him or make him feel better, he responded, "It seems to be a part of remembering how to talk in order to keep from forgetting how to talk." It could be that, when he feels afraid, it makes him feel as if he is going to forget how to talk. When asked about his coping strategies in cafés, Mark responded that he asks someone else whether his thought/fear is true, and they usually tell him that it is untrue.

Thus, although even highly verbal adults with ASD may not use words such as "anxious" or "afraid" or "worried" or "nervous" in describing their emotional states, they may still be able to articulate a feared outcome—i.e., that something bad will happen to them—and describe behaviors they engage in to make themselves feel better. However, in addition to limiting the usefulness of self-report, the difficulty of describing their mental states/ experiences and signaling their emotions to others might cause caretakers to be unaware of these individuals' thoughts, feelings, and behaviors, which could also limit the usefulness of other-informant reports and interviews.

Idiosyncratic Behavioral Expression

A second reason why anxiety is so difficult to assess in this population is because the actual behavioral expression of anxiety may differ from the expression of anxiety in TD individuals, making it more difficult for caretakers or providers to identify the symptoms of anxiety, which further limits the usefulness of other-informant reports. In other words, the symptoms of anxiety may present differently in people with ASD. In our clinical experience, individuals with ASD may express their anxiety in idiosyncratic ways, such as, for one child, plugging his ears, or, for someone else, using the perseverative phrase, "C'mon everybody!" or, for a third child, humming in a very specific way that escalates in volume and speed as his anxiety increases.

Not only is the behavioral expression or manifestation of anxiety often different, but the content of the anxiety may differ for some individuals with ASD. Indeed, Kerns *et al.* (2014) reported the prevalence of atypical symptoms of anxiety (e.g., fears of bears, graffiti, running water, mechanical noise) in some youth with ASD, in addition to the more common or traditional displays. Moreover, people with ASD are more likely than TD individuals to express fear and anxiety through "acting out" or "problem behaviors" such as aggression, self-injurious behaviors, and tantrums (White *et al.*, 2009). For example, Evans *et al.* (2005) found that the fears of children with ASD were more related to problem behaviors than the fears of children with Down syndrome and mental-age-matched and chronological-age-matched TD children. Many parents or teachers of children with ASD may attribute such "acting out" behavior to anger, irritability, frustration, boredom, noncompliance, disobedience, or oppositionality, rather than recognizing that the behavior is a sign of anxiety. Anecdotally, parents and teachers of children with ASD frequently report that the problem behavior often seems to "come out of nowhere," with no reliable antecedents and no apparent function or cause. One explanation for this unpredictable behavior is that psychological distress, in particular anxiety, may be an internal, and thus often unobservable, antecedent to problem behavior (Romanczyk and Matthews, 1998). It is important for parents, teachers, and practitioners to recognize that fear or anxiety may be causally or functionally related to problem behavior in many children with ASD (which was supported by Moskowitz *et al.*, 2013), in that some may engage in problem behavior to avoid, escape, reduce, or otherwise alleviate their anxiety. In other words, many children with ASD may engage in problem behavior *because* they are anxious and do not know how to cope with this anxiety, or because problem behavior *is* in fact their way of coping with anxiety (see Moskowitz and Ritter, 2016).

Symptom Overlap and Diagnostic Overshadowing

Given the current diagnostic classification system (the DSM-5), practitioners often have difficulty determining if certain symptoms are part of the ASD itself or a separate comorbid anxiety disorder (White *et al.*, 2009). For example, it can be difficult to distinguish whether a symptom such as social avoidance is due to social phobia (especially if the person cannot or does not articulate fear of being embarrassed) or is simply due to the deficits in social interaction that are characteristic of ASD (e.g., "abnormal social approach," "failure to initiate or respond to social interactions"; DSM-V; American Psychiatric Association, 2013). Similarly, it can be difficult to disentangle whether a symptom such as compulsive checking should be classified as a ritual related to obsessive-compulsive disorder (OCD) or as a "ritualized pattern of verbal or nonverbal behavior" (DSM-V; American Psychiatric Association, 2013) related to ASD. Ultimately, as Wood and Gadow (2010) suggested, the only way to distinguish between the overlapping symptoms of ASD and anxiety disorders may be to assess the function of the symptom —for example, to assess the function of the ritual (i.e., whether it is to obtain pleasure by engaging in a preferred ritual or routine, or to escape/avoid or reduce anxiety or distress by engaging in a ritual) or to assess the function of the social avoidance (i.e., whether the child is avoiding social interaction because he does not enjoy it versus because he is afraid of being scrutinized or rejected). Still, it may be difficult or even impossible to assess these functions if a child cannot talk, or if he cannot accurately report his own mental state.

Related to the difficulty of disentangling symptoms of anxiety disorders from symptoms of ASD, another reason that anxiety is often overlooked is because of "diagnostic overshadowing." Diagnostic overshadowing refers to the tendency for practitioners to attribute symptoms of anxiety and other psychopathology to the cognitive impairments of the child or to the autism itself (Reiss, Levitan, and Szyszko, 1982). In other words, the symptoms of anxiety may be minimized or "overshadowed" by the child's autism or ID. For example, White *et al.* (2009) noted that anxiety disorders are seldom diagnosed in ASD due to a general clinical consensus that symptoms of these disorders are "better explained by the ASD itself."

Intellectual Disability (ID)

Many researchers have suggested that individuals with ASD who are "higher functioning" (e.g., those who have average or above average intelligence and/or verbal ability) may experience more anxiety than those who are "lower functioning" (e.g., those who have an ID and/or are nonverbal or minimally verbal) (e.g., Weisbrot *et al.*, 2005). For instance, Sukhodolsky *et al.* (2008) found that children without cognitive impairment (IQ ≥ 70) were rated by their parents to display more anxiety than were those with cognitive impairment (IQ < 70). One common explanation for these findings is that children without ID are likely to have a greater understanding of their difficulties as compared with peers, which leads to increased anxiety. However, another reason for the findings that children without ID are reported to display more anxiety than children with ID could be due to the difficulty of recognizing, assessing, or measuring anxiety in children with ASD who have a cognitive impairment, given that they are even more likely than cognitively able children with ASD to lack the ability to self-report or communicate their fear or anxiety, and may express their fear or anxiety in idiosyncratic ways. Thus, it may be that parents, teachers, or clinicians may not recognize fear or anxiety in children with ASD who are minimally verbal and/or have ID, and may even attribute their problem behavior (e.g., aggression, self-injury, tantrums) to noncompliance, disobedience, oppositionality, or anger/irritability rather than attributing their problem behavior to fear or anxiety.

About This Book

Experts from many different fields have contributed to this book, offering insight into the complicated relationship between ASD and anxiety as well as the importance of treating anxiety using a multi-pronged approach.

Chapter 1 provides an in-depth overview of the neurological systems involved in anxiety and puts forth an argument as to how these systems, which are impaired in autism, are interrelated in a dysregulated manner. It also describes objective measures clinicians and researchers can use to assess many of the biological components of anxiety.

Chapter 2 analyzes the bi-directional relationship between the autonomic nervous system and the immune system, both of which are dysregulated in autism, and describes how their interaction may contribute to anxiety.

Chapter 3 discusses immune activation and its association with both common environmental toxins and autism. It also describes how immune activation, along with its effects on the autonomic nervous system, may be associated with an anxious condition.

Chapter 4 describes the gastrointestinal system and how it relates to other biological systems in the framework of anxiety. It also discusses how the microbiome, which is known to be dysregulated in autism, may contribute to anxiety.

Chapter 5 addresses the important role that healthy eating, supplement use, and avoidance of harmful ingredients can play in reducing anxiety, and explores the effects of diet on the microbiome.

Chapter 6 reviews eight sensory processing systems and three dysregulated processing (modulation) patterns, and explains how dysfunctional processing of internal and external sensations may be associated with anxiety.

Chapter 7 discusses a multi-disciplinary approach to understanding and treating anxiety. This includes evaluating medical issues, sensory processing disorders, and challenging behaviors. In addition, Temple Grandin comments on her personal experiences with anxiety, many of which relate to the topics discussed in the book.

Chapter 8 provides an overview of pharmacological interventions commonly prescribed to treat anxiety in autism, and shows how these medications affect specific neurochemical systems that contribute to an anxious state.

Chapter 9 discusses many of the cognitive and behavioral impairments associated with anxiety in autism, as well as interventions that are known to control stress and anxiety across the spectrum.

Chapter 10 provides a thorough review of several multi-component constructs of anxiety. In addition, it describes how to tailor cognitive and behavioral therapies to an individual's level of functioning.

Finally, the conclusion of the book argues that to best understand and treat anxiety in individuals with ASD, we need to evaluate its numerous biological and behavioral elements. It describes how quantitative assessment measures, obtained prior to and after implementing treatments, can enable us to optimize treatment plans for individuals across the entire spectrum.

References

American Psychiatric Association (2013). *Diagnostic and Statistical Manual of Mental Disorders* (5th ed.). Washington, DC: American Psychiatric Association.

Barlow, D. H. (2000). Unraveling the mysteries of anxiety and its disorders from the perspective of emotion theory. *American Psychologist, 55*, 1247–1263.

Evans, D. W., Canavera, K., Kleinpeter, F. L., Maccubbin, E., and Taga, K. (2005). The fears, phobias, and anxieties of children with autism spectrum disorders and Down syndrome: Comparisons with developmentally and chronologically age matched children. *Child Psychiatry and Human Development, 36*, 3–26.

Hagopian, L. P., and Jennett, H. K. (2008). Behavioral assessment and treatment of anxiety in individuals with intellectual disabilities. *Journal of Developmental and Physical Disabilities, 20*, 467–483.

Hollocks, M. J., Lerh, J. W., Magiati, I., Meiser-Stedman, R., Brugha, T. S. (2019). Anxiety and depression in adults with autism spectrum disorder: A systematic review and meta-analysis. *Psychological Medicine, 49*, 559–572.

Kanner, L. (1943). Autistic disturbances of affective contact. *Nervous Child, 2*, 217–250.

Kanner, L. (1951). The conception of wholes and parts in early infantile autism. *The American Journal of Psychiatry, 108*, 23–26.

Kerns, C. M., Kendall, P. C., Berry, L., Souders, M. C., Franklin, M. E., Schultz, R. T., ... Herrington, J. (2014). Traditional and atypical presentations of anxiety in youth with autism spectrum disorder. *Journal of Autism and Developmental Disorders, 44*, 2851.

Leyfer, O., Folstein, S. E., Bacalman, S., Davis, N. O., Dinh, E., Morgan, J., ... Lainhart, J. E. (2006). Comorbid psychiatric disorders in children with autism: Interview development and rates of disorders. *Journal of Autism and Developmental Disorders, 36*, 849–861.

Moskowitz, L. J., Mulder, E., Walsh, C., McLaughlin, D. M., Zarcone, J., Hajcak, G., and Carr, E. G. (2013). A multimethod assessment of anxiety and problem behavior in children with autism spectrum disorders and intellectual disability. *American Journal on Intellectual and Developmental Disabilities, 118*, 419–434.

Moskowitz, L. J., and Ritter, A. B. (2016). Assessment and intervention for self-injurious behavior related to anxiety. In S. M. Edelson and J. Johnson (Eds.), *Understanding and Treating Self-Injurious Behavior in Autism: A Multidisciplinary Perspective*. London: Jessica Kingsley Publishers.

Reiss, S., Levitan, G. W., and Szyszko, J. (1982). Emotional disturbance and mental retardation: Diagnostic overshadowing. *American Journal of Mental Deficiency, 86*, 567–574.

Rodgers, J. (2018, February 22). Anxiety in autistic people. Retrieved from https://network.autism.org.uk/good-practice/evidence-base/anxiety-autistic-people.

Rogers, S. J. (1998). Neuropsychology of autism in young children and its implications for early intervention. *Mental Retardation and Developmental Disabilities Research Reviews, 4*, 104–112.

Romanczyk, R. G., and Matthews, A. L. (1998). Physiological state as antecedent: Utilization in functional analysis. In J. Luiselli and M. Cameron (Eds.), *Antecedent Control: Innovative Approaches to Behavioral Support*. Baltimore: Brookes.

Sukhodolsky, D. G., Scahill, L., Gadow, K. D., Arnold, L. E., Aman, M. G., McDougle, C. J., ... Vitiello, B. (2008). Parent rated anxiety symptoms in children with pervasive developmental disorders: Frequency and association with core autism symptoms and cognitive functioning. *Journal of Abnormal Child Psychology, 36*, 117.

Tager-Flusberg, H., and Kasari, C. (2013). Minimally verbal school-aged children with autism spectrum disorder: The neglected end of the spectrum. *Autism Research, 6*, 468–478.

van Steensel, F. J. A., Bogels, S. M., and Perrin., S. (2011). Anxiety disorders in children and adolescents with autistic spectrum disorders: A meta-analysis. *Clinical Child and Family Psychology Review, 14*, 302–317.

Weisbrot, D. M., Gadow, K. D., DeVincent, C. J., and Pomeroy, J. (2005). The presentation of anxiety in children with pervasive developmental disorders. *Journal of Child and Adolescent Psychopharmacology, 15*, 477–496.

White, S. W., Oswald, D., Ollendick, T., and Scahill, L. (2009). Anxiety in children and adolescents with autism spectrum disorders. *Clinical Psychology Review, 29*, 216–229.

Wolpe, J. (1958). *Psychotherapy by Reciprocal Inhibition*. Stanford, CA: Stanford University Press.

Wood, J. J., and Gadow, K. D. (2010). Exploring the nature and function of anxiety in youth with autism spectrum disorders. *Clinical Psychology: Science and Practice, 17*, 281–292.

CHAPTER 1

Psychophysiological Markers of Arousal and Anxiety in Children with Autism Spectrum Disorder

Estate M. Sokhadze, Ph.D., Emily L. Casanova, Ph.D., Eva V. Lamina, Ph.D., and Desmond Kelly, M.D., University of South Carolina School of Medicine, Greenville, South Carolina, and Manuel F. Casanova, M.D., University of South Carolina School of Medicine, Greenville and Prisma Health System, Greenville, South Carolina

Introduction

Autism Spectrum Disorder (ASD) is characterized by severe disturbances in establishing reciprocal social relations, varying degrees of language and communication difficulties, and restricted, repetitive, and stereotyped behavioral patterns. Diagnostic manuals (e.g., DSM-IV-TR, DSM-5, ICD-10, ADI-R, and ADOS-2) also include, as a defining feature, qualitative impairments in emotional competence. Disturbances of affective reactivity and innate inability to perceive and respond to the social and emotional signals in a typical and appropriate manner are well-known deficits of ASD. No individual sign is pathognomonic of autism, and there is marked clinical heterogeneity among patients. When assessing children within the autism spectrum, it is therefore necessary to examine for accessory symptoms and comorbidities that, although not considered core features, are common, and may be a major handicap to the individual. Indeed, though the core symptoms of ASD have been the focus of research for many years, less is known about anxiety in ASD. Addressing it is a challenge, but understanding its pathophysiology can lead to more efficacious treatments and improved outcomes. Another frequent symptom of ASD is autonomic nervous system (ANS) dysfunction, observed both during the resting state and during exposure to stressors. There are reasons to believe that the stated symptoms of ASD do not happen coincidentally, but rather are intertwined by common pathology. The present chapter aims to review different paradigms for the investigation and understanding of ASD symptomatology. In particular, we consider investigation of emotional reactivity in children with ASD using psychophysiological methods, as a launching pad to study its relationship to other symptomatology, while simultaneously probing the possible neural substrates. This chapter suggests a model wherein indices of resting anterior electroencephalographic (EEG) asymmetry as well as frontal event-related EEG gamma oscillations asymmetry, i.e., measures reflecting brain processes associated with individual differences in approach and avoidance motivation, help explain differences in the expression of core autistic symptoms (Maxwell *et al.*, 2015; Sutton *et al.*, 2005). Our review will also discuss specifics of autonomic balance dysregulation as correlates to core symptoms of autism. One of the primary purposes of our chapter is the discussion of how application of affective psychophysiological tests can be used for in-depth analysis of the patterns of central and autonomic activity related to the experienced emotion in children with ASD and in typically developing (TD) children.

Autonomic Nervous System Activity in Autism

A series of current studies have shown an exponentially increasing interest in the investigation of the ANS activity abnormalities in children with ASD (Cohen *et al.*, 2015; Kleberg, 2015; Klusek *et al.*, 2015; Kushki *et al.*, 2013; Smeekens *et al.*, 2015; Sokhadze *et al.*, 2016a, 2017, 2019). Considering that sympathetic activation is often associated with autonomic arousal and anxiety, investigation of impairments of arousal regulation definitely deserves to become one of the main goals of autism research. Stereotyped and repetitive motor behaviors, among the core features of autism, might represent an attempt to reduce hyper-responsive sympathetic activity (Hirstein *et al.*, 2001; Toichi and Kamio, 2003; Spielmann and Miller, Chapter 6). Symptoms suggestive of a deficiency in autonomic control in ASD indicate the feasibility of developing a set of biomarkers defining autonomic phenotypes. It is possible to propose that clearly defined autonomic arousal phenotypes may open a new perspective for behavioral, pharmacological, and neuromodulation (e.g., heart rate variability (HRV) biofeedback) interventions in autism. Eventually, as noted by Rees (2014), there is an urgent need to accelerate recognition of the importance of ANS activity investigation in pediatrics, not limiting it to neurodevelopmental disorders.

Electroencephalographic Asymmetry in Autism

Recent studies linking frontal EEG asymmetry, specifically in high frequency (> th 30 Hz) EEG bands, are compatible with findings of excessive cortical excitation/inhibition (E/I) ratio, reduced GABAergic activity, and abnormal EEG gamma (30–80 Hz) activity in autism, wherein fast-spiking interneurons (responsible for gamma oscillations) are primarily affected. Studies in this research area may help us to better understand the etiology of this disorder, specifically in terms of the emotional and social communication impairments typical for ASD. We believe that knowledge of the link between E/I imbalance, atypical laterality, coherence and power of spontaneous and induced gamma-band activity, autonomic dysfunctions, and social functioning can also contribute to evaluating the effect of neuromodulation (e.g., transcranial magnetic stimulation (TMS), neurofeedback, etc.) pharmacological, and behavioral interventions for children with ASD.

This chapter attempts to examine the possibility that spontaneous resting-state and induced gamma-band power or hemispheric gamma asymmetry in individuals with ASD may predict the severity of autistic symptoms. In particular, we consider the possibility that atypically high induced gamma-band power, low hemispheric coherence, and left-dominant gamma asymmetry would be predictive of more severe presentation of core autistic symptoms. There is growing evidence in the literature that atypical hemispheric specialization may be a neurobiological marker for ASD (de Groot and van Strien, 2018; Heunis *et al.*, 2016, 2018). Atypical lateralization of the electrophysiological indices (e.g., EEG and event-related potentials (ERP)) of face processing have been reported in children (Webb *et al.*, 2006), adolescents, and adults (McPartland *et al.*, 2004) with ASD. The specific interest in this direction should be focused on investigation of event-related inter- and intra-hemispheric spontaneous and induced gamma-band oscillations phase coherence in TD and ASD children. Variations in induced gamma power using intracranial recording are believed to represent coherent synchronized activity of local neural assemblies (Lachaux *et al.*, 2007a, 2007b). The gamma-band coherence among discrete cortical regions may therefore represent the coupling of distributed rhythm generators that is necessary for the large-scale integration of cortical regions associated as functional networks (Keehn *et al.*, 2015).

Emotional Deficits in ASD, Autonomic Activity, and Anxiety

Anxiety is one of the most common clinical comorbidities in this population. There is no denying that more research is needed to understand the specifics of anxiety etiology in the context of ASD. It is possible to suggest that impairments both in emotional reactivity and in the ability to regulate affective states represent a risk factor for anxiety in ASD. One of the reasons why anxiety disorders are so frequently comorbid with ASD is because emotional self-regulation impairments are so typical of this condition. Emotion dysregulation is a well-known contributor to the development of anxiety in TD children, which might also apply to children with ASD. It is thus important to understand what factors contribute to abnormal emotional reactivity in ASD.

Data from numerous studies suggest the presence of autonomic hyperarousal and atypical reactivity to social tasks in ASD (Klusek *et al.*, 2015; Kushki *et al.*, 2013; Sokhadze *et al.*, 2019). Anxiety in autism was recognized as being directly linked with atypical autonomic control and excessive sympathetic arousal (Gillott *et al.*, 2001). Developmental deficits in autonomic regulation of cardiac activity may result in a lower ability to engage in social communication in children with autism (Porges, 2003). Cardiac parasympathetic hypofunction has often been reported in ASD in association with evidence of increased sympathetic tone (Ming *et al.*, 2005, 2011; Kushki *et al.*, 2013). The respiratory dysrhythmia in children with ASD, according to Ming *et al.* (2016), is a phenomenon associated with lower cardiac vagal activity. Both respiratory and cardiac vagal control hypofunction in ASD may suggest a brainstem dysfunction or diminished "top-down" control of the cortex over limbic and subcortical structures. Low parasympathetic activity can help explain the chronic sensory hyperarousal state and some of the social communication difficulties in ASD. This hypothesis is in agreement with Porges' "polyvagal theory" (2003), which emphasizes the important role of efferents and afferents of the vagus nerve in support of social engagement and communication.

Dysfunctions of the parasympathetic system negatively affect social behavior in children with ASD by impacting heart rate (HR) modulation. The inhibitory parasympathetic vagus nerve acts as a "brake," slowing heart rate (Porges, 2003; Porges *et al.*, 1996). Functionally, the vagal "brake," which modulates HR, enables rapid engagement and disengagement with objects and people, a skill important for promoting social behaviors (Porges, 1995, 2003). Spectral analysis of HRV represents a measure commonly used in psychopathology research (Cohen *et al.*, 2000; Thayer and Friedman, 2002) for assessment of cardiac autonomic control (Berntson *et al.*, 1997). Reduced HRV, and in particular attenuated power of the high frequency (HF) component of the HRV (index of parasympathetic control), is an indicator of limited psychophysiological flexibility (Berntson *et al.*, 1997; Cohen *et al.*, 2000; Movius and Allen, 2005; Thayer *et al.*, 2012). Deficits in the modulation of the HRV in the HF range (i.e., respiratory sinus arrhythmia (RSA)) in different social tasks have been found in autism. Typical children more effectively suppress the HF in HRV (Althaus *et al.*, 2004; Hutt *et al.*, 1975); autistic children, on the other hand, demonstrate dampened HR reactivity, unusually small deceleratory HR responses, and generally low cardiac reactions to auditory stimulation, including socially relevant speech, phrases, and tones (Coronoa *et al.*, 1998; Palkovitz and Wiesenfeld, 1980; Zahn *et al.*, 1987). Analysis of the HRV, and specifically the HF of HRV, and short-term (phasic) HR responses associated with dynamic parasympathetic activity may provide very important information about the autonomic dysfunctions in autism.

Studies of skin conductance level (SCL) and skin conductance response (SCR) in autism have demonstrated several manifestations of over-arousal (Ming *et al.*, 2005, 2016). Since electrodermal activity (EDA) is controlled solely by sympathetic inputs (Boucsein, 2012), the above effects are indications of high sympathetic tone. However, EDA cannot function as the sole indicator of sympathetic activity when taking into account Lacey's theory of "directional fractionation" between cardiovascular and electrodermal activity. Thus, the addition of cardiac measures of sympathetic arousal seems to be a logical approach. Because the heart is dually innervated by the sympathetic nervous system (SNS) and the parasympathetic nervous system (PNS), which accelerate or decelerate HR—either in coupled (reciprocal, coactivated, or coinhibited) or uncoupled modes—HR is not informative of the respective autonomic branch's influence upon cardiac functioning (Berntson *et al.*, 1993). Berntson *et al.* (1991) pointed out that chronotropic and inotropic influences on the heart might be mediated by separate efferent pathways controlled by different central mechanisms.

Therefore, it is useful to use both electrodermal (SCL, SCR) and cardiac indices (e.g., the low frequency (LF) component of HRV or the ratio of low vs. high frequency (HF) of HRV) of sympathetic arousal to better judge the level of sympathetic activation. In particular, reports of patterns of physiological activity during anxiety indicate increased HR, and decreased peak-to-valley RSA, as well as increases in LF and LF/HF, systolic blood pressure, diastolic blood pressure and total peripheral resistance, electrodermal activity (SCR, frequency of non-specific SCRs (NS.SCR), and tonic SCL), and respiratory variables indicative of increased respiration rate.

Exploring the relationship of autonomic activity with social competence in ASD is one example of the efforts indicating that autonomic activity may be related to social functioning in individuals with ASD (Smeekens *et al.*, 2015). Data from numerous studies suggest autonomic hyperarousal in ASD and atypical reactivity to social tasks (Kushki *et al.*, 2014). Anxiety in people diagnosed with autism needs to be recognized as directly linked with atypical autonomic control and excessive sympathetic arousal (Gillott *et al.*, 2001). The ANS is responsible for multiple physiological responses, and dysfunction of this system is often hypothesized as contributing to cognitive, affective, and behavioral responses in this population (Benevides and Lane, 2015). Kleberg (2015) emphasized that atypical autonomic arousal has been used to explain some of the core symptoms of ASD. In effect, it has been hypothesized that either elevated or attenuated tonic arousal was a causal factor behind some of the core autism symptoms, such as repetitive behaviors (Hirstein *et al.*, 2001) and avoidance of social interaction (Rogers and Ozonoff, 2005). According to other current theories, atypical regulation of arousal could cause impairment in attention functions, yet another feature associated with ASD (Orekhova and Stroganova, 2014).

Cardiac Autonomic Balance and Emotional Reactivity

Current views challenge the sympathetic over-arousal model of anxiety that overlooks the role of a hypofunctional parasympathetic system. According to Thayer *et al.*'s model for anxiety (2012), along with sympathetic over-arousal there is also reduced HRV and hypofunctional vagal activity. From this perspective, ASD presenting with anxiety and dysregulated autonomic control can involve varying degrees of sympathetic over-activation and parasympathetic under-activation, giving rise to the possibility of several distinct autonomic arousal phenotypes. Reduced cardiac vagal tone and labile respiration in autism was interpreted as a phenomenon associated with lower parasympathetic activity (Ming *et al.*, 2005, 2016; Porges, 2003; Sohn *et al.*, 2001). Both respiratory and cardiac vagal control hypofunction and sympathetic over-arousal in ASD may suggest a diminished "top-down" control of the prefrontal cortex (PFC) over limbic and subcortical structures (Loveland *et al.*, 2008). Multiple areas of the frontal lobe (dorsolateral, dorsal medial, anterior cingulate, orbital) couple their activity to the amygdala and downstream to the hypothalamus. The prefrontal cortex–amygdala–hypothalamic system is therefore well positioned to exert cognitive control over behavior. In this regard, atypical autonomic control due to frontal disinhibition may explain some of the core symptoms and comorbid conditions of ASD, such as anxiety (Kleberg, 2015). In autism, ANS dysfunction includes blunted cardiac responses to visual and auditory social stimuli (Hirstein *et al.*, 2001; Palkovitz and Wiesenfeld, 1980), important to the understanding of social situations. Cardiac parasympathetic hypofunction, decreased baroreflex sensitivity, and labile respiration have often been reported in ASD in association with evidence of increased sympathetic tone (Kushki *et al.*, 2013; Julu *et al.*, 2001; Matsushima *et al.*, 2016; Ming *et al.*, 2016).

To describe emotions, one of the most commonly used approaches is a dimensional model of emotion in which a few independent dimensions are considered on discrete or continuous scales (Kreibig, 2010). In this approach, two dimensions are usually chosen, namely arousal and valence. One more, dominance, is used only in rare cases. Taking a functional approach to autonomic response in emotion, Stemmler (2003, 2004; Stemmler and Wacker, 2009) stressed the importance of studying autonomic regulation patterns in emotion rather than single-response measures. Only a comprehensive assessment of cardiovascular, electrodermal, and respiratory measures can provide complementary information on ANS functioning in emotion. Cardiac chronotropic activity measures provide possible biomarkers for the identification of individuals with ASD at risk for the development of comorbid anxiety symptoms. Cardiac deceleration has been linked to impaired fear conditioning, while low HRV has been associated with elevated contextual anxiety and enhanced startle potentiation to affective stimuli. Most emotion theories consider autonomic activity responses as main components of emotional reactions. However, degree of ANS response specificity is quite diverse, and can be manifested as a general less differentiated arousal or very specific pattern of response typical for a certain emotion in a defined context (e.g., school setting). Stemmler and Wacker (2009) emphasized the need to include several variables that reflect both specific and unspecific effects of emotion in analysis. Unspecific emotion effects distinguish between control (i.e., neutral) and emotion conditions, but not between emotions, whereas a specific set of autonomic variables may distinguish between emotions.

Central coordination of autonomic activity represents a popular current view for integrating nervous system functioning (central autonomic network, CAN; Benarroch, 1997; see also Thayer and Lane, 2000). Unlike the original conceptualization of the ANS as functioning independently of the rest of the nervous system (e.g., involuntary, automatic, and autonomous control), close interactions between the central and autonomic nervous systems exist in various ways, and should be recognized during the interpretation of affective psychophysiological tests. Complementing autonomic responses with relevant EEG measures is one of the most appropriate approaches when evaluating affect in children with ASD.

EEG Gamma Activity in Autism

In psychophysiological studies using EEG, gamma activity (30–80 Hz, and more specifically 35–45 Hz sub-band, 40 Hz centered gamma (Sheer, 1989; Spydell et al., 1979)) received special attention as an EEG pattern related to social functioning and emotional responsiveness abnormalities in autism (de Groot and Van Strien, 2018). Besides being linked to higher cognitive functions such as perceptual binding (the pairing of different aspects of perception into a common object or experience), gamma plays an important role in the synchronization of cortical networks (Rojas and Wilson, 2014). There are studies showing that children with ASD have increased spontaneous gamma oscillations (Coben et al., 2008; Cornew et al., 2012; Orekhova et al., 2007), but at the same time they have low coherence between distal networks and show atypical laterality (Maxwell et al., 2015; Stroganova et al., 2007; Sun et al., 2012). Enhanced but at the same time incoherent gamma-band activity can therefore be considered a putative biomarker in autism. In addition, atypical stimulus-related oscillations in the gamma-band have been observed in individuals with ASD (Rojas and Wilson, 2014; Sokhadze et al., 2016b). These findings have several implications according to de Groot and van Strien (2018), suggesting that resting state and evoked gamma-band oscillation dysfunctions, as well as atypical gamma laterality, not only may serve as biomarkers, but could be considered as candidates for ASD endophenotyping. We propose that analysis of gamma oscillations evoked by affective stimuli may serve as a useful way of assessing emotional reactivity abnormalities in autism.

A possible relation between fast EEG activity and autism comes from data on genetically mediated abnormalities in GABAergic and glutamatergic systems. The morphological integrity of GABAergic interneuron connections within cortical minicolumns is important for the generation of normal gamma oscillations (Tamas et al., 2000; Uhlhaas et al., 2010; Whittington et al., 2000). Casanova et al. (2003) suggested that such abnormal minicolumnar organization may result in a deficit of inhibitory GABAergic fiber projections, which in turn may facilitate the occurrence of epilepsy, sensory disorders, and gamma-related abnormalities in autism. The presence of fast rhythms in EEG is usually considered an electrophysiological index of cortical activation. Therefore, excess of beta and gamma rhythms in EEGs of children with autism supports the hypothesis of abnormally high E/I ratio in cortical structures (Casanova et al., 2003; Rubenstein and Merzenich, 2003).

The underlying neurobiological mechanisms of cortical gamma function are well studied. A widely accepted mechanistic model for disrupted gamma generation is linked to cortical E/I imbalance known to be biased toward over-excitation in autism (Uzunova et al., 2016). This model states that suppressed GABAergic inhibition is a common factor in ASD, and that high levels of excitatory compared with inhibitory (GABAergic) activity might even be involved in the pathogenesis of the disorder (Casanova et al., 2003; Rubenstein and Merzenich, 2003). The mechanistic model and its theoretical background are supported by studies in which individuals with ASD show deviant GABA levels and a disrupted E/I balance. As such, enhanced gamma activity can be explained by a biological mechanism proven to be altered in ASD.

There are only a few EEG studies employing resting-state gamma examinations in individuals with ASD, and practically all of them report oscillatory anomalies (Castelhano *et al.*, 2015; Lajiness-O'Neil *et al.*, 2014, 2018; Maxwell *et al.*, 2015; Menassa *et al.*, 2017; Schwartz *et al.*, 2017; van Diessen *et al.*, 2015). Analysis of functional connectivity patterns using EEG coherence may provide a way to probe the resulting differences in cognitive functions and behavior between children with and without autism. There is general consensus that EEG coherence patterns differ between individuals with and without ASD (Schwartz *et al.*, 2017). In this regard, it is important to note that reduced interhemispheric gamma-band coherence in autism was found to be associated with perceptual integration deficits in a study by Peiker *et al.* (2015). According to a recent study of Lajiness-O'Neil *et al.* (2018), disrupted neural synchrony can be considered a primary electrophysiological abnormality in ASD, altering communication between discrete cortical regions and contributing to abnormalities in patterns of connectivity within identified neural networks. The brains of children with ASD as compared with TD children show less coherence in gamma-band between areas that are important for social information processing. The amount of communication between these areas was associated with social communication difficulties (Maxwell *et al.*, 2015). It is important to note that reduced synchrony in gamma during exposure to stimulation was often reported, along with increased amplitude of gamma modulation. This type of combination of low coherence despite increased power of gamma points to the importance of analyzing both power and synchrony of gamma-band during perception and cognitive activity (van Diessen *et al.*, 2015). It is therefore unsurprising that gamma-band activity is associated with sensory, perceptual, and cognitive functions that are compromised in autism.

Despite all the evidence, the utility of gamma variables as diagnostic biomarkers is currently under-explored, suggesting an urgent need for using gamma oscillation measures as biomarkers of response to interventions (e.g., TMS-based neuromodulation or neurofeedback). Differences in resting-state frontal EEG alpha and gamma asymmetry as well as emotional stimuli-related frontal EEG gamma oscillation asymmetry and coherence may affect the expression of autism symptoms, and could be used for investigation of the associations between anterior hemispheric asymmetry and behavioral-symptoms severity and social and emotional functioning in children with ASD (Sutton *et al.*, 2005).

Hemispheric Asymmetry of Gamma

It has been proposed that atypicality of hemispheric specialization is a potential biomarker for ASD. For gamma asymmetry studies, most models included resting-state, eyes-closed, and eyes-open conditions as potentially predictive of autism symptoms, with higher left dominant gamma asymmetry being predictive of more autistic traits. However, it is possible that the link between spontaneous resting-state gamma power asymmetry and autistic traits is not sufficiently strong, and that stimulus-related gamma activity may provide much stronger links. Differences in resting state frontal EEG gamma asymmetry as well as emotional stimuli-related frontal EEG gamma oscillation asymmetry and coherence may affect the expression of autism symptoms, and could be used for investigating possible associations between asymmetry and behavioral-symptoms severity and social and emotional functioning in children with ASD (Sutton *et al.*, 2005). The rationale for linking frontal EEG gamma asymmetry indices with severity of autism symptoms is based on the associations between approach behaviors and relatively more left than right resting frontal cortical activity, and between avoidant/withdrawal behaviors and relatively greater right than left resting activation (e.g., Balconi *et al.*, 2015; Davidson, 2002; Harmon-Jones, 2004).

Studies have found relationships between individual differences in resting anterior (frontal) brain activity asymmetry and characteristic levels of emotional responsiveness (Harmon-Jones, 2004). For example, individuals with relatively greater left-sided anterior activity while at rest report higher levels of dispositional positive affect, whereas those with relatively greater right-sided anterior activity report higher levels of dispositional negative affect (Tomarken *et al.*, 1992). Frontal resting EEG asymmetry has also been related to affective reactions to pertinent emotional stimuli. Individuals exhibiting relatively greater left anterior activity while at rest report stronger tendencies to engage in appetitive motivated approach behavior (Harmon-Jones, 2004). Stroganova *et al.* (2007) showed predominantly leftward EEG asymmetry in three- to eight-year-old children with autism. Right hemisphere deficits in EEG in autism were also reported by other authors (Lazarev *et al.*, 2004). Frontal EEG asymmetry changes in response to affective stimuli in individuals with autism are not sufficiently explored, and more studies are needed in this direction of EEG research.

Sutton *et al.* (2005) proposed that if approach-avoidance tendencies modify the expression of autism, then measures of resting anterior EEG asymmetry may be expected to be associated with significant differences in symptom expression in autism. We propose that links between anterior EEG gamma asymmetry and autistic symptoms will be even stronger in response to affective stimuli as compared with spontaneous resting-state frontal gamma oscillations. There are both theoretical models and experimental observations (Burnette *et al.*, 2011) that differences in approach and avoidance tendencies may represent an important base of variability in autism symptoms. Dominance of right frontal EEG asymmetry is proposed to reflect relatively greater activation of a neural network including the frontal cortex, amygdala, septo-hippocampal system, and brainstem that controls responses to stimuli of punishment, negative reinforcement, and non-reward. Consequently, individuals with relatively greater right anterior versus left anterior brain activity tend to exhibit inhibition of movement toward goals and withdrawal from novel situations and social interactions (e.g., see Davidson, 2002).

Left anterior EEG asymmetry is thought to involve a dopaminergically mediated network of the left middle-superior frontal and pre-central gyrus and the left inferior parietal lobe, as well as bilateral activation in the dorsolateral PFC, orbital frontal, and anterior cingulate cortices. It functions to regulate responses to signals of reward by initiating and modifying movement toward goals. Individuals with relatively heightened left frontal activity tend to exhibit more activation of goal-directed, reward-seeking behavior, and to anticipate positive affective states when exposed to cues of potential reward, as well as anger and frustration when approach-related goals are blocked (Harmon-Jones and Allen, 1998).

The study of Sutton *et al.* (2005) reported left frontal asymmetry in autistic children that was associated with increases in self-reports of outward expressions of anger and heightened symptoms of obsessive compulsive disorder. The former observation is consistent with a theory suggesting that the presence of greater goal-directed and reward-seeking patterns of behavior in people with left anterior EEG asymmetry may lead them to become more easily frustrated. It is this frustration that contributes to their increased tendency to express anger (Harmon-Jones and Allen, 1998). Sutton *et al.* (2005) also reported that social anxiety was more prominent in high-functioning children with left rather than right frontal EEG asymmetry. One possible explanation raised in the discussion of the data was based on the proposal by Heller *et al.* (1997) that symptoms of anxiety associated with anxious apprehension, such as worry, are related to left anterior cortical functioning, whereas anxious arousal including panic is associated with right cortical functioning. It was suggested that left frontal asymmetry is associated with a greater tendency toward active cognitive worry, including obsessive compulsive symptoms, among high-functioning children with autism.

Connection Between Central and Autonomic Nervous Systems

Thayer and Lane (2009) reviewed neuroanatomical and neuroimaging studies that implicate inhibitory GABAergic pathways from the prefrontal lobe to the limbic system, and inhibitory pathways between the amygdala and the sympathetic and parasympathetic neurons in the medulla known to be involved in the modulation of HRV. This group of authors (Lane, 2008; Lane et al., 2007; Thayer and Lane, 2000, 2005) described a neurovisceral integration model that is directly involved in the regulation of emotion, and proposed a role for dysregulation that may result in various psychopathologies, including anxiety disorder (Friedman, 2007), and potentially anxiety symptoms that are typical of children with ASD. Benarroch (1997) used the term "the central autonomic network (CAN)," and proposed connections of the CAN with the sinoatrial node of the heart via the stellate ganglia and the vagus nerve. As outlined by Thayer (2015), decreased tonic inhibitory output of the PFC can lead to disinhibition of the tonically inhibited structures under central autonomic control (i.e., CAN), and result in a simultaneous disinhibition of sympatho-excitatory neurons and an inhibition of parasympatho-excitatory neurons accompanied by an increase in HR and a concomitant decrease of vagally mediated HRV. Thayer et al. (2012) outlined that connections between the amygdala and medial PFC, which evaluate threat and safety, regulate HRV through their connections with the nucleus of the solitary tract (NST).

Furthermore, the CAN model proposes that vagally mediated HRV is linked to prefrontal executive functions, and that HRV reflects the functional capacity of the PFC to support emotional and physiological self-regulation. They hypothesize that parasympathetically mediated HRV is positively correlated with prefrontal cortical performance. More specifically, when the prefrontal cortical functioning is decreased, HR increases and HRV decreases. Prolonged prefrontal cortical inactivity can lead to hypervigilance, defensiveness, and social isolation (Thayer *et al.*, 2009). The CAN model predicts reduced HRV and hypofunctional vagal activity in anxiety, as it might be associated with abnormal ANS cardiac control (Friedman, 2007). This challenges the sympathetic over-activation model of anxiety that under-estimates the role of a hypofunctional parasympathetic system. From this perspective, disorders such as autism presenting with anxiety and dysregulated autonomic control can involve varying degrees of sympathetic over-activation and parasympathetic under-activation. Bal *et al.* (2010) suggested that children with ASD rely mostly on down-regulation of sympathetic arousal as they fail to engage the parasympathetic system for self-regulation. Analysis of both central (e.g., frontal asymmetry indices) and autonomic (HRV, SCR, respiration, etc.) biomarkers during exposure to affective stimuli allows for a better understanding of their contribution to emotional deficits and anxiety in autism.

Lateralization, Visceral Perception, and Interoceptive Representation

Several studies suggest hemispheric lateralization of autonomic cardiovascular control. There is a controversy regarding which hemisphere dominates sympathetic or parasympathetic activity. The results of Hilz *et al.'s* (2001) study showed sympathetic lateralization in the right hemisphere and also demonstrated parasympathetic predominance and up-regulation of baroreflex sensitivity in the left hemisphere. In addition, it is necessary to consider that the cortical representation of bodily arousal has been linked to social cognition and may be important to disorders such as ASD. According to Critchley *et al.* (2004), emotional and cognitive processes evoke patterned changes in profiles of physiological measures that may signal a particular emotional state. The discrete cortical substrates for these representations include the anterior regions of the insula and orbitofrontal cortex. The misperception of heightened arousal level may evoke changes in emotional behavior in ASD (Garfinkel *et al.*, 2016). Emotions are influenced by assessment of bodily arousal via interoception, which refers to the sensing of visceral signals from the inner body and contrasts with exteroceptive senses (including vision, hearing, touch, etc.) and with proprioceptive signals (Ewing *et al.*, 2017; Garfinkel and Critchley, 2013; Garfinkel *et al.*, 2016). Emotional manifestations are dependent on central representations of bodily arousal and share common neural substrates—in particular, the anterior insula subserves both interoceptive accuracy (Critchley *et al.*, 2004) and emotion processing (Terasawa *et al.*, 2013). Aberrant activation of the insula during emotional processing is noted as a feature of ASD (Ebisch *et al.*, 2011; Francis *et al.*, 2018; Hadjikhani *et al.*, 2009).

Brain functions involved in the generation and representation of arousal have been linked to social cognition in typical development (Critchley, 2005), suggesting that they may be important to disorders of social interaction such as ASD.

The modulation of the visceral state is mediated by the sympathetic and parasympathetic divisions of the ANS. Moreover, neural afferents support and convey representations of the internal state of the body to the brain, further influencing emotion and cognition. Feedback from the viscera is mapped in the brain to influence efferent neural signals, and at the cortical level reinforce affective responses and emotional states. The discrete cortical substrates for these representations include the anterior regions of the insula and the orbitofrontal cortex. The misperception of heightened arousal level may evoke changes in emotional behavior. Either poor perception of arousal or excessive sensitivity to signs of arousal is capable of influencing emotional experiences and behavior in individuals with ASD. Cognitive processes such as decision-making are guided by central feedback of bodily arousal responses (Damasio, 1996).

Autonomic arousal is generally understood as a shift in visceral state to facilitate ongoing or anticipated motor action, through an increase in cardiac output and blood flow to musculature and a parallel reduction in blood supply to the internal organs. This process is associated with a general increase in sympathetic activity, particularly to the heart, blood vessels, and skin, and is typically preceded by a more rapid withdrawal of parasympathetic activity. This "fight or flight" pattern of bodily response is produced stereotypically to a range of perceived environmental threats. The influence of transient arousal responses on aspects of affect and cognition is embodied within Damasio's "Somatic Marker Hypothesis" (1996), which proposes that emotional feelings originate in representations within the somatosensory cortices. Empirical studies have implicated the insular cortex as the substrate for emotional states, supported by activity within the amygdala, anterior cingulate cortex (ACC), and orbital prefrontal regions. The anterior insula and ventromedial prefrontal cortex contribute to the integration of visceral afferent information. Emotional deficits in children with ASD are associated not only with difficulties in recognizing others' emotions, but also in recognition and regulation of one's own emotions. Garfinkel *et al.* (2016) demonstrated that individuals with ASD have reduced interoceptive accuracy and exaggerated interoceptive sensibility, reflecting an impaired ability to objectively detect bodily signals alongside an over-inflated subjective perception of bodily sensations. Consequently, it is possible to propose that emotional deficits expressed by children with ASD may originate in impaired interoceptive processing and misjudgment related to their own arousal level.

Emotions draw on central representations of bodily arousal and share common neural substrates: in particular, the anterior insula both subserves interoceptive accuracy (Critchley *et al.*, 2004) and underscores deficits in emotion processing, thus lending support to the proposal that integrative processing within the anterior insula permits the detection of bodily state to inform emotional experience (Terasawa *et al.*, 2013). Atypical activation of the insula during affect states has been reported in ASD (Hadjikhani *et al.*, 2009). Moreover, the functional connectivity of the insula is impaired in ASD, including the observation that there is less efficient crosstalk between the anterior insula and somatosensory cortices (Ebisch *et al.*, 2011).

The anterior insula and ventromedial prefrontal cortex contribute to the integration of visceral afferent information. These observations also led to the "insula theory of anxiety" of Paulus and Stein (2006), who proposed that feelings of anxiety result from mismatched representation of anticipated and perceived bodily states within the insula cortex. The central and autonomic nervous systems are involved in the perception of affective stimuli, recognition of emotional salience, and generation of psychophysiological responses, which could be detected and compared in terms of differences in children with ASD and TD children.

Areas of Interest in Affective Psychophysiology and Anxiety Studies in Autism

Our chapter addresses only some of the critical needs of ASD research in several areas of interest: (1) exploration of psychophysiological reactivity subtypes underlying anxiety conditions frequently co-occurring in children with ASD; (2) identification of a subgroup of children with ASD with atypical emotional responsiveness using potential EEG asymmetry and ANS biomarkers; (3) review of experimental data showing differences in psychophysiological reactivity during exposure to emotional stimuli of various modalities between ASD and TD children; and (4) discussion of links between excessive sympathetic arousal, reduced parasympathetic activity, altered frontal asymmetry, and symptoms of autism such as anxiety and stereotyped behaviors, thus contributing to a better understanding of the neurobiology of aberrant behaviors and low emotional and social competence in ASD.

One of the major goals of the review was to examine how autonomic arousal and frontal asymmetry in children with autism are different from those of typically developing children, whether there are distinct autonomic and EEG arousal phenotypes in ASD, and how they may correlate with the clinical symptoms of autism. Understanding specifics of autonomic imbalance, atypical EEG symmetry, coherence, emotional responsiveness, and anxiety phenotypes closely follows the "Research Domain Criteria (RDoC)" initiative of the National Institute of Mental Health (NIMH).

The analysis of the current state of research in this area is guided by theoretical concepts developed in our laboratory, namely the neurodevelopmental "minicolumnopathy" hypothesis of autism that predicts an abnormal E/I ratio, GABA deficits, and gamma oscillation abnormality in autism (Casanova et al., 2002, 2003, 2014, 2015).

The pilot and current studies of our group (Casanova et al., 2014; Sokhadze et al., 2017; Wang et al., 2016) provided us with an opportunity to link a variety of phenomena in ways that had not been previously explored. Ties between E/I imbalance, GABAergic deficiency, gamma-band amplitude, coherence/laterality atypicalities, autonomic imbalance, and emotional competence and social communication impairments in children with autism will promote our understanding of the link between patterns of psychophysiological indices (e.g., gamma asymmetry, cardiac sympathovagal balance, skin conductance, respiration measures, etc.) with symptoms of autism (e.g., anxiety).

Acknowledgment

This study was partially supported by the Greenville Health System Transformative Research Award.

References

Althaus, M., Van Roon, A. M., Mulder, L. J., Mulder, G., Aarnoudse, C., and Minderaa, R. (2004). Autonomic response patterns observed during the performance of an attention-demanding task in two groups of children with autistic-type difficulties in social adjustment. *Psychophysiology, 41*(6), 893–904.

Bal, E., Harden, E., Lamb, D., Van Hecke, A. V., Denver, J. W., and Porges, S. W. (2010). Emotion recognition in children with autism spectrum disorders: Relations to eye gaze and autonomic state. *Journal of Autism and Developmental Disorders, 40*(3), 358–370.

Balconi, M., Grippa, E., and Vanutelli, M. E. (2015). What hemodynamic (fNIRS), electrophysiological (EEG) and autonomic integrated measures can tell us about emotional processing. *Brain and Cognition, 95*, 67–76.

Benarroch, E. E. (1997). The central autonomic network. In P. A. Low (Ed.), *Clinical Autonomic Disorders* (2nd ed.). Philadelphia, PA: Lippincott-Raven.

Benevides, T. W., and Lane, S. J. (2015). A review of cardiac autonomic measures: Considerations for examination of physiological response in children with autism spectrum disorder. *Journal of Autism and Developmental Disorders, 45*(2), 560–575.

Berntson, G. G., Cacioppo, J. T., and Quigley, K. S. (1991). Autonomic determinism: The modes of autonomic control, the doctrine of autonomic space, and the laws of autonomic constraint. *Psychological Review, 98*(4), 459–487.

Berntson, G., Cacippo, J. Y., and Quigley, K. (1993). Cardiac psychophysiology and autonomic space in humans: Empirical perspectives and implications. *Psychological Bulletin, 114*, 296–322.

Berntson, G., Bigger, J. T., Eckberg, D., Grossman, P., Kaufmann, P. G., Malik, M., ... Van der Molen, M. W. (1997). Heart rate variability: Origins, methods and interpretive caveates. *Psychophysiology, 34*, 623–648.

Boucsein, W. (2012). *Electrodermal Activity* (2nd ed.). New York, NY: Springer.

Burnette, C. P., Henderson, H. A., Inge, A. P., Zahka, N. E., Schwartz, C. B., and Mundy, P. C. (2011). Anterior EEG asymmetry and the Modifier model of autism. *Journal of Autism and Developmental Disorders, 41*(8), 1113–1124.

Casanova, M. F., Buxhoeveden, D. P., and Brown, C. (2002). Clinical and macroscopic correlates of minicolumnar pathology in autism. *Journal of Child Neurology, 17*(9), 692–695.

Casanova, M. F., Buxhoeveden, D., and Gomez, J. (2003). Disruption in the inhibitory architecture of the cell minicolumn: Implications for autism. *The Neuroscientist, 9*(6), 496–507.

Casanova, M. F., Hensley, M. K., Sokhadze, E. M., El-Baz, A. S., Wang, Y., Li, X., and Sears, L. (2014). Effects of weekly low-frequency rTMS on autonomic measures in children with autism spectrum disorder. *Frontiers in Human Neuroscience, 8*, 851.

Casanova, M. F., Sokhadze, E., Opris, I., Wang, Y., and Li, X. (2015). Autism spectrum disorders: Linking neuropathological findings to treatment with transcranial magnetic stimulation. *Acta Pediatrica, 104*(4), 346–355.

Castelhano, J., Bernardino, I., Rebola, J., Rodriguez, E., and Castelo-Branco, M. (2015). Oscillations or synchrony? Disruption of neural synchrony despite enhanced gamma oscillations in a model of disrupted perceptual coherence. *Journal of Cognitive Neuroscience, 27*(12), 2416–2426.

Coben, R., Clarke, A. R., Hudspeth, W., and Barry, R. J. (2008). EEG power and coherence in autistic spectrum disorder. *Clinical Neurophysiology, 119*(5), 1002–1009.

Cohen, N., Benjamin, J., Geva, A. B., Matar, M. A., Kaplan, Z., and Kotler, M. (2000). Autonomic dysregulation in panic disorder and in post-traumatic stress disorder: Application of power spectrum analysis of heart rate variability at rest and in response to recollection of trauma or panic attack. *Psychiatry Research, 96*(1), 1–13.

Cohen, S., Masyn, K., Mastergeorge, A., and Hessl, D. (2015). Psychophysiological responses to emotional stimuli in children and adolescents with autism and fragile X syndrome. *Journal of Clinical Child and Adolescent Psychology, 44*(2), 250–263.

Cornew, L., Roberts, T. P., Blaskey, L., and Edgar, J. C. (2012). Resting-state oscillatory activity in autism spectrum disorders. *Journal of Autism and Developmental Disorders, 42*(9), 1884–1894.

Coronoa, R., Dissanayake, C., Arbelle, S., Wellington, P., and Sigman, M. (1998). Is affect aversive to young children with autism? Behavioral and cardiac responses to experimenter distress. *Child Development, 69*(6), 1494–1502.

Critchley, H. D. (2005). Neural mechanisms of autonomic, affective, and cognitive integration. *Journal of Comparative Neurology, 493*(1), 154–166.

Critchley, H. D., Wiens, S., Rotshtein, P., Ohman, A., and Dolan, R. J. (2004). Neural systems supporting interoceptive awareness. *Nature Neuroscience, 7*(2), 189–195.

Damasio, A. R. (1996). The somatic marker hypothesis and the possible functions of the prefrontal cortex. *Philosophical Transactions of the Royal Society of London, Biological Sciences, 351*(1346), 1413–1420.

Davidson, R. J. (2002). Anxiety and affective style: Role of prefrontal cortex and amygdala. *Biological Psychiatry, 51*(1), 68–80.

de Groot, K., and van Strien, J. W. (2018). Spontaneous resting-state gamma oscillations are not predictive of autistic traits in the general population. *The European Journal of Neuroscience, 48*(8), 2928–2937.

Ebisch, S. J. H., Gallese, V., Willems, R. M., Mantini, D., Groen, W. B., Romani, G. L., … Bekkering, H. (2011). Altered intrinsic functional connectivity of anterior and posterior insula regions in high-functioning participants with autism spectrum disorder. *Human Brain Mapping, 32*(7), 1013–1028.

Ewing, D., Manassei, M., Gould van Praag, C., Philippides, A. O., Critchley, H. D., and Garfinkel, S. N. (2017). Sleep and the heart: Interoceptive differences linked to poor experiential sleep quality in anxiety and depression. *Biological Psychology, 127*, 163–172.

Francis, S. M., Camchong, J., Brickman, L., Goelkel-Garcia, L., Mueller, B. A., Tseng, A., … Jacob, S. (2018). Hypoconnectivity of insular resting-state networks in adolescents with autism spectrum disorder. *Psychiatry Research: Neuroimaging, 283*, 104–112.

Friedman, B. H. (2007). An autonomic flexibility–neurovisceral integration model of anxiety and cardiac vagal tone. *Biological Psychology, 74*(2), 185–199.

Garfinkel, S. N., and Critchley, H. D. (2013). Interoception, emotion and brain: New insights link internal physiology to social behaviour. Commentary on: "Anterior insular cortex mediates bodily sensibility and social anxiety" by Terasawa *et al.* (2012). *Social Cognitive and Affective Neuroscience, 8*(3), 231–234.

Garfinkel, S. N., Tiley, C., O'Keeffe, S., Harrison, N. A., Seth, A. K., and Critchley, H. D. (2016). Discrepancies between dimensions of interoception in autism: Implications for emotion and anxiety. *Biological Psychology, 114*, 117–126.

Gillott, A., Furniss, F., and Walter, A. (2001). Anxiety in high-functioning children with autism. *Autism, 5*(3), 277–286.

Hadjikhani, N., Joseph, R. M., Manoach, D. S., Naik, P., Snyder, J., Dominick, K., … Gelder, B. (2009). Body expressions of emotion do not trigger fear contagion in autism spectrum disorder. *Social Cognitive and Affective Neuroscience, 4*(1), 70–78.

Harmon-Jones, E. (2004). Contributions from research on anger and cognitive dissonance to understanding the motivational functions of asymmetrical frontal brain activity. *Biological Psychology, 67*(1–2), 51–76.

Harmon-Jones, E., and Allen, J. J. (1998). Anger and frontal brain activity: EEG asymmetry consistent with approach motivation despite negative affective valence. *Journal of Personality and Social Psychology, 74*(5), 1310–1316.

Heller, W., Nitschke, J. B., Etienne, M. A., and Miller, G. A. (1997). Patterns of regional brain activity differentiate types of anxiety. *Journal of Abnormal Psychology, 106*(3), 376–385.

Heunis, T. M., Aldrich, C., and de Vries, P. J. (2016). Recent advances in resting-state electroencephalography biomarkers for autism spectrum disorder: A review of methodological and clinical challenges. *Pediatric Neurology, 61*, 28–37.

Heunis, T., Aldrich, C., Peters, J. M., Jeste, S. S., Sahin, M., Scheffer, C., and de Vries, P. J. (2018). Recurrence quantification analysis of resting state EEG signals in autism spectrum disorder: A systematic methodological exploration of technical and demographic confounders in the search for biomarkers. *BMC Medicine, 16*(1), 101.

Hilz, M. J., Dütsch, M., Perrine, K., Nelson, P. K., Rauhut, U., and Devinsky, O. (2001). Hemispheric influence on autonomic modulation and baroreflex sensitivity. *Annals of Neurology, 49*(5), 575–584.

Hirstein, W., Iversen, P., and Ramachandran, V. S. (2001). Autonomic responses of autistic children to people and objects. *Proceedings: Biological Sciences/The Royal Society, 268*(1479), 1883–1888.

Hutt, C., Forrest, S. J., and Richer, J. (1975). Cardiac arrhythmia and behavior in autistic children. *Acta Psychiatrica Scandinavica, 51*(5), 361–372.

Julu, P. O., Kerr, A. M., Apartipoulos, F., Al-Rawas, S., Engerström, I. W., Engerström, L., ... Hansen, S. (2001). Characterization of breathing and associated central autonomic dysfunction in the Rett disorder. *Archives of Disease in Childhood, 85*(1), 29–37.

Keehn, B., Vogel-Farley, V., Tager-Flusberg, H., and Nelson, C. (2015). Atypical hemispheric specialization for faces in infants at-risk for Autism Spectrum Disorder. *Autism Research, 8*(2), 187–198.

Kleberg, J. L. (2015). Resting arousal state and functional connectivity in autism spectrum disorder. *Journal of Neurophysiology, 113*(9), 3035–3037.

Klusek, J., Roberts, J. E., and Losh, M. (2015). Cardiac autonomic regulation in autism and fragile X syndrome: A review. *Psychology Bulletin, 141*, 141–175.

Kreibig, S. D. (2010). Autonomic nervous system activity in emotion: A review. *Biological Psychology, 84*(3), 394–421.

Kushki, A., Drumm, E., Mobarak, M. P., Tanel, N., Dupius, A., Chau, T., and Anagnostou, E. (2013). Investigating the autonomic nervous system response to anxiety in children with autism spectrum disorders. *PLoS One, 8*(4), e59730.

Kushki, A., Brian, J., Dupius, A., and Anagnostou, E. (2014). Functional autonomic nervous system profile in children with autism spectrum disorder. *Molecular Autism, 5*, 39.

Lachaux, J. P., Fonlupt, P., Kahane, P., Minotti, L., Hoffmann, D., Bertrand, O., and Baciu, M. (2007a). Relationship between task-related gamma oscillations and BOLD signal: New insights from combined fMRI and intracranial EEG. *Human Brain Mapping, 28*(12), 1368–1375.

Lachaux, J. P., Jerbi, K., Bertrand, O., Minotti, L., Hoffmann, D., Schoendorff, B., and Kahane, P. (2007b). A blueprint for real-time functional mapping via human intracranial recordings. *PloS One, 2*(10), e1094.

Lajiness-O'Neill, R., Richard, A. E., Moran, J. E., Olszewski, A., Pawluk, L., Jacobson, D., ... Bowyer, S. M. (2014). Neural synchrony examined with magnetoencephalography (MEG) during eye gaze processing in autism spectrum disorders: Preliminary findings. *Journal of Neurodevelopmental Disorders, 6*(1), 15.

Lajiness-O'Neill, R., Brennan, J. R., Moran, J. E., Richard, A. E., Flores, A. M., Swick, C., ... Bowyer, S. M. (2018). Patterns of altered neural synchrony in the default mode network in autism spectrum disorder revealed with magnetoencephalography (MEG): Relationship to clinical symptomatology. *Autism Research, 11*(3), 434–449.

Lane, R. D. (2008). Neural substrates of implicit and explicit emotional processes: A unifying framework for psychosomatic medicine. *Psychosomatic Medicine, 70*(2), 214–231.

Lane, R. D., McRae, K., Reiman, E. M., Ahern, G. L., and Thayer, J. F. (2007). Neural correlates of vagal tone during emotion. *Psychosomatic Medicine, 69*, A-8.

Lazarev, V. V., Pontes, A., and de Azevedo, L. C. (2004). EEG photic driving: Right-hemisphere reactivity deficit in childhood autism. A pilot study. *International Journal of Psychophysiology, 71*(2), 177–183.

Loveland, K. A., Bachevalier, J., Pearson, D. A., and Lane, D. M. (2008). Fronto-limbic functioning in children and adolescents with and without autism. *Neuropsychologia, 46*(1), 49–62.

Matsushima, K., Matsubayashi, J., Toichi, M., Funabiki, Y., Kato, T., Awaya, T., and Kato, T. (2016). Unusual sensory features are related to resting-state cardiac vagus nerve activity in autism spectrum disorders. *Research in Autism Spectrum Disorders, 25*, 37–46.

Maxwell, C. R., Villalobos, M. E., Schultz, R. T., Herpertz-Dahlmann, B., Konrad, K., and Kohls, G. (2015). Atypical laterality of resting gamma oscillations in autism spectrum disorders. *Journal of Autism and Developmental Disorders, 45*(2), 292–297.

McPartland, J., Dawson, G., Webb, S. J., Panagiotides, H., and Carver, L. J. (2004). Event-related brain potentials reveal anomalies in temporal processing of faces in autism spectrum disorder. *Journal of Child Psychology and Psychiatry, and Allied Disciplines, 45*(7), 1235–1245.

Menassa, D. A., Braeutigam, S., Bailey, A., and Falter-Wagner, C. M. (2017). Frontal evoked γ activity modulates behavioural performance in autism spectrum disorders in a perceptual simultaneity task. *Neuroscience Letters, 665*, 86–91.

Ming, X., Julu, P. O., Brimacombe, M., Connor, S., and Daniels, M. L. (2005). Reduced cardiac parasympathetic activity in children with autism. *Brain and Development, 27*(7), 509–516.

Ming, X., Bain, J. M., Smith, D., Brimacombe, M., Gold von-Simson, G., and Axelrod, F. B. (2011). Assessing autonomic dysfunction symptoms in children: A pilot study. *Journal of Child Neurology, 26*(4), 420–427.

Ming, X., Patel, R., Kang, V., Chokroverty, S., and Julu, P. O. (2016). Respiratory and autonomic dysfunction in children with autism spectrum disorders. *Brain and Development, 38*(2), 225–232.

Movius, H. L., and Allen, J. J. (2005). Cardiac vagal tone, defensiveness, and motivational style. *Biological Psychology, 68*(2), 147–162.

Orekhova, E. V., Stroganova, T. A., Nygren, G., Tsetlin, M. M., Posikera, I. N., Gillberg, C., and Elam, M. (2007). Excess of high frequency electroencephalogram oscillations in boys with autism. *Biological Psychiatry, 62*(9), 1022–1029.

Orekhova, E. V., and Stroganova, T. A. (2014). Arousal and attention re-orienting in autism spectrum disorders: Evidence from auditory event-related potentials. *Frontiers in Human Neuroscience, 8*, 34.

Palkovitz, R. J., and Wiesenfeld, A. R. (1980). Differential autonomic responses of autistic and normal children. *Journal of Autism and Developmental Disorders, 10*(3), 347–360.

Paulus, M. P., and Stein, M. B. (2006). An insular view of anxiety. *Biological Psychiatry, 60*, 383–387.

Peiker, I., David, N., Schneider, T. R., Nolte, G., Schöttle, D., and Engel, A. K. (2015). Perceptual integration deficits in autism spectrum disorders are associated with reduced interhemispheric gamma-band coherence. *Journal of Neuroscience, 35*(50), 16352–16361.

Porges, S. W. (1995). Orienting in defensive world: Mammalian modifications of our evolutionary heritage. A polyvagal theory. *Psychophysiology, 32*(4), 301–318.

Porges, S. W. (2003). The polyvagal theory: Phylogenetic contributions to social behavior. *Physiology and Behavior, 79*(3), 503–513.

Porges, S. W., Daussard-Roosevelt, J. A., Portales, L., and Greenspan, S. I. (1996). Infant regulation of the vagal "brake" predicts child behavioral problems: A psychobiological model of social behavior. *Developmental Psychobiology, 29*(8), 697–712.

Rees, C. A. (2014). Lost among trees? The autonomic nervous system and paediatrics. *Archives of Disease in Childhood, 99*(6), 552–562.

Rogers, S. J., and Ozonoff, S. (2005). Annotation: What do we know about sensory dysfunction in autism? A critical review of the empirical evidence. *Journal of Child Psychology and Psychiatry, and Allied Disciplines, 46*(12), 1255–1268.

Rojas, D. C., and Wilson, L. B. (2014). γ-band abnormalities as markers of autism spectrum disorders. *Biomarkers in Medicine, 8*(3), 353–368.

Rubenstein, J. L., and Merzenich, M. M. (2003). Model of autism: Increased ratio of excitation/inhibition in key neural systems. *Genes, Brain, and Behavior, 2*(5), 255–267.

Schwartz, S., Kessler, R., Gaughan, T., and Buckley, A. W. (2017). Electroencephalogram coherence patterns in autism: An updated review. *Pediatric Neurology, 67*, 7–22.

Sheer, D. E. (1989). Focused arousal and the cognitive 40-Hz event-related potentials: Differential diagnosis of Alzheimer's disease. *Progress in Clinical and Biological Research, 317*, 79–94.

Smeekens, I., Dibben, R., and Verhoeven, E. W. (2015). Exploring the relationship of autonomic and endocrine activity with social functioning in adults with autism spectrum disorders. *Journal of Autism and Developmental Disorders, 45*(2), 495–505.

Sohn, J. H., Sokhadze, E., and Watanuki, S. (2001). Electrodermal and cardiovascular manifestations of emotions in children. *Journal of Physiological Anthropology and Applied Human Science, 20*(2), 55–64.

Sokhadze, E. M., Casanova, M. F., Kelly, D. L., Sokhadze, G. E., Li, Y., Elmaghraby, A., and El-Baz, A. (2016a). Virtual reality with psychophysiological monitoring as an approach to evaluate emotional reactivity, social skills and joint attention in autism spectrum disorder. In M. F. Casanova, A. S. El-Baz and J. Suri (Eds.), *Autism Imaging and Devices*. London and New York, NY: Taylor & Francis.

Sokhadze, E., El-Baz, A., Tasman, A., Sokhadze, G., Farag, H., and Casanova, M. F. (2016b). Repetitive transcranial magnetic stimulations (rTMS) effects on evoked and induced gamma frequency EEG oscillations in autism spectrum disorder. In M. F. Casanova, A. S. El-Baz and J. Suri (Eds.), *Autism Imaging and Devices*. London and New York, NY: Taylor & Francis.

Sokhadze, G. E., Casanova, M. F., Kelly, D. P., Casanova, E. L., Russell, B., and Sokhadze, E. M. (2017). Neuromodulation based on rTMS affects behavioral measures and autonomic nervous system activity in children with autism. *NeuroRegulation, 4*(2), 65–78.

Sokhadze, E. M., Casanova, M. F., Casanova, E. L., Klusek, J., and Roberts, J. (2019). Autonomic nervous system dysfunctions in children with autism spectrum disorder. In E. M. Sokhadze and M. F. Casanova (Eds.), *Autism Spectrum Disorder: Neuromodulation, Neurofeedback and Sensory Integration Approaches to Research and Treatment.* Murfreesboro, TN: FNNR.

Spydell, J. D., Ford, M. R., and Sheer, D. E. (1979). Task dependent cerebral lateralization of the 40 Hertz EEG rhythm. *Psychophysiology, 16*(4), 347–350.

Stemmler, G. (2003). Methodological considerations in the psychophysiological study of emotion. In R. J. Davidson, K. R. Scherer and H. Goldsmith (Eds.), *Handbook of Affective Sciences.* New York, NY: Oxford University Press.

Stemmler, G. (2004). Physiological processes during emotion. In P. Philippot and R. S. Feldman (Eds.), *The Regulation of Emotion.* Mahwah, NJ: Erlbaum.

Stemmler, G., and Wacker, J. (2009). Personality, emotion, and individual differences in physiological responses. *Biological Psychology, 84*(3), 541–551.

Stroganova, T. A., Nygren, G., Tsetlin, M. M., Posikera, I. N., Gillberg, C., Elam, M., and Orekhova, E. V. (2007). Abnormal EEG lateralization in boys with autism. *Clinical Neurophysiology, 118*(8), 1842–1854.

Sun, L., Grützner, C., Bölte, S., Wibral, M., Tozman, T., Schlitt, S., ... Uhlhaas, P. J. (2012). Impaired gamma-band activity during perceptual organization in adults with autism spectrum disorders: Evidence for dysfunctional network activity in frontal-posterior cortices. *Journal of Neuroscience, 32*(28), 9563–9573.

Sutton, S. K., Burnette, C. P., Mundy, P. C., Meyer, J., Vaughan, A., Sanders, C., and Yale, M. (2005). Resting cortical brain activity and social behavior in higher functioning children with autism. *Journal of Child Psychology and Psychiatry, and Allied Disciplines, 46*(2), 211–222.

Tamas, G., Buhl, E. H., Lorincz, A., and Somogyi, P. (2000). Proximally targeted GABAergic synapses and gap junctions synchronize cortical interneurons. *Nature Neuroscience, 3*(4), 366–371.

Terasawa, Y., Shibata, M., Moriguchi, Y., and Umeda, S. (2013). Anterior insular cortex mediates bodily sensibility and social anxiety. *Social Cognitive and Affective Neuroscience, 8*(3), 259–266.

Thayer, J. F. (2015). A neurovisceral integration perspective. The 46th annual meeting of the Association for Applied Psychophysiology and Biofeedback. Austin, TX, March 14.

Thayer, J. F., and Lane, R. D. (2000). A model of neurovisceral integration in emotion regulation and dysregulation. *Journal of Affective Disorders, 61*(3), 201–216.

Thayer, J. F., and Friedman, B. H. (2002). Stop that: Inhibition, sensitization, and their neurovisceral concomitants. *Scandinavian Journal of Psychology, 43*(2), 123–130.

Thayer, J. F., and Lane, R. D. (2005). The importance of inhibition in dynamical systems models of emotion and neurobiology. *Brain and Behavioral Sciences, 28*(2), 218–219.

Thayer, J. F., Hansen, A. L., Saus-Rose, E., and Johnsen, B. H. (2009). Heart rate variability, prefrontal neural function, and cognitive performance: The neurovisceral integration perspective on self-regulation, adaptation, and health. *Annals of Behavioral Medicine, 37*(2), 141–153.

Thayer, J. F., and Lane, R. D. (2009). Claude Bernard and the heart–brain connection: Further elaboration of a model of neurovisceral integration. *Neuroscience and Biobehavioral Reviews, 33*(2), 81–88.

Thayer, J. F., Ahs, F., Fredrikson, M., Sollers, J. J., and Wager, T. D. (2012). A meta-analysis of heart rate variability and neuroimaging studies: Implications for heart rate variability as a marker of stress and health. *Neuroscience and Biobehavioral Reviews, 36*(2), 747–756.

Toichi, M., and Kamio, Y. (2003). Paradoxical autonomic response to mental task in autism. *Journal of Autism and Developmental Disorders, 33*(4), 417–426.

Tomarken, A. J., Davidson, R. J., Wheeler, R. E., and Kinney, L. (1992). Psychometric properties of resting anterior EEG asymmetry: Temporal stability and internal consistency. *Psychophysiology, 29*(5), 576–592.

Uhlhaas, P. J., Roux, F., Rodriguez, E., Rotarska-Jagiela, A., and Singer, W. (2010). Neural synchrony and the development of cortical networks. *Trends in Cognitive Sciences, 14*(2), 72–80.

Uzunova, G., Pallanti, S., and Hollander, E. (2016). Excitatory/inhibitory imbalance in autism spectrum disorders: Implications for interventions and therapeutics. *World Journal of Biological Psychiatry, 17*(3), 174–186.

van Diessen, E., Senders, J., Jansen, F. E., Boersma, M., and Bruining, H. (2015). Increased power of resting-state gamma oscillations in autism spectrum disorder detected by routine electroencephalography. *European Archives of Psychiatry and Clinical Neuroscience, 265*(6), 537–540.

Wang, Y., Hensley, M., Tasman, A., Sears, L., Casanova, M. F., and Sokhadze, E. M. (2016). Heart rate variability and skin conductance during repetitive TMS course in children with autism. *Applied Psychophysiology and Biofeedback, 41*(1), 47–60.

Webb, S. J., Dawson, G., Bernier, R., and Panagiotides, H. (2006). ERP evidence of atypical face processing in young children with autism. *Journal of Autism and Developmental Disorders, 36*(7), 881–890.

Whittington, M. A., Traub, R. D., Kopell, N., Ermentrout, B., and Buhl, E. (2000). Inhibition-based rhythms: Experimental and mathematical observations on network dynamics. *International Journal of Psychophysiology, 38*(3), 315–336.

Zahn, T. P., Rumsey, J. M., and Van Kammen, D. P. (1987). Autonomic nervous system activity in autistic, schizophrenic, and normal men: Effects of stimulus significance. *Journal of Abnormal Psychology, 96*(2), 135–144.

CHAPTER 2

Crosstalk Between the Immune and Autonomic Nervous Systems and Their Relationship to Anxiety in Autism

Emily L. Casanova, Ph.D., University of South Carolina School of Medicine, Greenville, South Carolina, Manuel F. Casanova, M.D., University of South Carolina School of Medicine, Greenville and Prisma Health System, Greenville, South Carolina, and Estate M. Sokhadze, Ph.D. and Eva V. Lamina, Ph.D., University of South Carolina School of Medicine, Greenville, South Carolina

Introduction

The peripheral nervous system and the immune system are evolutionarily designed to communicate with one another and with other organ systems across a wide range of bodily territory, helping to integrate incoming signals and mount adaptive responses. The peripheral nervous system is comprised of two main branches, the motor and sensory branches—here we will focus on a subset of the former.

The motor branch of the peripheral nervous system is further subdivided into the somatic nervous system, which controls voluntary movements, and the autonomic nervous system (ANS), which regulates the body's involuntary responses. The ANS is comprised of sympathetic and parasympathetic branches. Although a gross generalization of its function, the sympathetic nervous system (SNS) is largely responsible for the "fight or flight" response, stimulating the adrenal glands and triggering a release of catecholamines like epinephrine and norepinephrine. This leads to symptoms such as increased heart rate and sweating, fast and shallow breathing, pupil dilation, muscle tension, and slowing of digestion and peristalsis (intestinal contractions)—many of the features associated with anxiety states. Meanwhile, the parasympathetic nervous system (PSNS) is sometimes referred to as the "rest and digest" response and often, though not always, helps to suppress sympathetic activation.

The ANS is comprised of components of both the central and peripheral nervous systems. Within the central nervous system (CNS), the ANS consists of portions of the prefrontal cortex, the limbic system (especially the hypothalamus), parts of the brainstem, and tracts within the spinal cord (Kenney and Ganta, 2014). These regions directly or indirectly synapse onto dorsal root ganglia stemming from the spinal cord, which provide continuity with the peripheral nervous system and its many contacts.

The SNS and the immune system communicate with one another at a variety of locations within the body and through a range of means. The SNS directly innervates both primary and secondary lymphoid organs, such as bone marrow, thymus, spleen, and lymph nodes and other lymphatic tissue, strongly influencing their development and function (Kenny and Ganta, 2014). Many of these peripheral nerve fibers share subsequent communication with the CNS, providing a feedback loop to the brain concerning peripheral immune system activity.

In addition, there are two locations at the junction between the periphery and the CNS that lack the protective blood–brain barrier (BBB) and allow a freer communication between circulating immunomodulators and the brain. These occur at sites of the third and fourth ventricles and are known as the circumventricular organs (CVO). However, some immune mediators, such as tumor necrosis factor alpha (TNF-α) and interleukin 1 (IL-1), are also able to cross the strict BBB present at most sites within the CNS vasculature with the help of their complementary receptors. Finally, other immunomodulators can trigger the production of cyclooxygenase 2 (COX-2) and prostaglandin E2 (PGE2) within endothelial and perivascular macrophages lining the BBB. PGE2 then influences activation of the hypothalamic–pituitary–adrenal (HPA) axis, fever induction, and further regulation of the SNS (Kenny and Ganta, 2014).

In order to foster direct communication between the immune and nervous systems, immune cells such as lymphocytes (e.g., T and B cells) and granulocytes/phagocytes all maintain a variety of neurotransmitter receptors (cholinergic, catecholaminergic, peptidergic, etc.), which allow them to respond to the nervous system in a process known as the "inflammatory reflex" (Tracey, 2009; Levite, 2000; Straub *et al.*, 2000; Csaba, 2011). Cytokine receptors are also present on the visceral organs, allowing a means for indirect and even complementary crosstalk between these two systems (Kenny and Ganta, 2014). Meanwhile, both the CNS and the peripheral nervous system express a variety of cytokine receptors, closing the circle of communication (Hopkins and Rothwell, 1995).

As a prime example of immune and nervous system crosstalk, mast cells, a type of granulocyte, are closely juxtaposed to nerves within most tissues, forming cell–nerve junctions that are maintained through adhesion molecules, providing constant feedback to the nervous system (Suzuki *et al.*, 2004). Distributed throughout connective tissue and mucosal surfaces, mast cells are the immune system's first line of defense to invading pathogens, parasites, noxious stimuli, and injury, and as such are ideally placed to foster communication directly with the nervous system (Suzuki *et al.*, 1999). Mast cells synthesize and release a wide variety of pro- and anti-inflammatory mediators, including histamines, prostaglandins, leukotrienes, and various cytokines (Van der Kleij and Bienenstock, 2005). In addition, both tumor necrosis factor (TNF) and nerve growth factor (NGF) released by mast cells have sensitizing effects on pain-associated C-fibers, lowering their threshold for excitation (Nicol *et al.*, 1997; Kakurai *et al.*, 2006; Van Houwelingen *et al.*, 2002; Leon *et al.*, 1994). It is possible that the release of these growth factors into the local surround that promotes increased nerve growth seen during inflammation may be responsible for some chronic pain syndromes (Woolf *et al.*, 1994; Landry *et al.*, 2017; Martinov *et al.*, 2013).

The inflammatory reflex mentioned earlier is a series of reflexive arcs in which the ANS directly regulates immune system activity. Although once more a gross oversimplification, epinephrine and norepinephrine released from the SNS typically drive inflammation, while cholinergic signaling from the vagus nerve (i.e., PSNS) attenuates the inflammatory response (Tracey, 2002). A number of chronic inflammatory-related diseases have, in part, been associated with weak vagal tone and activation of the sympathetic branch, suggesting that nervous system-derived dysregulation may drive some of the exaggerated pro-inflammatory responses in these conditions (e.g., Hansson, 2005; Triposkiadis *et al.*, 2009). Interestingly, traumatic brain injury (TBI) and stroke have likewise been associated with weak vagal tone and sympathoactivation, leading to increased inflammatory responses in peripheral organs, susceptibility to infection, and alterations to intestinal permeability (Griffin, 2011; Hang *et al.*, 2003; Macrez *et al.*, 2011). As you continue reading this chapter it will become clearer that there is significant crosstalk between the nervous and immune systems.

The Immune and Autonomic Nervous Systems in Autism
The Immune System

We will not go into extensive detail on the immune system in autism, as that topic will be covered in Chapter 3 by Edelson, Van de Water and Edelson. However, we will briefly review some of the basic findings so that we can better understand how they may relate to dysregulation of the ANS in this condition.

A variety of immunological findings have been reported in autism, which together suggest that immune dysregulation is a common feature of the condition and that it may play a role in the etiologies of at least a subset of cases. Some of the reported findings include: familial clustering of autoimmune disorders; abnormal cytokine levels in children with autism; abnormal T cell populations and functional dysregulation; the presence of brain-specific autoantibodies (including those maternally derived); occasional immunoglobulin deficiencies; and the sometimes successful amelioration of behavioral symptoms via intravenous infusion of immunoglobulins (IVIG) (Comi et al., 1999; Ashwood et al., 2011a, 2011b; Singh et al., 1997; Braunschweig et al., 2013; Warren et al., 1997; Gupta et al., 1996; Plioplys, 1998). The innate immune system has been implicated in autism (particularly mast cells), but their involvement is currently theoretical—though promising (Theoharides et al., 2016; Casanova et al., 2018).

Maternal immune activation (MIA) during pregnancy, either from acute or chronic illness, has also been implicated as a mechanism in the development of autism (reviewed in Onore et al., 2012). MIA has been tested using various animal models, which suggest that MIA has long-lasting effects not only on offspring behavior, but in the developing immune system as well (Hsiao et al., 2012).

The Autonomic Nervous System

As we see with the immune system, it is uncertain whether functional abnormalities of the ANS in autism are primary (i.e., due to dysfunction within the ANS itself) or secondary, and responding to an abnormality in one of its communicating systems. Due to this uncertainty, we refer to "dysregulation" rather than "dysfunction" in these two important systems.

Cardiac and electrodermal activities are the most frequently used indices in the study of the ANS in autism. Heart rate (HR) and heart rate variability (HRV) are used to estimate sympathetic and parasympathetic influences. Mean HR is a reflection of the conjoined effects of sympathetic and parasympathetic inputs, while evoked HR is due to fluctuations in overall vagal tone. The high frequency range of HRV, otherwise known as respiratory sinus arrhythmia (RSA), reflects the role of the PSNS. Finally, electrodermal activity (EDA) refers to the activity of sweat glands in the skin, which are believed to be innervated solely by the SNS and are used as a reliable indicator of activation of that system (reviewed in Sokhadze *et al.*, 2018).

Numerous studies on autism have reported similar results, agreeing that the condition is typified by SNS hyperarousal and weak PSNS vagal tone (Klusek *et al.*, 2015; Patriquin *et al.*, 2013; Ming *et al.*, 2016). People with autism often exhibit blunted cardiac responses to various novel and social stimuli compared with controls, yet do not habituate well to stimuli overall (Hirstein *et al.*, 2001; Palkovitz and Wiesenfeld, 1980; Barry and James, 1988; van Engeland, 1984). Interestingly, the severity of ANS dysregulation correlates with severity of the core symptoms of autism and general cognitive level, indicating a poorly understood yet promising relationship between these symptoms (Klusek *et al.*, 2013; Watson *et al.*, 2010, 2012; Patriquin *et al.*, 2013). Meanwhile, stereotypies have been proposed as a mechanism by which an individual may reduce sympathetic hyperarousal, suggesting these behaviors are functional adaptations to a poorly regulated nervous system (Condy *et al.*, 2017; Hirstein *et al.*, 2001).

The Immune or Nervous Systems?

While we cannot determine whether the seat of dysfunction in autism lies within the immune or nervous systems, we do see evidence of chronic inflammatory processes in the condition. This inflammation is theoretically capable of influencing activity of the ANS both directly through its contacts with innate immune cells and indirectly through the communicating cerebrovasculature. Likewise, decreased vagal tone associated with autism suggests a means by which ANS dysregulation can lead to inflammation, as evidenced by cases of stroke and TBI. While this unfortunately doesn't answer the chicken-versus-egg question, it does give us an appreciation of how complex their etiologies may be, and the possibility that that answer may vary on a case-by-case basis.

Anxiety and Autonomic Dysregulation

Anxiety can often lead to symptoms associated with sympathetic arousal, such as increased HR, reduced HRV, sweaty palms, shallow breathing, nausea, and even lightheadedness (Mayo Clinic, 2019). Numerous studies have found an association between autonomic dysregulation and the presence of anxiety disorders, although, as with autism, it is difficult to discern whether the anxiety leads to autonomic dysregulation or vice versa (Hoehn-Saric and McLeod, 1988). We do know, however, that a falsely elevated HR can trigger a panic attack in anxiety sufferers, suggesting that some of the cognitive effects of anxiety may be precipitated or even triggered by the physical symptoms of autonomic dysregulation (Ehlers *et al.*, 1988). Interestingly, aerobic exercise, a technique used to treat certain autonomic disorders such as postural orthostatic tachycardia syndrome (POTS), also reduces anxiety sensitivity in those with generalized anxiety disorder (GAD), suggesting that feedback from the peripheral nervous system can improve cognitive symptoms of anxiety (Broman-Fulks *et al.*, 2004; Fu *et al.*, 2011). The method of exercise's effectiveness on ANS function is currently uncertain, although it may partly reflect increases in baroreflex sensitivity and its subsequent effects on the PSNS (Ueno and Moritani, 2003).

Certain classes of drugs that are commonly used in conditions like anxiety or depression may also influence the ANS and, counter to intuition, drive poor vagal tone. A study done in the Netherlands reported that while low RSA (i.e., low vagal tone) was associated with anxiety and depression, the use of tricyclics, selective serotonin reuptake inhibitors (SSRIs), and other antidepressants may have promoted low RSA (Licht *et al.*, 2009). Therefore, while we are attempting to treat anxiety and depression with these drugs, they may have untoward effects on the peripheral nervous system that, ironically, help to exacerbate symptoms of the conditions, thus suggesting that alternative drug therapies may be warranted.

Similar to autism, chronic anxiety sufferers exhibit reduced HRV and vagal tone compared with controls (Miu *et al.*, 2009). As discussed above, individuals with depression also show a similar trend and, like those with anxiety and presumably those with autism, are at increased risk for sudden death due to coronary heart disease and arrhythmias, possibly due to the amount of chronic sympathetic stress that is placed on the cardiovascular system (Gorman and Sloan, 2000; Roest *et al.*, 2010). For these reasons in particular, and with the current aging autism spectrum population, it is vital that we better understand these risk factors and provide means for relief so as to extend length and quality of life for those on the spectrum.

Anxiety in Autism

It appears that the majority of youth with autism experience some form of significant anxiety, whether it is in the form of social phobia, generalized anxiety, or specific phobias (Kerns *et al.*, 2014; White *et al.*, 2009). This trend continues into adulthood, with reports of anxiety related especially to difficulties coping with change, sensory over-responsivity, and unpleasant events (Gillot and Standen, 2007). Meanwhile, neither cognitive ability nor sex appears to be a significant determinant of anxiety risk in autism, the latter despite the fact that women on the spectrum report greater sensory over-responsivity and fewer socio-communication problems than their male counterparts (Bradley *et al.*, 2004; Hofvander *et al.*, 2009; Lai *et al.*, 2011). Therefore, anxiety prevalence in autism knows no bounds when it comes to major demographic breakdowns. Interestingly, however, according to Davis *et al.* (2011), anxiety increases in autism from toddlerhood to childhood, decreases into adolescence and into young adulthood, but increases once again into older adulthood—a trend potentially reflective of the changing demands that occur across the lifespan. While this study looked at individuals diagnosed with autistic disorder, it is uncertain if the same trend is seen in individuals who fall into the Asperger's range of cognitive functioning or whether they exhibit their own unique pattern of anxiety across the lifespan.

As mentioned earlier, individuals with anxiety often exhibit low RSA, indicative of poor vagal tone, and autistic people are little different. In autism, RSA shares a positive relationship with social skills ability (i.e., the lower the vagal tone, the poorer the social skills), as well as internalizing symptoms such as anxiety/depression, withdrawal, and somatic complaints (Neuhaus *et al.*, 2014). Individuals with autism also often exhibit blunted heart rate response and HRV compared with controls—however, these results appear to be largely related to the presence of anxiety in autism. In other words, individuals with autism without an anxiety disorder do not differ from typical controls in terms of heart rate response. Meanwhile, autistic individuals with anxiety differ significantly and likewise produce lower levels of cortisol during psychosocial stress (Hollocks *et al.*, 2014). Other studies in autism have found an inverse relationship between overall levels of stress and cortisol production, as well as some aspects of sensory over-responsivity (Corbett *et al.*, 2009).

Stereotypic behavior and sensory over-responsivity are common symptoms of autism. Interestingly, while arousal states can be associated with increased sensory responsiveness, motor behaviors such as stereotypies can provide strong suppression of incoming somatosensory information (Chapin and Woodward, 1981). For this and other reasons, it has been proposed that autistic people may often intuitively use stereotypic behavior to regulate incoming sensory input and reduce overall sympathetic activation (Condy *et al.*, 2017; Hirstein *et al.*, 2001). And, as mentioned above, it has been suggested that some aspects of sensory over-responsivity and anxiety may be causally related (Green and Ben-Sasson, 2010; Spielmann and Miller, Chapter 6).

When measured during anxiety-provoking tasks such as the Stroop task,[1] autistic individuals exhibit elevated EDA (sympathetic activation) while doing the baseline task during which they should otherwise be calm, but then blunted activation while doing the anxiety tasks (Kushki *et al.*, 2013). This suggests that autistic individuals experience chronic sympathoactivation and also that they do not adjust to the demands of a given task. The same can be seen during social tasks, such as the judgment of emotional facial expressions: those with autism exhibit lower skin conductance response than controls (Hubert *et al.*, 2009). In addition, autistic children with higher RSA (better vagal tone) not only identify facial emotions more accurately, but also spend an increased amount of time looking at the eyes compared with autistic children with reduced vagal tone (Bal *et al.*, 2010).

Interestingly, autistic children exhibit heightened skin conductance responses compared with controls when shown facial stimuli with a straight

---

1 In psychology, the Stroop task is a test that illustrates cognitive interference in which a delay in response occurs due to mismatch in stimuli. A common example includes color words, such as the word "red," in which the color of the text is mismatched with the meaning of the word.

gaze (i.e., direct eye contact) versus an averted gaze (Kylliäinen and Hietanen, 2006). This is one of the major social stimuli in which autistic people tend to experience an exaggerated autonomic response, undoubtedly explaining many autistic people's aversion to eye contact. Whether this aversion is related to overall anxiety in autism is uncertain, although a similar feature in social anxiety disorder suggests this could be the case and that autistic people with higher RSA may not experience the same aversion to eye contact as their more anxious autistic counterparts (Schneier et al., 2011).

Discussion

While ANS dysregulation may not exist in all cases of autism, it is clear that it occurs in a significant majority. Whether dysregulation is linked primarily with high comorbidity rates of anxiety/depression in autism is unclear, some studies suggest that anxiety disorders are a predictive factor for the occurrence of autonomic disorders. How medication exposure complicates this complex phenotype in autism is currently uncertain.

Immune dysregulation is also very common in the condition and may share links with ANS function, given the varied feedback loops these systems share with one another. Interestingly, some studies suggest there are links between anxiety and inflammation, particularly in men, indicating once again that the presence of anxiety may be a risk factor (Vogelzangs et al., 2013). However, whether anxiety disorders drive immune dysregulation or vice versa remains to be seen.

Because the CNS, PSNS, and immune system share extensive feedback loops with one another, therapeutically targeting any one component of this larger multisystem network may theoretically provide relief from anxiety, autonomic, and immune disorders. Therapeutic methods that target vagal tone, improve sensitivity to changes in blood pressure (e.g., aerobic exercise) or lower blood pressure (e.g., propranolol), and reduce inflammation, may all provide relief of associated symptoms. Future studies will determine to what extent these therapies improve quality of life in autism and, hopefully, extend the lifespan.

References

Ashwood, P., Krakowiak, P., Hertz-Picciotto, I., Hansen, R., Pessah, I., and Van de Water, J. (2011a). Elevated plasma cytokines in autism spectrum disorders provide evidence of immune dysfunction and are associated with impaired behavioral outcome. *Brain, Behavior, and Immunity, 25*, 40–45.

Ashwood, P., Krakowiak, P., Hertz-Picciotto, I., Hansen, R., Pessah, I., and Van de Water, J. (2011b). Altered T cell responses in children with autism. *Brain, Behavior, and Immunity, 25*, 840–849.

Bal, E., Harden, E., Lamb, D., Van Hecke, A. V., Denver, J. W., and Porges, S. W. (2010). Emotion recognition in children with autism spectrum disorders: Relationship to eye gaze and autonomic state. *Journal of Autism and Developmental Disorders, 40*, 358–370.

Barry, R. J., and James, A. L. (1988). Coding of stimulus parameters in autistic, retarded, and normal children: Evidence for a two-factor theory of autism. *International Journal of Psychophysiology, 6*, 139–149.

Bradley, E. A., Summers, J. A., Wood, H. L., and Bryson, S. E. (2004). Comparing rates of psychiatric and behavior disorders in adolescents and young adults with severe intellectual disability with and without autism. *Journal of Autism and Developmental Disorders, 34*, 151–161.

Braunschweig, D., Krakowiak, P., Duncanson, P., Boyce, R., Hansen, R. L., Ashwood, P., *et al.* (2013). Autism-specific maternal autoantibodies recognize critical proteins in developing brain. *Translational Psychiatry, 3*, e277.

Broman-Fulks, J., Berman, M. E., Rabian, B. A., and Webster, M. J. (2004). Effects of aerobic exercise on anxiety sensitivity. *Behaviour Research and Therapy, 42*, 125–136.

Casanova, E. L., Sharp, J. L., Edelson, S. M., Kelly, D. P., and Casanova, M. F. (2018). A cohort study comparing women with autism spectrum disorder with and without generalized joint hypermobility. *Behavioral Sciences, 8*, 35.

Chapin, J. K., and Woodward, D. J. (1981). Modulation of sensory responsiveness of single somatosensory cortical cells during movement and arousal behaviors. *Experimental Neurology, 72*, 164–178.

Comi, A. M., Zimmerman, A. W., Frye, V. H., Law, P. A., and Peeden, J. N. (1999). Familial clustering of autoimmune disorders and evaluation of medical risk factors in autism. *Journal of Child Neurology, 14*, 388–394.

Condy, E., Scarpa, A., and Friedman, B. H. (2017). Respiratory sinus arrthythmia predicts restricted repetitive behavior severity. *Journal of Autism and Developmental Disorders, 47*, 2795–2804.

Corbett, B. A., Schupp, C. W., Levine, S., and Mendoza, S. (2009). Comparing cortisol, stress, and sensory sensitivity in children with autism. *Autism Research, 2*, 39–49.

Csaba, G. (2011). The immune-endocrine system: Hormones, receptors and endocrine function of immune cells. The packed-transport theory. *Advances in Neuroimmune Biology, 1*, 71–85.

Davis, T. E., Hess, J. A., Moree, B. N., Fodstad, J. C., Dempsey, T., Jenkins, W. S., and Matson, J. L. (2011). Anxiety symptoms across the lifespan in people diagnosed with autistic disorder. *Research in Autism Spectrum Disorders, 5*, 112–118.

Ehlers, A., Margraf, J., Rother, W. T., Taylor, C. B., and Birbaumer, N. (1988). Anxiety induced by false heart rate feedback in patients with panic disorder. *Behaviour Research and Therapy, 26*, 1–11.

Fu, Q., VanGundy, T. B., Shibata, S., Auchus, R. J., Williams, G. H., and Levine, B. D. (2011). Exercise training versus propranolol in the treatment of the postural orthostatic tachycardia syndrome. *Hypertension, 58*, 167–175.

Gillot, A., and Standen, P. J. (2007). Levels of anxiety and souces of stress in adults with autism. *Journal of Intellectual Disabilities, 11*, 359–370.

Gorman, J. M., and Sloan, R. P. (2000). Heart rate variability in depressive and anxiety disorders. *American Heart Journal, 140*, S77–S83.

Green, S. A., and Ben-Sasson, A. (2010). Anxiety disorders and sensory over-responsivity in children with autism spectrum disorders: Is there a causal relationship? *Journal of Autism and Developmental Disorders, 12*, 1495–1504.

Griffin, G. D. (2011). The injured brain: TBI, mTBI, the immune system, and infection: Connecting the dots. *Military Medicine, 176*, 364–368.

Gupta, S., Aggarwal, S., and Heads, C. (1996). Brief report: Dysregulated immune system in children with autism: Beneficial effects of intravenous immune globulin on autistic characteristics. *Journal of Autism and Developmental Disorders, 26*, 439–452.

Hang, C.-H., Shi, J.-X., Li, J.-S., Wu, W., and Yin, H.-X. (2003). Alterations of intestinal mucosa structure and barrier function following traumatic brain injury in rats. *World Journal of Gastroenterology, 9*, 2776.

Hansson, G. K. (2005). Inflammation, atherosclerosis, and coronary artery disease. *New England Journal of Medicine, 352*, 1685–1695.

Hirstein, W., Iversen, P., and Ramachandran, V. S. (2001). Autonomic responses of autistic children to people and objects. *Proceedings of the Royal Society of London, B Biological Sciences, 268*, 1883–1888.

Hoehn-Saric, R. and McLeod, D. R. (1988). The peripheral sympathetic nervous system: Its role in normal and pathologic anxiety. *Psychiatric Clinics, 11*, 375–386.

Hofvander, B., Delorme, R., Chaste, P., Nydén, A., Wentz, E., Ståhlberg, O., *et al.* (2009). Psychiatric and psychosocial problems in adults with normal-intelligence autism spectrum disorders. *BMC Psychiatry, 9*, 35.

Hollocks, M. J., Howlin, P., Papadopoulos, A. S., Khondoker, M., and Simonoff, E. (2014). Differences in HPA-axis and heart rate responsiveness to psychosocial stress in children with autism spectrum disorders with and without co-morbid anxiety. *Psychoneuroendocrinology, 46*, 32–45.

Hopkins, S. J., and Rothwell, N. J. (1995). Cytokines and the nervous system I: Expression and recognition. *Trends in Neurosciences, 18*, 83–88.

Hsiao, E. Y., McBride, S. W., Chow, J., Mazmanian, S. K., and Patterson, P. H. (2012). Modeling an autism risk factor in mice leads to permanent immune dysregulation. *Proceedings of the National Academy of Sciences, 109*, 12776–12781.

Hubert, B. E., Wicker, B., Monfardini, E., and Deruelle, C. (2009). Electrodermal reactivity to emotion processing in adults with autistic spectrum disorders. *Autism, 13*, 9–19.

Kakurai, M., Monteforte, R., Suto, H., Tsai, M., Nakae, S., and Galli, S. J. (2006). Mast cell-derived tumor necrosis factor can promote nerve fiber elongation in the skin during contact hypersensitivity in mice. *The American Journal of Pathology, 169*, 1713–1721.

Kenney, M. J., and Ganta, C. K. (2014). Autonomic nervous system and immune system interactions. *Comprehensive Physiology, 4*, 1177–1200.

Kerns, C. M., Kendall, P. C., Berry, L., Souders, M. C., Franklin, M. E., Schultz, R. T., *et al.* (2014). Traditional and atypical presentations of anxiety in youth with autism spectrum disorder. *Journal of Autism and Developmental Disorders, 44*, 2851–2861.

Klusek, J., Martin, G. E., and Losh, M. (2013). Physiological arousal in autism and fragile X syndrome: Group comparisons and links with pragmatic language. *American Journal on Intellectual and Developmental Disabilities, 118*, 475–495.

Klusek, J., Roberts, J. E., and Losh, M. (2015). Cardiac autonomic regulation in autism and fragile X syndrome: A review. *Psychology Bulletin, 141*, 141–175.

Kushki, A., Drumm, E., Mobarak, M. P., Tanel, N., Dupuis, A., Chau, T., *et al.* (2013). Investigating the autonomic nervous sytem response to anxiety in children with autism spectrum disorders. *PLoS One, 8*, e59730.

Kylliäinen, A., and Hietanen, J. K. (2006). Skin conductance responses to another person's gaze in children with autism. *Journal of Autism and Developmental Disorders, 36*, 517–525.

Lai, M. C., Lombardo, M. V., Pasco, G., Ruigrok, A. N., Wheelwright, S. J., Sadek, S. A., *et al.* (2011). A behavioral comparison of male and female adults with high functioning autism spectrum conditions. *PLoS One, 6*, e20835.

Landry, J., Martinov, T., Mengistu, H., Dhanwada, J., Benck, C. J., Kline, J., *et al.* (2017). Repeated hapten exposure induces persistent tactile sensitivity in mice modeling localized provoked vulvodynia. *PLoS One, 12*, e0169672.

Leon, A., Buriani, A., Dal Toso, R., Fabris, M., Romanello, S., Aloe, L., and Levi-Montalcini, R. (1994). Mast cells synthesize, store, and release nerve growth factor. *Proceedings of the National Academy of Sciences USA, 91*, 3739–3743.

Levite, M. (2000). Nerve-driven immunity. The direct effects of neurotransmitters on T-cell function. *Annals of the New York Academy of Sciences, 917*, 307–321.

Licht, C. M., De Geus, E. J., Van Dyck, R., and Penninx, B. W. (2009). Association between anxiety disorders and heart rate variability in The Netherlands Study of Depression and Anxiety (NESDA). *Psychosomatic Medicine, 71*, 508–518.

Macrez, R., Ali, C., Toutirais, O., Le Mauff, B., Defer, G., Dirnagl, U., and Vivien, D. (2011). Stroke and the immune system: From pathophysiology to new therapeutic strategies. *The Lancet Neurology, 10*, 471–480.

Martinov, T., Glenn-Finer, R., Burley, S., Tonc, E., Balsells, E., Ashbaugh, A., *et al.* (2013). Contact hypersensitivity to oxazolone provokes vulvar mechanical hyperalgesia in mice. *PLoS One, 8*, e78673.

Mayo Clinic. (2019). Anxiety disorders. Accessed on 4/16/19 from: www.mayoclinic.org/diseases-conditions/anxiety/symptoms-causes/syc-20350961.

Ming, X., Patel, R., Kang, V., Chokroverty, S., and Julu, P. O. (2016). Respiratory autonomic dysfunction in children with autism spectrum disorders. *Brain and Development, 38*, 225–232.

Miu, A. C., Heilman, R. M., and Miclea, M. (2009). Reduced heart rate variability and vagal tone in anxiety: Trait versus state, and the effects of autogenic training. *Autonomic Neuroscience, 145*, 99–103.

Neuhaus, E., Bernier, R., and Beauchaine, T. P. (2014). Brief report: Social skills, internalizing and externalizing symptoms, and respiratory sinus arrhythmia in autism. *Journal of Autism and Developmental Disorders, 44*, 730–737.

Nicol, G. D., Lopshire, J. C., and Pafford, C. M. (1997). Tumor necrosis factor enhances the capsaicin sensitivity of rat sensory neurons. *Journal of Neuroscience, 17*, 975–982.

Onore, C., Careaga, M., and Ashwood, P. (2012). The role of immune dysfunction in the pathophysiology of autism. *Brain, Behavior, and Immunity, 26*, 383–392.

Palkovitz, R. J., and Wiesenfeld, A. R. (1980). Differential autonomic responses of autistic and normal children. *Journal of Autism and Developmental Disorders, 10*, 347–360.

Patriquin, M. A., Scarpa, A., Friedman, B. H., and Porges, S. W. (2013). Respiratory sinus arrhythmia: A marker for positive social functioning and receptive language skills in children with autism spectrum disorders. *Developmental Psychobiology, 55*, 101–112.

Plioplys, A. V. (1998). Intravenous immunoglobulin treatment of children with autism. *Journal of Child Neurology, 13*, 79–82.

Roest, A. M., Martens, E. J., de Jonge, P., and Denollet, J. (2010). Anxiety and risk of incident coronary heart disease: A meta-analysis. *Journal of the American College of Cardiology, 56*, 38–46.

Schneier, F. R., Rodebaugh, T. L., Blanco, C., Lewin, H., and Liebowitz, M. R. (2011). Fear and avoidance of eye contact in social anxiety disorder. *Comprehensive Psychiatry, 52*, 81–87.

Singh, V. K., Warren, R., Averett, R., and Ghaziuddin, M. (1997). Circulating autoantibodies to neuronal and glial filament proteins in autism. *Pediatric Neurology, 17*, 88–90.

Sokhadze, E. M., Casanova, M. F., Casanova, E. L., Klusek, J., and Roberts, J. (2018). Autonomic nervous system dysfunctions in children with autism spectrum disorder. In E. M. Sokhadze and M. F. Casanova (Eds.), *Autism Spectrum Disorder: Neuromodulation, Neurofeedback and Sensory Integration Approaches to Research and Treatment.* Murfreesboro, TN: FNNR.

Straub, R. H., Mayer, M., Kreutz, M., Leeb, S., Schölmerich, J., and Falk, W. (2000). Neurotransmitters of the sympathetic nerve terminal are powerful chemoattractants for monocytes. *Journal of Leukocyte Biology, 67*, 553–558.

Suzuki, R., Furuno, T., McKay, D. M., Wolvers, D., Teshima, R., Nakanishi, M., *et al.* (1999). Direct neurite-mast cell communication *in vitro* occurs via the neuropeptide substance P. *The Journal of Immunology, 163*, 2410–2415.

Suzuki, A., Suzuki, R., Furuno, T., Teshima, R., and Nakanishi, M. (2004). N-cadherin plays a role in the synapse-like structures between mast cells and neurites. *Biological and Pharmaceutical Bulletin, 27*, 1891–1894.

Theoharides, T. C., Stewart, J. M., Panagiotidou, S., and Melamed, I. (2016). Mast cells, brain inflammation and autism. *European Journal of Pharmacology, 778*, 96–102.

Tracey, K. J. (2002). The inflammatory reflex. *Nature, 420*, 853–859.

Tracey, K. J. (2009). Reflex control of immunity. *Nature Reviews Immunology, 9*, 418.

Triposkiadis, F., Karayannis, G., Giamouzis, G., Skoularigis, J., Louridas, G., and Butler, J. (2009). The sympathetic nervous system in heart failure: Physiology, pathophysiology, and clinical implications. *Journal of the American College of Cardiology, 54*, 1747–1762.

Ueno, L. M., and Moritani, T. (2003). Effects of long-term exercise training on cardiac autonomic nervous activities and baroreflex sensitivity. *European Journal of Applied Physiology, 89*, 109–114.

Van der Kleij, H. P. M., and Bienenstock, J. (2005). Significance of conversation between mast cells and nerves. *Allergy, Asthma, and Clinical Immunology, 1*, 65–80.

van Engeland, H. (1984). The electrodermal orienting response to auditive stimuli in autistic children, normal children, mentally retarded children, and child psychiatric patients. *Journal of Autism and Developmental Disorders, 14*, 261–279.

Van Houwelingen, A. H., Kool, M., de Jager, S. C., Redegeld, F. A., van Heuven-Nolsen, D., Kraneveld, A. D., *et al.* (2002). Mast cell-derived TNF-alpha primes sensory nerve endings in a pulmonary hypersensitivity reaction. *Journal of Immunology, 168*, 5297–5302.

Vogelzangs, N., Beekman, A. T. F., De Jonge, P., and Penninx, B. W. J. H. (2013). Anxiety disorders and inflammation in a large adult cohort. *Translational Psychiatry, 3*, e249.

Warren, R. P., Odell, J. D., Warren, W. L., Burger, R. A., Maciulis, A., Daniels, W. W., *et al.* (1997). Brief report: Immunoglobulin A deficiency in a subset of autistic subjects. *Journal of Autism and Developmental Disorders, 27*, 187–192.

Watson, L. R., Baranek, G. T., Roberts, J. E., David, F. J., and Perryman, T. Y. (2010). Behavioral and physiological responses to child-directed speech as predictors of communication outcomes in children with autism spectrum disorders. *Journal of Speech, Language, and Hearing Research, 53*, 1052–1064.

Watson, L. R., Roberts, J. E., Baranek, G. T., Mandulak, K. C., and Dalton, J. C. (2012). Behavioral and physiological responses to child-directed speech of children with autism spectrum disorders or typical development. *Journal of Autism and Developmental Disorders, 42*, 1616–1629.

White, S. W., Oswald, D., Ollendick, T., and Scahill, L. (2009). Anxiety in children and adolescents with autism spectrum disorders. *Clinical Psychology Review, 29*, 216–229.

Woolf, C. J., Safieh-Garabedian, B., Ma, Q.-P., Crilly, P., and Winter, J. (1994). Nerve growth factor contributes to the generation of inflammatory sensory hypersensitivity. *Neuroscience, 62*, 327–331.

CHAPTER 3

The Immune System and Anxiety
A Case for Toxic Exposure

Stephen M. Edelson, Ph.D., Autism Research Institute, California, Judy Van de Water, Ph.D., Department of Internal Medicine and U.C. Davis MIND Institute, and Micaela S. G. Edelson, M.Sc., Leeds University, UK

Introduction

Anxiety is one of the most common and disabling conditions suffered by individuals on the autism spectrum (Gordon-Lipkin *et al.*, 2018; McVey, 2019; Postorino *et al.*, 2017; Simonoff *et al.*, 2008). In this chapter, we will first discuss several immunological impairments often associated with autism, and then suggest how environmental toxicants may trigger an inflammatory response which, in turn, may play an instrumental role in anxiety.

Cytokines are the signaling molecules of the immune system, and there are now numerous reports of cytokine imbalances in autism spectrum disorder (ASD). Such dysregulation could have a pathogenic role, or, alternatively, could be an indication of genetic and environmental underpinnings. While cytokines act primarily as mediators of immune cell function, they also have a significant role in development and maintenance of the nervous system. For example, appropriate cytokine levels are critical for normal neural development and function, and changes in homeostatic levels can have a variety of neurological implications both during gestation and early in childhood. Further, circulating levels of cytokines can differ dramatically in the context of infection, disease, and toxicant exposures. Cytokines implicated in ASD include IL-1B, IL-6, IL-4, IFN-gamma, and TGF-Beta, and while their direct role in ASD is not clear, the implications based on their functional roles suggest an imbalance in some children between the inflammatory and regulatory cytokines (Goines and Ashwood, 2013; Meltzer and Van de Water, 2017).

It is possible that a cascade of events resulting from an immunological response to environmental toxicants could lead to anxiety in individuals with autism. Several toxic substances can trigger the release of pro-inflammatory cytokines, many of which have been linked to autism. Furthermore, such immune activation has a direct impact on the autonomic nervous system (ANS), and both immune function and the ANS are dysregulated in autism. The physiological changes caused by the sympathetic nervous system (SNS), a branch of the ANS, may be perceived in an exaggerated manner due to an impairment in the anterior insula, the primary site of interoception and a region known to be dysfunctional in autism. This could result in heightened awareness of one's own internal sensations, triggering an anxious state of arousal. We will provide supporting evidence for this proposed cascade of events in the remainder of this chapter.

Environmental Toxicants, Autism, and Immune Activation

Numerous biomedical studies have documented a relationship between autism and exposure to various classes of toxicants, including air pollution, persistent organic pollutants, pesticides, and heavy metals.

Air Pollution

For more than a decade, researchers have documented high prevalence rates of autism near dense traffic regions, such as highways (Volk *et al.*, 2011; von Ehrenstein *et al.*, 2014). See Flores-Pajot *et al.* (2016) for a review and meta-analysis of this research.

Traffic pollution consists of several components, including particulate matter (PM), halogenated/polycyclic aromatic hydrocarbons, and gaseous compounds (Saraswathy *et al.*, 2018). Regarding the first, PM consists of ammonia, black carbon, mineral dust, nitrates, sodium chloride, and sulfate. Although researchers have often focused their attention on the relationship between PM and neurotoxicity and asthma (Costa *et al.*, 2017), it is also known to trigger pro-inflammatory cytokine activity. Many of these cytokines have been associated with autism; research shows elevated levels of pro-inflammatory cytokines IL-1B, IL-6, and GM-CSF in autism as well as a reduction in the anti-inflammatory cytokine IL-10 (Barth *et al.*, 2017; Gruzieva *et al.*, 2017; Latzin *et al.*, 2011; van Eeden *et al.*, 2001).

Note: Gruzieva *et al.* (2017) found elevated levels of IL-10 associated with PM, which is generally in response to elevated inflammatory cytokines.

Persistent Organic Pollutants (POPs)

Halogenated/polycyclic aromatic hydrocarbons are highly toxic chemicals and include polychlorinated biphenyls (PCBs) and polybrominated diphenyl ethers (PBDEs). The latter were commonly used to make flame retardant materials. Relatively high levels of these persistent organic pollutants have been found in autistic individuals. See Vuong *et al.* (2018), Hertz-Picciotto *et al.* (2011), and Ye *et al.* (2017) for reviews.

Similar to PM, these POPs have been shown to trigger inflammatory cytokine activity. PCBs have been associated with elevations in IL-1B, IL-6, IL-10, IL-12, and TNF-alpha (Hayley *et al.*, 2011), and PBDEs have been associated with elevations in IL-1B (Ashwood *et al.*, 2009).

Pesticides

Research has documented increased rates of autism in communities located near regions using large amounts of pesticides (Shelton *et al.*, 2014; von Ehrenstein *et al.*, 2019). Three types of pesticides—organochlorines, organophosphates, and pyrethroids—are associated with inflammatory cytokine activity. Many of these cytokines, including IL-1B, IL-2, IL-4, IL-6, IL-8, and IFN-gamma, have also been linked to autism. See Goines and Ashwood (2013) for a discussion and review.

Heavy Metals

Levels of metals such as lead and mercury have been shown to be elevated in autism (Adams *et al.*, 2013; Adams *et al.*, 2007). These metals are known to trigger cytokine activity. Elevated lead levels are associated with high levels of IL-1B, IL-6, and TNF-alpha, which are also seen in autism (Machoń-Grecka *et al.*, 2017). Elevated mercury levels are associated with high levels of IL-6 and TNF-alpha as well as reduced levels of IL-10, also documented in autism (Gump *et al.*, 2014; Hui *et al.*, 2016).

The Autonomic Nervous System and Anxiety

Our discussion below is consistent with the previous two chapters by Sokhadze, Casanova, and their colleagues (Chapters 1 and 2), in which they summarize research on dysregulation in the ANS, a compromised immune system, and impairment in neural structures and processing in relation to both autism and anxiety. In addition, they outline a coherent multistage process to account for the biological underpinnings of anxiety in autistic individuals. However, they do not discuss the possible role of environmental toxicants in relation to this cascade of events.

As discussed in detail by Sokhadze *et al.* (Chapter 1) and Casanova *et al.* (Chapter 2), the immune system has a direct relationship with the ANS. That is, inflammation is associated with both the SNS and the peripheral nervous system (PNS), and both are dysregulated in autism. Activation of the SNS is known to trigger increases in heart rate, breathing, and muscle tension as well as lead to perspiration, pupil dilation, and gastrointestinal (GI) dysregulation (e.g., altered peristalsis and a deceleration of digestion).

With regard to the ANS and emotions, Sokhadze *et al.* (Chapter 1) stated: "Emotions are influenced by assessment of bodily arousal via interoception, which refers to the sensing of visceral signals from the inner body..." (page 36); and "Consequently, it is possible to propose that emotional deficits expressed by children with ASD may originate in impaired interoceptive processing and misjudgment related to their own arousal level" (page 38).

The perception of internal sensations occurs in the anterior insula. Research in the areas of both neuropathology and sensory processing has documented abnormalities in interoception in autistic children and adults, especially with regard to hyper-responsive interoception or an exaggerated awareness of internal sensations (Garfinkel *et al.*, 2016; Palser *et al.*, 2018).

Hyper-responsive interoception has been associated directly with anxiety (Garfinkel *et al.*, 2016; Krautwurst *et al.*, 2016). It is important to note that a substantial amount of research has also demonstrated a relationship between hyper-responsive interoception and anxiety in the neurotypical population (Owens *et al.*, 2017; Mallorquí-Bagué *et al.*, 2016; Paulus and Stein, 2010).

Situation-Specific vs. Generalized Anxiety

Numerous studies on emotions in autism have examined fears and social anxiety, both of which can be viewed as situation-specific anxiety. Substantially less attention has been centered on understanding a more generalized long-term form of anxiety, such as Generalized Anxiety Disorder (GAD) (Bitsika and Sharpley, 2017). We suggest that prolonged high levels of toxicants in the body may be responsible for GAD in autism. Interestingly, research on GAD has linked it to cytokine activity, including elevated levels of IL-4, IFN-gamma, and TNF-alpha, and decreased levels of IL-10, all of which, again, have been found to be altered in individuals with autism (Hou *et al.*, 2017).

Gastrointestinal Distress and Anxiety

An in-depth discussion of GI issues in relation to anxiety is located in Chapter 4 by Law, Ferguson, Margolis, and Beversdorf. One source of GI distress is microbial dysbiosis (Ge *et al.*, 2017; Ni *et al.*, 2017), and exposure to pesticides, air pollution, heavy metals, or hydrocarbons may alter the microbiome (Jin *et al.*, 2017; Laue *et al.*, 2019; Mutlu *et al.*, 2018).

Prolonged exposure during constipation would allow for a greater likelihood of digesting such toxic substances, which may not be simple to absorb. This could trigger a cascade of neurological, autonomic, and immune reactions, as outlined by Sokhadze, Casanova *et al.*, and in this chapter. Furthermore, prolonged or chronic activation of the SNS may exacerbate constipation by causing altered peristalsis and slowed digestion. And lastly, awareness of discomfort and pain, which are often associated with constipation, may be further heightened and contribute to anxiety.

Behavioral and Sensory Perspectives Regarding Autism

The arguments outlined above are consistent with both behavioral and sensory perspectives on autism. With respect to the former, one type of contextual variable is referred to as a "setting event." Setting events have been shown to account for much of the variability in a child's behavior, especially in familiar settings (see Chapter 10 of this book, and Carr and Smith, 1995). An example is a child who typically enters a classroom and is greeted by the teacher. Both acknowledge one another. However, on days when the child has a headache, he or she may ignore the teacher or suddenly become upset soon after entering the classroom. In this case, the child's headache has changed the dynamics of an antecedent–consequence behavioral relationship. With respect to anxiety, the physical and emotional components of a heightened sense of arousal would be viewed as setting events.

With regard to the sensory approach to autism, a heightened arousal level, such as in the case of SNS activation, would impact a dysregulated sensory system. The processing of sensory sensations, such as in interoception, can have a significant impact on anxiety. Spielmann and Miller (Chapter 6) discuss arousal levels with respect to sensory responsivity in anxiety and autism.

Future Directions for Research

It is important to mention that at the present time, there are only correlational studies linking specific toxicants to immune dysregulation in autism. That is, research studies have demonstrated links between autism and environmental toxicant exposure, and between autism and inflammatory cytokine activity. Research examining a causal relationship among these factors will provide much-needed insight into the role of environmental exposure in autism.

In their chapters, Casanova, Sokhadze, and their colleagues recommend studying brain and immune function as well as their bi-directional relationship with the ANS. In addition, we suggest including measures of interoceptive function and toxic burden as well as a functional behavioral analysis.

The potential causal relationship between toxicant exposure and autism, possibly general anxiety, warrants awareness in the scientific community and health-related government agencies as well as the general public. Furthermore, toxicant exposure of minority and low-income communities needs to be addressed directly (Rickenbacker *et al.*, 2019). That is, researchers have demonstrated a disproportionate exposure to traffic pollution (Pratt *et al.*, 2015), exposure to agricultural pesticides (Dilworth-Bart and Moore, 2006), and proximity to U.S. Superfund sites (abandoned waste sites requiring long-term clean-up) within these communities (Kramer *et al.*, 2018). This issue is further exacerbated by the trend of autism underdiagnoses in minority communities. See Angell *et al.* (2018) for a review of disparities in both autism diagnoses and services for racial and ethnic minority children in the U.S.

Conclusion

As mentioned earlier and throughout this book, anxiety is one of the most common symptoms of autism. A number of biological impairments often reported in autism are directly or indirectly related to anxiety. Such findings should be of great interest to researchers studying anxiety in general, given that four major components of anxiety (i.e., neurological, ANS, immune, and sensory interoception) are all known to be impaired in many-to-most individuals with autism.

These first three chapters provide a roadmap for understanding the underlying biological processes involved in anxiety and autism. Research focusing on these processes will likely provide a clearer understanding of how to optimally treat this condition. This may include normalizing brain inhibition (e.g., transcranial magnetic stimulation or TMS), ANS arousal (e.g., deep pressure, relaxation methods), immune system modulation through the use of turmeric or curcumin, and interoception (e.g., teaching awareness of one's internal sensations such as heartbeats). In addition, if levels of certain toxicants are elevated, there are numerous medical and natural interventions known to detoxify the body.

References

Adams, J. B., Romdalvik, J., Ramanujam, V. M., and Legator, M. S. (2007). Mercury, lead, and zinc in baby teeth of children with autism versus controls. *Journal of Toxicology and Environmental Health, 70*(12), 1046–1051.

Adams, J. B., Audhya, T., McDonough-Means, S., Rubin, R. A., Quig, D., Geis, E., Gehn, E., Loresto, M., Mitchell, J., Atwood, S., Barnhouse, S., and Lee, W. (2013). Toxicological status of children with autism vs. neurotypical children and the association with autism severity. *Biological Trace Element Research, 151*(2), 171–180. doi: 10.1007/s12011-012-9551-1.

Angell, A. M., Empey, A., Zuckerman, K. E. (2018). A review of diagnosis and service disparities among children with autism from racial and ethnic minority groups in the United States. *International Review of Research in Developmental Disabilities, 55*, 145–180.

Ashwood, P., Schauer, J., Pessah, I. N., and Van de Water, J. (2009). Preliminary evidence of the in vitro effects of BDE-47 on innate immune responses in children with autism spectrum disorders. *Journal of Neuroimmunology, 208*, 130–135. doi: 10.1016/j.jneuroim.2008.12.012.

Barth, A., Brucker, N., Moro, A. M., Nascimento, S., Goethel, G., *et al.* (2017). Association between inflammation processes, DNA damage, and exposure to environmental pollutants. *Environmental Science and Pollution Research International, 24*(1), 353–362. doi: 10.1007/s11356-016-7772-0.

Bitsika, V., and Sharpley, C. F. (2017). The association between parents' ratings of ASD symptoms and anxiety in a sample of high-functioning boys and adolescents with autism spectrum disorder. *Research in Developmental Disabilities, 63*, 38–45. doi: 10.1016/j.ridd.2017.02.010.

Carr, E. G., and Smith, C. E. (1995). Biological setting events for self-injury. *Mental Retardation and Developmental Disabilities Research Reviews, 1*(2), 94–98.

Costa, L. G., Cole, T. B., Coburn, J., Chang, Y. C., Dao, K., and Roqué, P. J. (2017). Neurotoxicity of traffic-related air pollution. *Neurotoxicology, 59*, 133–139. doi: 10.1016/j.neuro.2015.11.008.

Dilworth-Bart, J., and Moore, C. (2006). Mercy, mercy me: Social injustice and the prevention of environmental pollutant exposures among ethnic minority and poor children. *Child Development, 77*(22), 247–265. doi: 10.1111/j.1467-8624.2006.00868.x.

Flores-Pajot, M. C., Ofner, M., Do, M. T., Lavigne, E., and Villeneuve, P. J. (2016). Childhood autism spectrum disorders and exposure to nitrogen dioxide, and particulate matter air pollution: A review and meta-analysis. *Environmental Research, 151*, 763–776. doi: 10.1016/j.envres.2016.07.030.

Garfinkel, S. N., Tiley, C., O'Keeffe, S., Harrison, N. A., Seth, A. K., and Critchley, H. D. (2016). Discrepancies between dimensions of interoception in autism: Implications for emotion and anxiety. *Biological Psychology, 114*, 117–126.

Ge, X., Zhao, W., Ding, C., Tian, H., Xu, L., Wang, H., Ni, L., Jiang, J., Gong, J., Zhu, W., Zhu, M., and Li, N. (2017). Potential role of fecal microbiota from patients with slow transit constipation in the regulation of gastrointestinal motility. *Scientific Reports, 7*(1), 441. doi: 10.1038/s41598-017-00612-y.

Goines, P. E., and Ashwood, P. (2013). Cytokine dysregulation in autism spectrum disorders (ASD): Possible role of the environment. *Neurobehavioral Toxicology and Teratology, 36*, 67–81. doi: 10.1016/j.ntt.2012.07.006.

Gordon-Lipkin, E., Marvin, A. R., Law, J. K., and Lipkin, P. H. (2018). Anxiety and mood disorder in children with autism spectrum disorder and ADHD. *Pediatrics, 141*(4), 1–8. pii: e20171377. doi: 10.1542/peds.2017-1377.

Gruzieva, O., Merid, S. K., Gref, A., Gajulapuri, A., Lemonnier, N., *et al.* (2017). Exposure to traffic-related air pollution and serum inflammatory cytokines in children. *Environmental Health Perspectives, 125*(6), 067007. doi: 10.1289/EHP460.

Gump, B.B., Gabrikova, E., Bendinskas, K., Dumas, A. K., Palmer, C. D., *et al.* (2014). Low-level mercury in children: Associations with sleep duration and cytokines TNF-α and IL-6. *Environmental Research, 134*, 228–232. doi: 10.1016/j.envres.2014.07.026.

Hayley, S., Mangano, E., Crowe, G., Li, N., and Bowers, W. J. (2011). An in vivo animal study assessing long-term changes in hypothalamic cytokines following perinatal exposure to a chemical mixture based on Arctic maternal body burden. *Environmental Health, 10*, 65. doi: 10.1186/1476-069X-10-65.

Hertz-Picciotto, I., Bergman, A., Fängström, B., Rose, M., Krakowiak, P., Pessah, I., Hansen, R., and Bennett, D. H. (2011). Polybrominated diphenyl ethers in relation to autism and developmental delay: A case-control study. *Environmental Health, 10*(1), 1. doi: 1476-069X-10-1 [pii]. 10.1186/1476-069X-10-1. PubMed PMID: 21205326; PMCID: PMC3029221.

Hou, R., Garner, M., Holmes, C., Osmond, C., Teeling, J., *et al.* (2017). Peripheral inflammatory cytokines and immune balance in Generalised Anxiety Disorder: Case-controlled study. *Brain, Behavior, and Immunity, 62*, 212–218. doi: 10.1016/j.bbi.2017.01.021.

Hui, L. L., Chan, M. H. M., Lam, H. S., Chan, P. H. Y., Kwok, K. M., *et al.* (2016). Impact of fetal and childhood mercury exposure on immune status in children. *Environmental Research, 144*(Pt A), 66–72. doi: 10.1016/j.envres.2015.11.005.

Jin, Y., Wu, S., Zeng, Z., and Fu, Z. (2017). Effects of environmental pollutants on gut microbiota. *Environmental Pollution, 222*, 1–9. doi: 10.1016/j.envpol.2016.11.045.

Kramer, D. E., Anderson, A., Hilfer, H., Branden, K., and Gutrich, J. J. (2018). A spatially informed analysis of environmental justice: Analyzing the effects of gerrymandering and the proximity of minority populations to U.S. Superfund sites. *Environmental Justice, 11*(1). doi: 10.1089/env.2017.0031.

Krautwurst, S., Gerlach, A. L., and Witthöft, M. (2016). Interoception in pathological health anxiety. *Journal of Abnormal Psychology, 125*(8), 1179–1184.

Latzin, P., Frey, U., Armann, J., Kieninger, E., Fuchs, O., *et al.* (2011). Exposure to moderate air pollution during late pregnancy and cord blood cytokine secretion in healthy neonates. *PLoS One, 6*(8), e23130. doi: 10.1371/journal.pone.0023130.

Laue, H. E., Brennan, K. J. M., Gillet, V., Abdelouahab, N., Coull, B. A., Weisskopf, M. G., Burris, H. H., Zhang, W., Takser, L., and Baccarelli, A. A. (2019). Associations of prenatal exposure to polybrominated diphenyl ethers and polychlorinated biphenyls with long-term gut microbiome structure: A pilot study. *Environmental Epidemiology, 3*(1), pii: e039. doi: 10.1097/EE9.0000000000000039.

Machoń-Grecka, A., Dobrakowski, M., Boroń, M., Lisowska, G., Kasperczyk, A., and Kasperczyk, S. (2017). The influence of occupational chronic lead exposure on the levels of selected pro-inflammatory cytokines and angiogenic factors. *Human and Experimental Toxicology, 36*(5), 467–473. doi: 10.1177/0960327117703688.

Mallorquí-Bagué, N., Bulbena, A., Pailhez, G., Garfinkel, S. N., and Critchley, H. D. (2016). Mind–body interactions in anxiety and somatic symptoms. *Harvard Review of Psychiatry, 24*(1), 53–60. doi: 10.1097/HRP.0000000000000085.

McVey, A. J. (2019). The neurobiological presentation of anxiety in autism spectrum disorder: A systematic review. *Autism Research, 12*(3), 346–369. doi: 10.1002/aur.2063.

Meltzer, A., and Van de Water, J. (2017). The role of the immune system in autism spectrum disorder. *Neuropsychopharmacology, 42*(1), 284–298. Epub 2016/08/19. doi: 10.1038/npp.2016.158. PubMed PMID: 27534269; PMCID: PMC5143489.

Mutlu, E. A, Comba, I. Y., Cho, T., Engen, P. A., Yazıcı, C., Soberanes, S., Hamanaka, R. B., Niğdelioğlu, R., Meliton, A. Y., Ghio, A. J., Budinger, G. R. S., and Mutlu, G. M. (2018). Inhalational exposure to particulate matter air pollution alters the composition of the gut microbiome. *Environmental Pollution, 240*, 817–830. doi: 10.1016/j.envpol.2018.04.130.

Ni, J., Wu, G. D., Albenberg, L., and Tomov, V. T. (2017). Gut microbiota and IBD: causation or correlation? *Nature Reviews: Gastroenterology and Hepatology, 14*(1), 573–584. doi: 10.1038/nrgastro.2017.88.

Owens, A. P., Low, D. A., Lodice, V., Critchley, H. D., and Mathias, C. J. (2017). The genesis and presentation of anxiety in disorders of autonomic overexcitation. *Autonomic Neuroscience: Basic and Clinical, 203*, 81–87. doi: 10.1016/j.autneu.2016.10.004.

Palser, E. R., Fotopoulou, A., Pellicano, E., and Kilner, J. M. (2018). The link between interoceptive processing and anxiety in children diagnosed with autism spectrum disorder: Extending adult findings into a developmental sample. *Biological Psychology, 136*, 13–21. doi: 10.1016/j.biopsycho.2018.05.003.

Paulus, M. P., and Stein, M. B. (2010). Interoception in anxiety and depression. *Brain Structure and Function, 214*(5–6), 451–463. doi: 10.1007/s00429-010-0258-9.

Postorino, V., Kerns, C. M., Vivanti, G., Bradshaw, J., Siracusano, M., and Mazzone, L. (2017). Anxiety disorders and obsessive-compulsive disorder in individuals with autism spectrum disorder. *Current Psychiatry Reports, 19*(12), 92. doi: 10.1007/s11920-017-0846-y.

Pratt, G. C., Vadali, M. L., Kvale, D. L., and Ellickson, K. M. (2015). Traffic, air pollution, minority and socio-economic status: Addressing inequities in exposure and risk. *International Journal of Environmental Research and Public Health, 12*(5), 5355–5372. doi: 10.3390/ijerph120505355.

Rickenbacker, H., Brown, F., and Bilec, M. (2019). Creating environmental consciousness in underserved communities: Implementation and outcomes of community-based environmental justice and air pollution research. *Sustainable Cities and Society, 47*. doi: 10.1016/j.scs.2019.101473.

Saraswathy, S., Dixit, R., Agrawal, P., and Krishnan, M. (2018). Air pollution and cytokines. *Journal of Medical Academics, 1*(1), 43–49.

Shelton, J. F., Geraghty, E. M., Tancredi, D. J., Delwiche, Schmidt, R. J., *et al.* (2014). Neurodevelopmental disorders and prenatal residential proximity to agricultural pesticides: The CHARGE study. *Environmental Health Perspectives, 122*(10), 1103–1109. doi: 10.1289/ehp.1307044.

Simonoff, E., Pickles, A., Charman, T., Chandler, S., Loucas, T., *et al.* (2008). Psychiatric disorders in children with autism spectrum disorders: Prevalence, comorbidity, and associated factors in a population-derived sample. *American Academy of Child Adolescence and Psychiatry, 47*(8), 921–929. doi: 10.1097/CHI.0b013e318179964f.

van Eeden, S. F., Tan, W. C., Suwa, T., Mukae, H., Terashima, T., *et al.* (2001). Cytokines involved in the systemic inflammatory response induced by exposure to particulate matter air pollutants (PM(10)). *American Journal of Respiratory and Critical Care Medicine, 164*(5), 826–830.

Volk, H. E., Hertz-Picciotto, I., Delwiche, L., Lurmann, F., and McConnell, R. (2011). Residential proximity to freeways and autism in the CHARGE study. *Environmental Health Perspectives, 119*(6), 873–877.

von Ehrenstein, O. S., Aralis, H., Cockburn, M., and Ritz, B. (2014). In utero exposure to toxic air pollutants and risk of childhood autism. *Epidemiology, 25*, 851–858.

von Ehrenstein, O. S., Ling, C., Cui, X., Cockburn, M., Park, A. S., *et al.* (2019). Prenatal and infant exposure to ambient pesticides and autism spectrum disorder in children: Population based case-control study. *British Medical Journal, 364*, l962. doi: 10.1136/bmj.l962.

Vuong, A. M., Yolton, K., Dietrich, K. N., Braun, J. M., Lanphear, B. P., and Chen, A. (2018). Exposure to polybrominated diphenyl ethers (PBDEs) and child behavior: Current findings and future directions. *Hormones and Behavior, 101*, 94–104. doi: 10.1016/j.yhbeh.2017.11.008.

Ye, B. S., Leung, A. O. W., and Wong, M. H. (2017). The association of environmental toxicants and autism spectrum disorders in children. *Environmental Pollution, 227*, 234–242. doi: 10.1016/j.envpol.2017.04.039.

CHAPTER 4
Gastrointestinal Symptoms, Anxiety, and Autism Spectrum Disorder

Kimberly M. Law, M.D., Columbia University Medical Center, Morgan Stanley Children's Hospital, Division of Pediatric Gastroenterology, Hepatology, and Nutrition, Brad J. Ferguson, Ph.D., University of Missouri, Departments of Health Psychology and Radiology, and Thompson Center for Autism and Neurodevelopmental Disorders, Kara Gross Margolis, M.D., Columbia University Medical Center, Morgan Stanley Children's Hospital, Division of Pediatric Gastroenterology, Hepatology, and Nutrition, and David Q. Beversdorf, M.D., University of Missouri, Departments of Radiology, Neurology, Psychological Sciences, and Thompson Center for Autism and Neurodevelopmental Disorders

Introduction

Gastrointestinal (GI) disorders are among the most common medical issues both nationally and internationally. Among the GI diagnoses, abdominal pain and constipation tend to be among the more common problems (Bharucha *et al.*, 2016). Up to 19 percent of children suffer from recurrent abdominal pain in the western world, and up to 29 percent suffer from constipation (Bharucha *et al.*, 2016; Rajindrajith *et al.*, 2016). Children with autism spectrum disorder (ASD) have been found, in a number of studies, to suffer from GI conditions more commonly than their neurotypical peers. In the largest meta-analysis to date, children with ASD are thought to be diagnosed with a GI problem almost four times more often than children without ASD (McElhanon *et al.*, 2014). However, the reported prevalence of GI symptoms ranges from 9 to 91 percent (Buie *et al.*, 2010), likely a result of different methods of GI assessment, highlighting the need for standardized assessment of GI disorders in this population. Regardless, constipation and diarrhea tend to be the most common diagnoses made in ASD (McElhanon *et al.*, 2014). Due to the fact that anxiety is associated with GI distress, it is imperative to make efficient diagnoses.

Diagnosis of Gastrointestinal Disorders in ASD

Although there appears to be a higher prevalence of GI disorders in children with ASD in the current studies, GI problems may be even more common because of the difficulty in making a diagnosis (McElhanon *et al.*, 2014; Doshi-Velez *et al.*, 2014; Chaidez *et al.*, 2014). Individuals with ASD often have limited communication ability, impairing their ability to communicate GI symptoms or discomfort (Holingue *et al.*, 2018). They often also manifest difficulty processing sensory abnormalities, making it difficult to localize pain even if their verbal ability is adequate (Buie *et al.*, 2010).

The current gold-standard method for the diagnosis of some common functional GI problems is based on the Rome IV criteria.[1] Many of the Rome IV criteria rely on the report of abdominal pain, so diagnosis may be challenging in individuals who cannot verbalize or localize discomfort from abdominal pain (Gorrindo *et al.*, 2012). These issues in the ASD population can result in delayed or missed diagnoses (Wasilewska and Klukowski, 2015). In some instances, children with abdominal pain have been shown to manifest difficult and distressing behaviors including, but not limited to, irritability, social withdrawal, stereotypy, and hyperactivity, as well as aggression and self-injurious behaviors (Chaidez *et al.*, 2014; Buie *et al.*, 2010; Wasilewska and Klukowski, 2015). Therefore, it is imperative to address GI problems in ASD, especially given their association with both internalizing and externalizing symptoms (Ferguson *et al.*, 2019).

A new GI screening measure was recently developed that may be able to detect common GI problems in ASD such as diarrhea, constipation, and gastroesophageal reflux disease with greater sensitivity than the Rome IV criteria. This screen relies more on caretaker's observations rather than the ability of a child with ASD to identify their symptoms (Margolis *et al.*, 2019). Though promising, this screen still requires validation in a larger clinical cohort of patients.

---

1 The Rome IV Diagnostic Questionnaires for Pediatric Functional Gastrointestinal Disorders include a child/adolescent version which has both parent- and self-report versions. The Rome IV questionnaire assesses the frequency, severity, and duration of functional (i.e., brain–gut) GI symptoms using a Likert scale and several Yes/No questions regarding the presence or absence of specific GI symptoms.

Though GI questionnaires and screening tools can help with the diagnosis of GI disorders in ASD, some cases may require a more thorough evaluation. In a clinical report of GI problems in ASD that was authored by clinical experts, including pediatric gastroenterologists, it was suggested that for children with chronic abdominal pain or diarrhea exceeding one month, evaluation with diagnostic tests including stool studies, blood work, imaging, or endoscopy should be considered (Buie *et al.*, 2010). As such, utilizing a variety of measures and diagnostic tests can be useful in the diagnosis of GI problems in ASD, and clinicians should be aware of special considerations, such as limited communication ability in some patients with ASD, that can complicate and sometimes delay diagnosis.

Treatment of Gastrointestinal Disorders in ASD

The most common GI diagnosis in children with ASD is constipation (Peeters *et al.*, 2013). Constipation results in a large proportion of emergency department visits and admissions to hospitals for children with ASD (Sparks *et al.*, 2018). Constipation is a common pediatric diagnosis, and the sensory processing abnormalities commonly observed in children with ASD may contribute to stool-withholding behaviors. However, given that many children with ASD are picky eaters and have altered diets (Cermak *et al.*, 2010), the cause of the constipation may be the result of a number of other factors such as limited water consumption or possibly microbial dysbiosis.

When evaluating any child with constipation, a thorough medical history should be taken. An important component is understanding what the family means by constipation, by determining how often the child has a bowel movement, what the stools look like, and whether the bowel movements are accompanied by pain. It is crucial to discuss the current medication history and recent dosage changes as some medications can contribute to constipation. Individuals with ASD are more commonly on anti-epileptic or psychiatric medications, many classes of which are associated with constipation. As in any patient with constipation, an abdominal and rectal exam should be performed (Rao and Meduri, 2011).

Once an individual with ASD has been diagnosed with a GI problem, beginning treatment is imperative. There has been only one set of guidelines published that are focused specifically on the diagnosis of a GI problem in ASD, and these guidelines are focused specifically on constipation. These guidelines, however, contain an algorithm consisting of evaluation and management (Furuta *et al.*, 2012). An important aspect of constipation management is frequent follow-up, in order to determine whether treatment is effective. This is particularly important for individuals with more severe forms of ASD, as they may be more likely to respond less optimally to what are often considered the first line therapies, including stool softeners such as lactulose or polyethylene glycol 3350 (Furuta *et al.*, 2012).

Relationship between Gastrointestinal Disorders and Other Comorbidities in ASD

Once an individual with ASD is diagnosed with a GI disorder, it is important to consider other comorbidities that have been demonstrated in the literature to occur more often in association with GI problems. These comorbidities commonly include seizures, anxiety, depressed mood, attention-deficit/hyperactivity disorder, oppositional defiant disorder, sleep problems, irritability, aggression, somatic complaints, and other problem behaviors (Doshi-Velez *et al.*, 2014; Aldinger *et al.*, 2015; Simonoff *et al.*, 2008; Mazurek *et al.*, 2013; Ferguson *et al.*, 2019). Problem behaviors may be indicative of GI distress in ASD, given that many individuals with ASD have limited language or are non-verbal (Buie *et al.*, 2010). This relationship may also vary by age, with younger individuals with ASD displaying more externalizing behaviors such as aggression, and older individuals with ASD displaying more internalizing symptoms such as anxiety and depression (Ferguson *et al.*, 2019). Stress has also been shown to be associated with GI symptoms in ASD through the measurement of heart rate variability (HRV), a measure of sympathetic and parasympathetic nervous system functioning that is derived from electrocardiogram data. Specifically, research has shown a positive relationship between the stress response, as measured by HRV, and constipation symptoms in children and adolescents with ASD (Ferguson *et al.*, 2017). Furthermore, anxiety has been shown to alter the relationship between HRV and symptoms of the lower GI tract, suggesting that a co-occurring anxiety disorder places an individual with ASD at a heightened risk of developing autonomic-related GI symptoms. This may be the result of alterations in sympathetic and parasympathetic responses from the body in response to an environmental stressor in some people with ASD (Ferguson *et al.*, 2017). Thus, when providers are treating GI disorders in individuals with ASD, the presence or absence of the aforementioned common comorbidities can provide further clues about underlying GI symptomatology. Furthermore, the relationship between anxiety and GI symptoms raises the possibility of benefit from treatment approaches targeting both altered stress reactivity and problem behavior.

Anxiety and Gastrointestinal Disorders in ASD

Anxiety disorders are one of the most common psychiatric disorders in children, with up to 20 percent being affected (Cartwright-Hatton *et al.*, 2006). In children who have anxiety disorders, 40 percent of them had symptoms of a functional GI disorder, versus only 5.9 percent of children without anxiety (Waters *et al.*, 2013). Children with ASD commonly have a psychiatric disorder, with anxiety being the most common diagnosis (Simonoff *et al.*, 2008).

The "brain–gut axis" may be a link between anxiety and the GI tract. The brain–gut axis is based on a continuous, bidirectional communication that occurs between the central nervous system and the GI tract (Costa *et al.*, 2000). Within the axis there are modulators known as neurotransmitters, including serotonin, norepinephrine, epinephrine, and dopamine (Mittal *et al.*, 2017). These neurotransmitters act on targeted receptors, communicating within the enteric nervous system (ENS), the nervous system within the GI tract. The hypothalamic–pituitary–adrenal (HPA) axis also has a role in communicating with the ENS. The HPA axis is critical to our body's response to any type of stress, with corticotrophin-releasing factor (CRF) acting on the pituitary gland to release adrenocorticotrophic hormone (ACTH), which eventually triggers the adrenal cortex to release cortisol (Tsigos and Chrousos, 2002). Stress, as well as cytokines, which cause inflammation, can activate the HPA axis with cortisol (Carabotti *et al.*, 2015). CRF pathway activation will interact within the ENS, causing increase in peristalsis within the colon (Taché and Million, 2015).

Another important component within the ENS is the immune system. Children with ASD and GI symptoms were found to have an imbalance in their immune response, having lower levels of regulatory cytokines and higher levels of inflammatory cytokines when compared with children without ASD (Rose *et al.*, 2018). One study did not find a relationship between GI problems and the inflammatory cytokine TNF-alpha and the pro- and anti-inflammatory cytokine IL-6, but did reveal a relationship between the cortisol response to a brief stressor and symptoms of the lower GI tract (Ferguson *et al.*, 2016), lending further support to the role of altered stress reactivity in GI problems. Further research is needed in the nature of the endocrine–immunological–GI relationship in ASD.

Serotonin and Gastrointestinal Disorders in ASD

There is ample data to suggest that the neurotransmitter serotonin is an important link between the brain and the intestine. Serotonin is produced in the brain as well as in the gut. Although most of the research on serotonin has been done in the brain, the vast majority of the body's serotonin (95%) is produced in the intestine (Gershon, 2013). In the brain, serotonin has been linked to central nervous system development and functions such as mood, including anxiety (Lin *et al.*, 2014). Polymorphisms in the promotor region of the serotonin transporter gene have been associated with altered reactivity of the amygdala to emotional stimuli (Hariri *et al.*, 2002). Furthermore, alterations in serotonin transporter genetics are associated with rigidity and compulsive behavior in ASD (McCauley *et al.*, 2004). In the gut, serotonin has been found to be critical in ENS development and functions such as mood (Jenkins *et al.*, 2016). Hence, when serotonin signaling is dysfunctional, both anxiety and GI dysfunction can result (Grzesiak *et al.*, 2017). In line with these findings, approximately 30 percent of patients with ASD have been found to have significantly higher levels of serotonin in their blood and hyperserotonemia (Gabriele *et al.*, 2014; Muller *et al.*, 2016). Interestingly, hyperserotonemia has also been associated with anxiety and anxiety-associated traits in individuals with ASD (Abdulamir *et al.*, 2018; Veenstra-VanderWeele *et al.*, 2012). A significant positive correlation between symptoms of the lower GI tract (e.g., functional constipation) and whole blood 5-HT concentrations has been observed in ASD; however, no relationship existed between 5-HT concentrations and functional constipation diagnosis (Marler *et al.*, 2016). Thus, more research examining the relationship between 5-HT and GI symptoms, including microbiome–gut interactions, is necessary.

The Microbiome and Gastrointestinal Disorders in ASD

The gut microbiome may also be a key link between the brain and the intestine (Khlevner *et al.*, 2018). The gut microbiome is a term used for the 100 trillion microorganisms (e.g., bacteria, viruses, and yeast) that reside within an individual's intestine (Turnbaugh *et al.*, 2007). The gut microbiome harbors approximately 150-fold more genes than the human body (Qin *et al.*, 2010), and there is increasing evidence to suggest that the gut microbiome plays an important role in multiple functions including the digestion, synthesis, and absorption of vitamins and other nutrients. This breakdown of some nutrients has been recently shown to potentially play critical roles in the modulation of the immune system. For example, microbial digestion of soluble fibers may lead to production of anti-inflammatory short-chain fatty-acids (e.g., butyrate), while ingestion of a high-fat diet may cause a microbial dysbiosis with subsequent systemic inflammation (Wang *et al.*, 2012; He *et al.*, 2018). Systemic inflammation has been associated with psychiatric conditions, including anxiety (Vogelzangs *et al.*, 2013; Pitsavos *et al.*, 2006; Yang *et al.*, 2016). Additionally, evidence is beginning to suggest potential benefit from manipulations of the microbiome for the treatment of anxiety (Lach *et al.*, 2018).

There have been multiple studies demonstrating that children with ASD harbor different microbial populations than neurotypical children (De Angelis *et al.*, 2015; Adams *et al.*, 2011; De Theije *et al.*, 2014). These studies have demonstrated variable results. The reasons for these variable results are based on the methodologies used for cultivating the bacteria, the small sample sizes, and the heterogeneity of ASD (e.g., types of GI disturbance, medications, medical comorbidities, or altered diets from either picky eating or dietary interventions) not having been considered.

Future Directions for the Treatment of Gastrointestinal Disorders in ASD

Besides treating a primary GI disorder, a more comprehensive brain–gut approach would ideally be used in the future in treating patients with ASD and GI problems. Given the important roles that serotonin modulates in CNS and gut function, drugs that target serotonin may be helpful in treating these patients. Prucalopride, a serotonin-4 receptor agonist, has been effective in treating constipation in humans. In mice with ASD-like behaviors and a serotonin-related genetic abnormality, administration of prucalopride prevented constipation (Margolis *et al.*, 2016). Of note, serotonin-4 receptor agonists have also been proposed to have anti-depressive effects (Lucas *et al.*, 2007; Samuels *et al.*, 2016).

Treating core ASD symptoms as well as co-occurring GI and behavioral problems might be possible through alterations in the gut microbiome (for a review, see Vuong and Hsiao, 2017). Looking at ways to reset the gut microbiome using probiotics or prebiotics may be an answer to treating both brain and gut dysfunction (Li *et al.*, 2017). In a maternal infection-driven ASD mouse model, administration of a probiotic including *Bacteroides fragilis* resulted in an improvement in both ASD-related behaviors and gut barrier function (Hsiao *et al.*, 2013). Successful results were also derived from a study in children given a probiotic containing *Lactobacillus rhamnosus*, who both improved behavior and decreased GI symptoms, including diarrhea and constipation (West *et al.*, 2013). Furthermore, it is possible that certain species of gut bacteria interact with the CNS to provide their effects on organ systems and behavior. For instance, one study using an animal model found that *Lactobacillus rhamnosus* has been shown to interact with the CNS via alterations in gamma-aminobutyric acid which resulted in reduced stress-induced corticosterone as well as anxiety- and depression-related behavior (Bravo *et al.*, 2011). Interestingly, these effects were not noted in mice when the vagus nerve, or the parasympathetic nerve, was surgically cut, suggesting a bidirectional line of communication from the gut to the brain via the vagus. However, it is not clear if this finding is also true in humans, and so more research is needed to determine if stress- and anxiety-related GI disorders in ASD can be treated with the supplementation of gut bacteria. Along these lines, a small open-label trial demonstrated the success of fecal transplant in improving ASD-related behavioral outcomes and also improvement in GI dysfunction in humans (Kang *et al.*, 2017). Symptoms were followed and sustained for eight weeks after treatment. However, the trial was not double-blinded, which limits the strength of the finding. Larger, double-blind, placebo-controlled human studies with more precise ASD subtyping may provide a more comprehensive understanding of how the microbiome differs in individuals with ASD and how this may contribute to the brain and behavioral manifestations, including anxiety disorders.

Furthermore, given the relationship between anxiety, an augmented stress response, and GI symptoms in ASD, it follows that research on pharmacotherapies that block the stress response might be a consideration. One possibility might be the beta-adrenergic antagonist propranolol, which has shown benefit for social communication, behavior, and anxiety in case series and single-dose psychopharmacological studies (Beversdorf *et al.*, 2008; Beversdorf *et al.*, 2011; Bodner *et al.*, 2012; Hegarty *et al.*, 2017; Ratey *et al.*, 1987; Sagar-Ouriaghli *et al.*, 2018; Zamzow *et al.*, 2016; Zamzow *et al.*, 2017). It is also undergoing a serial dose, double-blinded, placebo-controlled trial in ASD at this time (ClinicalTrials.gov Identifier: NCT02871349). It is also possible that the benefits of an agent blocking the stress response might extend beyond anxiety and social communication, and also positively impact GI function in individuals with dysregulated sympathetic/parasympathetic balance and anxiety (Ferguson *et al.*, 2017).

Conclusion

GI problems are very common in ASD, particularly constipation, and can result in problem behavior. Identification of these comorbid conditions can be challenging in ASD, and are often resistant to standard therapy. Additionally, GI problems in ASD are frequently associated with other comorbid issues, including anxiety. Many aspects of the pathophysiology of GI problems and anxiety are overlapping, including psychophysiological reactivity, the role of the serotonergic system, and the impact of the microbiome, raising the question of whether targeting these aspects might prove to be beneficial adjunctive or even primary approaches to treatment of GI problems in ASD.

References

Abdulamir, H. A., Abdul-Rasheed, O. F., and Abdulghani, E. A. (2018). Serotonin and serotonin transporter levels in autistic children. *Saudi Medical Journal, 39*(5), 487.

Adams, J. B., Johansen, L. J., Powell, L. D., Quig, D., and Rubin, R. A. (2011). Gastrointestinal flora and gastrointestinal status in children with autism—comparisons to typical children and correlation with autism severity. *BMC Gastroenterology, 11*(1), 22.

Aldinger, K. A., Lane, C. J., Veenstra-VanderWeele, J., and Levitt, P. (2015). Patterns of risk for multiple co-occurring medical conditions replicate across distinct cohorts of children with autism spectrum disorder. *Autism Research, 8*(6), 771–781.

Beversdorf, D. Q., Carpenter, A. L., Miller, R. F., Cios, J. S., and Hillier, A. (2008). Effect of propranolol on verbal problem solving in autism spectrum disorder. *Neurocase, 14*(4), 378–383.

Beversdorf, D. Q., Saklayen, S., Higgins, K. F., Bodner, K. E., Kanne, S. M., and Christ, S. E. (2011). Effect of propranolol on word fluency in autism. *Cognitive and Behavioral Neurology, 24*(1), 11–17.

Bharucha, A. E., Chakraborty, S., and Sletten, C. D. (2016). Common functional gastroenterological disorders associated with abdominal pain. *Mayo Clinic Proceedings, 91*(8), 1118–1132.

Bodner, K. E., Beversdorf, D. Q., Saklayen, S. S., and Christ, S. E. (2012). Noradrenergic moderation of working memory impairments in adults with autism spectrum disorder. *Journal of the International Neuropsychological Society, 18*(3), 556–564.

Bravo, J. A., Forsythe, P., Chew, M. V., Escaravage, E., Savignac, H. M., Dinan, T. G., ... Cryan, J. F. (2011). Ingestion of Lactobacillus strain regulates emotional behavior and central GABA receptor expression in a mouse via the vagus nerve. *Proceedings of the National Academy of Sciences, 108*(38), 16050–16055.

Buie, T., Campbell, D. B., Fuchs, G. J., Furuta, G. T., Levy, J., VandeWater, J., ... Carr, E. G. (2010). Evaluation, diagnosis, and treatment of gastrointestinal disorders in individuals with ASDs: A consensus report. *Pediatrics, 125*(Supplement 1), S1–S18.

Carabotti, M., Scirocco, A., Maselli, M. A., and Severi, C. (2015). The gut-brain axis: interactions between enteric microbiota, central and enteric nervous systems. *Annals of Gastroenterology, 28*(2), 203–209.

Cartwright-Hatton, S., McNicol, K., and Doubleday, E. (2006). Anxiety in a neglected population: Prevalence of anxiety disorders in pre-adolescent children. *Clinical Psychology Review, 26*(7), 817–833.

Cermak, S. A., Curtin, C., and Bandini, L. G. (2010). Food selectivity and sensory sensitivity in children with autism spectrum disorder. *Journal of the American Dietetic Association, 110*(2), 238–246.

Chaidez, V., Hansen, R. L., and Hertz-Picciotto, I. (2014). Gastrointestinal problems in children with autism, developmental delays or typical development. *Journal of Autism and Developmental Disorders, 44*(5), 1117–1127.

Costa, M., Brookes, S. J., and Hennig, G. W. (2000). Anatomy and physiology of the enteric nervous system. *Gut, 47*(Supplement 4), iv15–iv19.

De Angelis, M., Francavilla, R., Piccolo, M., De Giacomo, A., and Gobbetti, M. (2015). Autism spectrum disorders and intestinal microbiota. *Gut Microbes, 6*(3), 207–213.

De Theije, C. G., Wopereis, H., Ramadan, M., van Eijndthoven, T., Lambert, J., Knol, J., ... Oozeer, R. (2014). Altered gut microbiota and activity in a murine model of autism spectrum disorders. *Brain, Behavior, and Immunity, 37,* 197–206.

Doshi-Velez, F., Ge, Y., and Kohane, I. (2014). Comorbidity clusters in autism spectrum disorders: An electronic health record time-series analysis. *Pediatrics, 133*(1), e54–e63.

Ferguson, B. J., Marler, S., Altstein, L. L., Lee, E. B., Mazurek, M. O., McLaughlin, A., ... Gillespie, C. H. (2016). Associations between cytokines, endocrine stress response, and gastrointestinal symptoms in autism spectrum disorder. *Brain, Behavior, and Immunity, 58,* 57–62.

Ferguson, B. J., Marler, S., Altstein, L. L., Lee, E. B., Akers, J., Sohl, K., ... Macklin, E. A. (2017). Psychophysiological associations with gastrointestinal symptomatology in autism spectrum disorder. *Autism Research, 10*(2), 276–288.

Ferguson, B. J., Dovgan, K., Takahashi, N., and Beversdorf, D. Q. (2019). The relationship among gastrointestinal symptoms, problem behaviors, and internalizing symptoms in children and adolescents with autism spectrum disorder. *Frontiers in Psychiatry, 10,* 194.

Furuta, G. T., Williams, K., Kooros, K., Kaul, A., Panzer, R., Coury, D. L., and Fuchs, G. (2012). Management of constipation in children and adolescents with autism spectrum disorders. *Pediatrics, 130*(Supplement 2), S98–S105.

Gabriele, S., Sacco, R., and Persico, A. M. (2014). Blood serotonin levels in autism spectrum disorder: A systematic review and meta-analysis. *European Neuropsychopharmacology, 24*(6), 919–929.

Gershon, M. D. (2013). Hydroxytryptamine (serotonin) in the gastrointestinal tract. *Current Opinion in Endocrinology, Diabetes, and Obesity, 20*(1), 14–21.

Gorrindo, P., Williams, K. C., Lee, E. B., Walker, L. S., McGrew, S. G., and Levitt, P. (2012). Gastrointestinal dysfunction in autism: Parental report, clinical evaluation, and associated factors. *Autism Research, 5*(2), 101–108.

Grzesiak, M., Beszłej, J. A., Waszczuk, E., Szechiński, M., Szewczuk-Bogusławska, M., Frydecka, D., ... Mulak, A. (2017). Serotonin-related gene variants in patients with irritable bowel syndrome and depressive or anxiety disorders. *Gastroenterology Research and Practice, 2017.*

Hariri, A. R., Mattay, V. S., Tessitore, A., Kolachana, B., Fera, F., Goldman, D., ... Weinberger, D. R. (2002). Serotonin transporter genetic variation and the response of the human amygdala. *Science, 297*(5580), 400–403.

He, C., Cheng, D., Peng, C., Li, Y., Zhu, Y., and Lu, N. (2018). High-fat diet induces dysbiosis of gastric microbiota prior to gut microbiota in association with metabolic disorders in mice. *Frontiers in Microbiology, 9,* 639.

Hegarty, J. P., Ferguson, B. J., Zamzow, R. M., Rohowetz, L. J., Johnson, J. D., Christ, S. E., and Beversdorf, D. Q. (2017). Beta-adrenergic antagonism modulates functional connectivity in the default mode network of individuals with and without autism spectrum disorder. *Brain Imaging and Behavior, 11*(5), 1278–1289.

Holingue, C., Newill, C., Lee, L. C., Pasricha, P. J., and Daniele Fallin, M. (2018). Gastrointestinal symptoms in autism spectrum disorder: A review of the literature on ascertainment and prevalence. *Autism Research, 11*(1), 24–36.

Hsiao, E. Y., McBride, S. W., Hsien, S., Sharon, G., Hyde, E. R., McCue, T., ... Patterson, P. H. (2013). Microbiota modulate behavioral and physiological abnormalities associated with neurodevelopmental disorders. *Cell, 155*(7), 1451–1463.

Jenkins, T., Nguyen, J., Polglaze, K., and Bertrand, P. (2016). Influence of tryptophan and serotonin on mood and cognition with a possible role of the gut-brain axis. *Nutrients, 8*(1), 56.

Kang, D. W., Adams, J. B., Gregory, A. C., Borody, T., Chittick, L., Fasano, A., ... Pollard, E. L. (2017). Microbiota Transfer Therapy alters gut ecosystem and improves gastrointestinal and autism symptoms: An open-label study. *Microbiome, 5*(1), 10.

Khlevner, J., Park, Y., and Margolis, K. G. (2018). Brain–gut axis: Clinical implications. *Gastroenterology Clinics, 47*(4), 727–739.

Lach, G., Schellekens, H., Dinan, T. G., and Cryan, J. F. (2018). Anxiety, depression, and the microbiome: a role for gut peptides. *Neurotherapeutics, 15*(1), 36–59.

Li, Q., Han, Y., Dy, A. B. C., and Hagerman, R. J. (2017). The gut microbiota and autism spectrum disorders. *Frontiers in Cellular Neuroscience, 11,* 120.

Lin, S. H., Lee, L. T., and Yang, Y. K. (2014). Serotonin and mental disorders: A concise review on molecular neuroimaging evidence. *Clinical Psychopharmacology and Neuroscience, 12*(3), 196.

Lucas, G., Rymar, V. V., Du, J., Mnie-Filali, O., Bisgaard, C., Manta, S., ... Sadikot, A. F. (2007). Serotonin4 (5-HT4) receptor agonists are putative antidepressants with a rapid onset of action. *Neuron, 55*(5), 712–725.

Margolis, K. G., Buie, T. M., Turner, J. B., Silberman, A. E., Feldman, J. F., Murray, K. F., ... Whitaker, A. H. (2019). Development of a brief parent-report screen for common gastrointestinal disorders in autism spectrum disorder. *Journal of Autism and Developmental Disorders, 49*(1), 349–362.

Margolis, K. G., Li, Z., Stevanovic, K., Saurman, V., Israelyan, N., Anderson, G. M., ... Gershon, M. D. (2016). Serotonin transporter variant drives preventable gastrointestinal abnormalities in development and function. *The Journal of Clinical Investigation, 126*(6), 2221–2235.

Marler, S., Ferguson, B. J., Lee, E. B., Peters, B., Williams, K. C., McDonnell, E., ... Margolis, K. G. (2016). Brief report: Whole blood serotonin levels and gastrointestinal symptoms in autism spectrum disorder. *Journal of Autism and Developmental Disorders, 46*(3), 1124–1130.

Mazurek, M. O., Vasa, R. A., Kalb, L. G., Kanne, S. M., Rosenberg, D., Keefer, A., ... Lowery, L. A. (2013). Anxiety, sensory over-responsivity, and gastrointestinal problems in children with autism spectrum disorders. *Journal of Abnormal Child Psychology, 41*(1), 165–176.

McCauley, J. L., Olson, L. M., Dowd, M., Amin, T., Steele, A., Blakely, R. D., ... Sutcliffe, J. S. (2004). Linkage and association analysis at the serotonin transporter (SLC6A4) locus in a rigid-compulsive subset of autism. *American Journal of Medical Genetics Part B: Neuropsychiatric Genetics, 127*(1), 104–112.

McElhanon, B. O., McCracken, C., Karpen, S., and Sharp, W. G. (2014). Gastrointestinal symptoms in autism spectrum disorder: A meta-analysis. *Pediatrics, 133*(5), 872–883.

Mittal, R., Debs, L. H., Patel, A. P., Nguyen, D., Patel, K., O'Connor, G., ... Liu, X. Z. (2017). Neurotransmitters: The critical modulators regulating gut-brain axis. *Journal of Cellular Physiology, 232*(9), 2359–2372.

Muller, C. L., Anacker, A. M., and Veenstra-VanderWeele, J. (2016). The serotonin system in autism spectrum disorder: From biomarker to animal models. *Neuroscience, 321,* 24–41.

Peeters, B., Noens, I., Philips, E. M., Kuppens, S., and Benninga, M. A. (2013). Autism spectrum disorders in children with functional defecation disorders. *The Journal of Pediatrics, 163*(3), 873–878.

Pitsavos, C., Panagiotakos, D. B., Papageorgiou, C., Tsetsekou, E., Soldatos, C., and Stefanadis, C. (2006). Anxiety in relation to inflammation and coagulation markers, among healthy adults: The ATTICA study. *Atherosclerosis, 185*(2), 320–326.

Qin, J., Li, R., Raes, J., Arumugam, M., Burgdorf, K. S., Manichanh, C., ... Mende, D. R. (2010). A human gut microbial gene catalogue established by metagenomic sequencing. *Nature, 464*(7285), 59.

Rajindrajith, S., Devanarayana, N. M., Perera, B. J. C., and Benninga, M. A. (2016). Childhood constipation as an emerging public health problem. *World Journal of Gastroenterology, 22*(30), 6864.

Rao, S. S., and Meduri, K. (2011). What is necessary to diagnose constipation? *Best Practice and Research Clinical Gastroenterology, 25*(1), 127–140.

Ratey, J. J., Bemporad, J., Sorgi, P., Bick, P., Polakoff, S., O'Driscoll, G., and Mikkelsen, E. (1987). Brief report: Open trial effects of beta-blockers on speech and social behaviors in 8 autistic adults. *Journal of Autism and Developmental Disorders, 17*(3), 439–446.

Rose, D. R., Yang, H., Serena, G., Sturgeon, C., Ma, B., Careaga, M., ... Van de Water, J. (2018). Differential immune responses and microbiota profiles in children with autism spectrum disorders and co-morbid gastrointestinal symptoms. *Brain, Behavior, and Immunity, 70,* 354–368.

Sagar-Ouriaghli, I., Lievesley, K., and Santosh, P. J. (2018). Propranolol for treating emotional, behavioural, autonomic dysregulation in children and adolescents with autism spectrum disorders. *Journal of Psychopharmacology, 32*(6), 641–653.

Samuels, B. A., Mendez-David, I., Faye, C., David, S. A., Pierz, K. A., Gardier, A. M., ... David, D. J. (2016). Serotonin 1A and serotonin 4 receptors: Essential mediators of the neurogenic and behavioral actions of antidepressants. *The Neuroscientist, 22*(1), 26–45.

Simonoff, E., Pickles, A., Charman, T., Chandler, S., Loucas, T., and Baird, G. (2008). Psychiatric disorders in children with autism spectrum disorders: Prevalence, comorbidity, and associated factors in a population-derived sample. *Journal of the American Academy of Child and Adolescent Psychiatry, 47*(8), 921–929.

Sparks, B., Cooper, J., Hayes, C., and Williams, K. (2018). Constipation in children with autism spectrum disorder associated with increased emergency department visits and inpatient admissions. *The Journal of Pediatrics, 202,* 194–198.

Taché, Y., and Million, M. (2015). Role of corticotropin-releasing factor signaling in stress-related alterations of colonic motility and hyperalgesia. *Journal of Neurogastroenterology and Motility, 21*(1), 8.

Tsigos, C., and Chrousos, G. P. (2002). Hypothalamic–pituitary–adrenal axis, neuroendocrine factors and stress. *Journal of Psychosomatic Research, 53*(4), 865–871.

Turnbaugh, P. J., Ley, R. E., Hamady, M., Fraser-Liggett, C. M., Knight, R., and Gordon, J. I. (2007). The human microbiome project. *Nature, 449*(7164), 804.

Veenstra-VanderWeele, J., Muller, C. L., Iwamoto, H., Sauer, J. E., Owens, W. A., Shah, C. R., ... Ye, R. (2012). Autism gene variant causes hyperserotonemia, serotonin receptor hypersensitivity, social impairment and repetitive behavior. *Proceedings of the National Academy of Sciences, 109*(14), 5469–5474.

Vogelzangs, N., Beekman, A. T. F., De Jonge, P., and Penninx, B. W. J. H. (2013). Anxiety disorders and inflammation in a large adult cohort. *Translational Psychiatry, 3*(4), e249.

Vuong, H. E., and Hsiao, E. Y. (2017). Emerging roles for the gut microbiome in autism spectrum disorder. *Biological Psychiatry, 81*(5), 411–423.

Wang, L., Christophersen, C. T., Sorich, M. J., Gerber, J. P., Angley, M. T., and Conlon, M. A. (2012). Elevated fecal short chain fatty acid and ammonia concentrations in children with autism spectrum disorder. *Digestive Diseases and Sciences, 57*(8), 2096–2102.

Wasilewska, J., and Klukowski, M. (2015). Gastrointestinal symptoms and autism spectrum disorder: Links and risks – a possible new overlap syndrome. *Pediatric Health, Medicine and Therapeutics, 6,* 153.

Waters, A. M., Schilpzand, E., Bell, C., Walker, L. S., and Baber, K. (2013). Functional gastrointestinal symptoms in children with anxiety disorders. *Journal of Abnormal Child Psychology, 41*(1), 151–163.

West, R., Roberts, E., Sichel, L. S., and Sichel, J. (2013). Improvements in gastrointestinal symptoms among children with autism spectrum disorder receiving the Delpro® probiotic and immunomodulator formulation. *Journal of Probiotics and Health, 1*(2).

Yang, L., Wang, M., Guo, Y. Y., Sun, T., Li, Y. J., Yang, Q., ... Wu, Y. M. (2016). Systemic inflammation induces anxiety disorder through CXCL12/CXCR4 pathway. *Brain, Behavior, and Immunity, 56,* 352–362.

Zamzow, R. M., Ferguson, B. J., Stichter, J. P., Porges, E. C., Ragsdale, A. S., Lewis, M. L., and Beversdorf, D. Q. (2016). Effects of propranolol on conversational reciprocity in autism spectrum disorder: A pilot, double-blind, single-dose psychopharmacological challenge study. *Psychopharmacology, 233*(7), 1171–1178.

Zamzow, R. M., Ferguson, B. J., Ragsdale, A. S., Lewis, M. L., and Beversdorf, D. Q. (2017). Effects of acute beta-adrenergic antagonism on verbal problem solving in autism spectrum disorder and exploration of treatment response markers. *Journal of Clinical and Experimental Neuropsychology, 39*(6), 596–606.

CHAPTER 5

Dietary and Nutrition Intervention to Address Issues of Anxiety

Kelly McCracken Barnhill, M.B.A., C.N., C.C.N., The Johnson Center for Child Health and Development, Texas

Introduction

A significant amount of research acknowledges and verifies the relationship between poorer nutritional status and mental health concerns in pediatric and adolescent populations (Gonoodi *et al.*, 2018; Greuter *et al.*, 2018; Robertson *et al.*, 2017; Tahmasebi *et al.*, 2017; Tehrani *et al.*, 2018). A recent systematic review of nutritional aspects of depression in adolescents indicated that components of a Western diet or standard American diet (SAD) are implicated in greater risk for depression in the long term (Khanna *et al.*, 2019). Items such as baked goods, prepared cereals, and foods containing artificial flavors, colors, and preservatives are implicated in this work, and these are majority components of most Western diets. Additionally, the review concludes that some foods are inversely related to depression and anxiety, and these can be used to improve symptoms of depression. These include nuts and legumes, Omega-3 essential fatty acids, fish, olive oil, and fresh fruits and vegetables (Khanna *et al.*, 2019). As a clinical nutritionist with two decades of experience in the field of diet and nutrition, it is my firm belief that appropriate nutritional status can and does play a role in management of a child's stress and anxiety. My hope in this work is to provide clear information on what is reasonable intervention in terms of both diet and therapeutic nutritional supplementation to support individual children who suffer from anxiety.

Dietary Concerns

Western diets in developed countries are characterized by a high intake of compromised food items, leaning heavily toward those foodstuffs that are processed and preserved. This dietary pattern typically presents with high intake of processed carbohydrates and sucrose, additives, preservatives, artificial colors, and artificial flavors, coupled with low intake of fresh produce, resulting in significantly decreased fiber intake. This dietary approach can create an inflammatory process in the body, resulting in a variety of chronic, long-term health implications, including heart disease, metabolic syndrome, obesity, diabetes, inflammatory bowel disease, thyroid disease, and more. Research of the past decade offers observation of consistent cross-sectional associations between unhealthy dietary patterns and worse mental health in childhood and adolescence (O'Neil *et al.*, 2014). The theory that dietary quality also has an impact on the brain, then, with conditions such as autism spectrum disorder (ASD), attention deficit hyperactivity disorder (ADHD), anxiety, and depression also linked with poor dietary intake, is a reasonable assumption under these circumstances (Van Egmond-Fröhlich *et al.*, 2012).

Therefore, the first step in this process, addressing therapeutic nutrition for anxiety, is referral to a knowledgeable professional for comprehensive assessment. Consultation with a qualified professional to provide evaluation and guided dietary change, if warranted, is a reasonable approach to serving a child or adolescent with anxiety well. Professionally managed dietary protocols can enhance health for those children and adolescents suffering from anxiety, and are a reasonable and cost-effective step to consider in proactively addressing the symptoms children face. Trialing a reasonable diet plan for a period of 60–90 days, collecting extensive data, and also including subjective observations, can have a profound impact on an individual's overall health and well-being. It is important to emphasize here that standardized dietetic assessment and appropriate treatment and care for those requiring intervention is of primary importance in improving an individual's health and maximizing response to any given intervention.

From a dietary perspective, cleaning up intake by removing offending components and focusing on what is truly food is the first step in this plan. This would include focusing on ample clean water intake, sufficient protein, healthy fats, appropriate carbohydrates, and fiber. Adopting a diet that mirrors the Mediterranean Diet approach is recommended. These diets can include reasonable animal and plant-based protein, healthy fats and oils, freshly prepared vegetables, fresh fruits, and, when appropriate to individual dietary concerns, whole grains. Ideally, a diet free from exposure to non-organic commercially raised animal products (such as beef, chicken, pork, and eggs) is recommended, given the additional concerns associated with these dietary confounders. Safe, optimally sourced Omega-3 rich fish such as salmon can also be eaten. Further, healthy animal protein can be included in the diet, but the focus for ideal protein consumption is plant foods, including legumes, nuts, seeds, and some grains. For most individuals, a diet based on real food, ample fresh vegetables and fruits, lean protein, and healthy fats, without refined sugars, flours, and other processed foods is best.

Beyond this basic dietary change of removing harmful and inflammatory foods for general good health, it is also important to look at the specific dietary components of people facing anxiety. Assessment of dietary allergies and intolerances is an important next step. Food allergies and intolerances are increasing across the pediatric population, and the prevalence of anxiety disorders and comorbid allergic conditions is increasing as well (Gregory *et al.*, 2009; Friedman and Morris, 2006). This trend speaks to the importance of professional assessment to fully evaluate dietary considerations that may be contributing to or exacerbating anxiety. There are numerous specific examples of dietary additives or foods that are implicated in increasing anxiety. These include the sweetener aspartame (Wolraich *et al.*, 1994) as well as Red #40 and Yellow #5 dyes. Each is documented as a nervous system disruptor that increases anxiety symptoms (Arnold *et al.*, 2012).

Gastrointestinal Evaluation

It is also important to assess overall gastrointestinal (GI) systemic health, once dietary intake components have been fully explored and evaluated. Work published over the past decade has established that many children with ASD also have comorbid GI concerns (Alessandria *et al.*, 2019; Ibrahim *et al.*, 2009; McElhanon *et al.*, 2014). Further, these GI symptoms have the potential to manifest behavioral symptoms as well (Mazefsky *et al.*, 2014; Nikolov *et al.*, 2009). Those with ASD have been shown to experience GI symptoms more often than those without ASD. GI diagnoses evaluated and confirmed in those with ASD include eosinophilic esophagitis (Heifert *et al.*, 2016), gastroesophageal reflux (GERD), and abdominal pain, constipation, and/or diarrhea (Black *et al.*, 2002; Buie *et al.*, 2010a, 2010b; Ferguson *et al.*,

2019; Valicenti-McDermott *et al.*, 2006). Furthermore, a subset of children with ASD and comorbid GI concerns have been noted to present with a pattern of inflammatory mucosal pathology (Alessandria *et al.*, 2019; Garza-Gonzalez *et al.*, 2005; Horvath *et al.*, 1999; Valicenti-McDermott *et al.*, 2006).

Ample research published over the past two decades also substantiates functional GI abnormalities present in children with ASD. These concerns include low activities of disaccharidase enzymes (Melmed *et al.*, 2000), defective sulfation of ingested phenolic amines (Alberti *et al.*, 1999), bacterial overgrowth with greater diversity and number of clostridial species (Finegold *et al.*, 2002), and increased intestinal permeability (D'Eufemia *et al.*, 1996).

Additional factors also play a role in the health of the GI system in those with ASD. Concerns such as picky eating and problem feeding behavior, unmanaged restricted dietary protocols, nutrient malabsorption, and increased intestinal losses in children, through ongoing battles with diarrhea for those with ASD, compromise dietary intake and also cause nutritional depletion.

It has become more widely accepted in recent years that the microbiome-gut–brain axis can truly affect overall mental health, and anxiety in particular. Emerging research substantiates the idea that gastrointestinal health plays a role in multiple mental health concerns, including autism, ADHD, anxiety, and depression, among others. The bacterial, fungal, and viral components of the microbiome in the GI tract affect communication with the brain. The enteric nervous system (ENS) consists of over 100 trillion cells and communicates with the brain constantly. The information shared via this pathway is influenced by the various microbiota in the GI tract, with documented evidence that when the microbiome is burdened with bad bacteria, for example, anxiety, depression, and other neurological concerns can emerge in the pediatric population (Slattery *et al.*, 2016). Microbiome imbalances can lead to altered production of serotonin; with 90 percent of the body's serotonin produced in the GI tract, this shift can have a profound impact. As such, supporting healthy serotonin production and levels is another key to addressing anxiety in the children we serve.

Multiple factors can influence the GI tract in the short term, and also impact behavior for the long term. For example, a GI bacterial infection is associated with increased risk of anxiety disorder development within 24 months post infection (Bruch, 2016). Similarly, it is now also acknowledged in the research literature that the use of antibiotics to treat infection dramatically impacts the microbial makeup of the gut diversity, increasing the risk of an anxiety disorder later in life (Lurie *et al.*, 2015; Jernberg *et al.*, 2007).

Evaluating the overall health of the GI tract, then, is a reasonable step in comprehensive nutritional care for symptoms of anxiety. Beneficial probiotics, bacterial strains that are healthy for the GI tract, perform a variety of roles for the body—they support digestion, absorption, and energy production; support metabolic function; create neurotransmitters; and regulate the immune system (Valdes *et al.*, 2018; Hemarajata and Versalovic, 2013). The intestinal microbiome can and does prompt immune system cytokine production which then influences the neurological system, with both positive and negative effects (Lazar *et al.*, 2018). These cytokines are excreted from immune cells and promote inflammation. A healthy, balanced GI microbiotia can dampen production of cytokines, while a preponderance of bad bacteria can influence increased cytokine production. This inflammatory cascade is caused by the body's appropriate response to infection and illness. Cytokine-driven inflammation has been linked to anxiety in pediatric acute-onset neuropsychiatric syndrome (PANS) (Frankovich *et al.*, 2017) as well as bipolar disorder. With a bipolar diagnosis, cytokine markers have been shown to increase during depressive episodes and resolve when this depression is alleviated (Muneer, 2016).

In terms of supporting the overall health of the GI tract and microbiota, ample water intake is crucial. Probiotic foods such as fermented yogurt, kefir, cultured vegetables, kim chi, and lacto-fermented pickles are all beneficial in supporting a healthy microbiome. Foods such as avocadoes, bananas, garlic, onions, and nuts contain a prebiotic fiber called inulin, a chain of fructose molecules that provide energy for healthy bacteria of the GI tract. This type of fiber specifically helps support and maintain a beneficial balance of bacteria strains in the GI tract. Ultimately, the overall goal is breadth and depth of healthy bacteria of the GI system, so exposure to a variety of healthy strains through multiple sources can help achieve that mark.

From a treatment perspective, the effect of probiotics on treatment of anxiety in humans has yet to be fully established, though some probiotic strains have been shown to be useful in treatment of anxiety (Wang *et al.*, 2016; Pirbaglou *et al.*, 2016; Romijn and Rucklidge, 2015). *Lactobacillus rhamnosus* in particular has been shown to significantly reduce symptoms of anxiety (Reis *et al.*, 2018). Of interest here is very recent research on increased exposure to soil-based microorganisms for support and treatment in GI health. This has been touted in the probiotic industry as a way of improving current GI as well as overall health, and recent research indicates that a fatty acid in the bacterium *Mycobacterium vaccae*, which is found in the soil, inhibits inflammation by binding with a key receptor and effectively shutting down the cytokine inflammatory cascade (Smith *et al.*, 2019). In considering a treatment approach including probiotic supplementation, it is important to note that working with a professional who is aware of the quality of any probiotic recommended is key, as nutritional supplements are not an independently regulated industry. These can be expensive products, and it is important to be fully aware of the integrity of any product used.

Therapeutic Clinical Nutrition

A third avenue for exploration, once dietary intake and GI health have been addressed, is the use of nutrients to promote positive change in the symptoms of anxiety.

The mineral magnesium is a reasonable place to begin therapeutic nutritional treatment in this case. Magnesium plays myriad roles in the body (Schwalfenberg and Genuis, 2017). It acts as a natural muscle relaxant, and it assists with mitigating fear, anxiety, irritability, restlessness, fatigue, and inattention. When the body is physically or emotionally stressed or anxious, magnesium levels are quickly depleted, and in a vicious cycle, this in turn creates more stress and anxiety for the body at the cellular level (Cuciureanu and Vink, 2011). Reasonable oral doses of 250–400 mg of ionic magnesium citrate can have a beneficial effect in addressing symptoms of anxiety. Other forms of magnesium support can include Epsom salt baths, Epsom salt creams, and magnesium oil. These all allow the body access via the skin, and can further support magnesium levels in the body to mitigate anxiety symptoms. Additionally, Vitamin B6 is synergistic with magnesium in support of reducing anxiety and stress response. Research suggests that combining B6 and magnesium creates a greater reduction in anxiety than using magnesium alone (Pouteau *et al.*, 2018). B6 is also needed for GABA synthesis in the body, suggesting one mechanism of action for increased B6 support.

Vitamin B12 has also been acknowledged as affecting behaviors associated with autism as well as anxiety levels, with a handful of recent studies evaluating the impact of B12 support on anxiety and depression (Bertoglio *et al.*, 2010). One 2018 study reported statistically significant improvements from consumption of B12-enhanced foods on anxiety symptoms (Mikkelsen *et al.*, 2018).

Zinc is another mineral that has been identified as playing a role in anxiety concerns. It is now believed that zinc is a potent and crucial neuromodulator, supporting the glutamate/GABAergic balance in the body. If zinc is deficient, neurotransmitter balance is compromised and development of anxiety is one potential outcome.

Choline, which can be found in liver, eggs, and some cruciferous vegetables, is an essential nutrient that has only been recognized to be of primary nutritional importance since 1998. The human liver can only manufacture small amounts of it daily, so the need for choline must be met from dietary sources. Choline deficiency has been linked to concerns with cognitive function, brain development, and mood disorders. One study confirmed that deficient choline is also associated with higher levels of anxiety (Bieland *et al.*, 2009). Choline support can be found in most high-quality multivitamins, establishing an appropriate level of choline intake to remediate any dietary deficiencies.

Gamma-amino butyric acid (GABA) is an amino acid and neurotransmitter that balances and calms the nervous system. It is the brain's main inhibitory neurotransmitter, and it keeps the brain from becoming overstimulated and overactive. GABA's mechanism of action in anxiety and other mental health concerns has been well studied; fewer studies have evaluated its role in treatment. However, a 2009 review article concluded that the research supported the use of such supplements as GABA, l-theanine, and l-tryptophan to improve anxiety. L-theanine plays a role in GABA synthesis, with increased l-theanine improving GABA levels (Lopes-Sakamoto *et al.*, 2019; Sarris *et al.*, 2019; White *et al.*, 2016).

Another reasonable approach to therapeutic nutritional intervention for anxiety is Omega-3 essential fatty acids. Recent research confirms that dietary long chain Omega-3 fatty acids are inversely related to anxiety disorders (Jacka *et al.*, 2013), and another recent study noted that individuals consuming greater than 2000 mg of Omega-3s daily evidenced the greatest reduction in anxiety symptoms (Su *et al.*, 2018). Again, quality control is highly important with this type of nutritional supplementation, so confidence in the manufacturer is imperative.

Conclusion

The body of current research on the role of a variety of nutrient levels, along with the potential for nutritional intervention to alleviate symptoms of anxiety, speaks to the viability of dietary and nutritional support in treatment of ASD.

References

Alberti, A., Pirrone, P., Elia, M., Waring, R. H., and Romano, C. (1999). Sulphation deficit in "low-functioning" autistic children: A pilot study. *Biological Psychiatry, 46*(1), 420–424. doi: 10.1016/S0006-3223(98)00337-0.

Alessandria, C., Caviglia, G. P., Campion, D., Nalbone, F., Sanna, C., Musso, A., *et al.* (2019). HLA-DQ genotyping, duodenal histology, and response to exclusion diet in autistic children with gastrointestinal symptoms. *Journal of Pediatric Gastroenterology and Nutrition, 69*(1), 39–44. doi: 10.1097/MPG.0000000000002293.

Arnold, L. E., Lofthouse, N., and Hurt, E. (2012). Artificial food colors and attention-deficit/hyperactivity symptoms: Conclusions to dye for. *Neurotherapeutics, 9*(3), 599–609. doi: 10.1007/s13311-012-0133-x.

Bertoglio, K., James, S. J., Deprey, L., Brule, N., and Hendren, R. L. (2010). Pilot study of the effect of methyl B12 treatment on behavioral and biomarker measures in children with autism. *Journal of Alternative and Complementary Medicine, 16*(5). doi: 10.1089/acm.2009.0177

Bieland, I., Tell, G. S., Vollset, S. E., Konstantinova, S., and Ueland, P. M. (2009). Choline in anxiety and depression: The Hordaland Health Study. *American Journal of Clinical Nutrition, 90*(4), 1056–1060.

Black, C., Kaye, J. A., and Jick, H. (2002). Relation of childhood gastrointestinal disorders to autism: Nested case-control study using data from the UK General Practice Research Database. *BMJ, 325*, 419–421. doi: 10.1136/bmj.325.7361.419.

Bruch, J. D. (2016). Intestinal infection associated with future onset of an anxiety disorder: Results of a nationally representative study. *Brain, Behavior, and Immunity, 22*(3), 354–356. doi: 10.1016/j.bbi.2016.05.014.

Buie, T., Campbell, D. B., Fuchs, G. J., Furuta, G. T., Levy, J., Vandewater, J., ... Winter, H. (2010a). Evaluation, diagnosis, and treatment of gastrointestinal disorders in individuals with ASDs: A consensus report. *Pediatrics, 125*(1), 1–18. doi: 10.1542/peds.2009-1878C.

Buie, T., Fuchs, G. J., Furuta, G. T., Kooros, K., Levy, J., Lewis, J. D., ... Winter, H. (2010b). Recommendations for evaluation and treatment of common gastrointestinal problems in children with ASDs. *Pediatrics, 125*(1), 19–29. doi: 10.1542/peds.2009-1878D.

Cuciureanu, M. D., and Vink, R. (2011). Magnesium and stress. *Magnesium in the Central Nervous System, 1*(19), 251–268. doi: 10.1017/UPO9780987073051.

D'Eufemia, P., Celli, M., Finocchiaro, R., Pacifico, L., Viozzi, L., Zaccagnini, E., ... Giardini, O. (1996). Abnormal intestinal permeability in children with autism. *Acta Paediatrica, 85*(9). doi: 10.1111/j.1651-2227.1996.tb14220.x.

Ferguson, B. J., Dovgan, K., Takahashi, N., and Beversdorf, D. Q. (2019). The relationship among gastrointestinal symptoms, problem behaviors, and internalizing symptoms in children and adolescents with autism spectrum disorder. *Frontiers in Psychiatry, 10*.

Finegold, S. M., Molitoris, D., Song, Y., Liu, C., Vaisanen, M. L., Bolte, E., ... Kaul, A. (2002). Gastrointestinal microflora studies in late-onset autism. *Clinical Infectious Diseases, 35*(1), 6–16. doi: 10.1086/341914.

Frankovich, J., Swedo, S., Murphy, T., Dale, R. C., Agalliu, S., Williams, K., ... Thienemann, M. (2017). Clinical management of pediatric acute-onset neuropsychiatric syndrome: Part II—use of immunomodulatory therapies. *Journal of Child and Adolescent Psychopharmacology, 27*(7), 574–593. doi: 10.1089/cap.2016.0148.

Friedman, A. H., and Morris, T. L. (2006). Allergies and anxiety in children and adolescents: A review of the literature. *Journal of Clinical Psychology in Medical Setting, 13*(3), 323–336. doi: 10.1007/s10880-006-9026-7.

Garza-Gonzalez, E., Bosques-Padilla, F. J., El-Omar, E., Hold, G., Tijerina-Menchaca, R., Maldonado-Garza, H. J., and Pérez-Pérez, G. I. (2005). Role of the polymorphic IL-1B, IL-RN and TNF-A genes in distal gastric cancer in Mexico. *International Journal of Cancer, 114*(2), 237–241. doi: 10.1002/ijc.20718.

Gonoodi, K., Moslem, A., Ahmadnezhad, M., Darroudi, S., Mazloum, Z., Tayefi, M., ... Ghayour-Mobarhan, M. (2018). Relationship of dietary and serum zinc with depression score in Iranian adolescent girls. *Biological Trace Element Research, 186*(1), 91–97. doi:10.1007/s12011-018-1301-6.

Gregory, A. M., Caspi, A., Moffitt, T. E., Milne, B. J., Poulton, R., and Sears, M. R. (2009). Links between anxiety and allergies: Psychobiological reality or possible methodological bias? *Journal of Personality, 77*(2), 347–362. doi: 10.1111/j.1467-6494.2008.00550.x.

Greuter, T., Franc, Y., Kaelin, M., Schoepfer, A. M., Schreiner, P., Zeitz, J., ... Biedermann, L. (2018). Low serum zinc levels predict presence of depression symptoms, but not overall disease outcome, regardless of ATG16L1 genotype in Crohn's disease patients. *Therapeutic Advances in Gastroenterology, 11*(1), 1–15. doi: 10.1177/1756283X18757715.

Heifert, T. A., Susi, A., Hisle-Gorman, E., Erdie-Lalena, C. R., Gorman, G., Min, S. B., and Nylund, C. M. (2016). Feeding disorders in children with autism spectrum disorders are associated with Eosinophilic Escophagitis. *Journal of Pediatric Gastroenterology and Nutrition, 63*(4), 69–73. doi: 10.1097/MPG. 0000000000001282.

Hemarajata, P., and Versalovic, J. (2013). Effects of probiotics on gut microbiota: Mechanisms of intestinal immunomodulation and neuromodulation. *Therapeutic Advances in Gastroenterology, 6*(1), 39–51. doi: 10.1177/1756283X12459294.

Horvath, K., Papadimitriou, J. C., Rabsztyn, A., Drachenberg, C., and Tildon, J. T. (1999). Gastrointestinal abnormalities in children with autistic disorder. *The Journal of Pediatrics, 135*(5), 559–563. doi: 10.1016/S0022-3476(99)70052-1.

Ibrahim, S. H., Voigt, R. G., Katusic, S. K., Weaver, A. L., and Barbaresi, W. J. (2009). Incidence of gastrointestinal symptoms in children with autism: A population-based study. *Pediatrics, 124*(2), 680–686. doi: 10.1542/peds/2008-2933.

Jacka, F. N., Pasco, J. A., Williams, L. J., Meyer, B. J., Digger, R., and Berk, M. (2013). Dietary intake of fish and PUFA, and clinical depressive and anxiety disorders in women. *British Journal of Nutrition, 109*(11), 2059–2066. doi: 10.1017/S0007114512004102.

Jernberg, C., Löfmark, S., Edlund C., and Jansson, J. K. (2007). Long-term ecological impacts of antibiotic administration on the human intestinal microbiota. *The ISME Journal, 1*(1), 56–66. doi: 10.1038/ismej.2007.3.

Kazanci, S. Y., Saglam, N. O., and Omar, R. H. (2017). Vitamin B12 < 300 pg/mL in children and especially adolescents may predispose forgetfulness, anxiety, and unhappiness. *Iranian Journal of Pedeatrics, 27*(4), 1–7. doi: 10.5812/ijp.4663.

Khanna, P., Chattu, V. K., and Aeri, B. T. (2019). Nutritional aspects of depression in adolescents – a systematic review. *International Journal of Preventive Medicine, 10*(1), 42. doi: 10.4103/ijpvm.IJPVM_400_18.

Lazar, V., Ditu, L. M., Pircalabioru, G. G., Gheorghe, I., Curutiu, C., Holban, A. M., ... Chifiriuc, M. C. (2018). Aspects of gut microbiota and immune system interactions in infectious diseases, immunopathology, and cancer. *Frontiers in Immunology, 9*(1), 1830. doi: 10.3389/fimmu.2018.01830.

Lopes-Sakamoto, F., Pereira-Ribeiro, R. M., Bueno, A. A., and Santos, H. O. (2019). Psychotropic effects of L-theanine and its clinical properties: From the management of anxiety and stress to a potential use in schizophrenia. *Pharmacological Research, 147*(1). doi: 10.1016/j.phrs.2019.104395.

Lurie, I., Yang, Y. X., Haynes, K., Mamtani, R., and Boursi, B. (2015). Antibiotic exposure and risk for depression, anxiety, or psychosis: A nested case-control study. *Journal of Clinical Psychiatry, 76*(11), 1522–1528. doi: 10.4088/JCP.15m09961.

Mazefsky, C. A., Schreiber, D. R., Olino, T. M., and Minshew, N. (2014). The association between emotional and behavioral problems and gastrointestinal symptoms among children with high-functioning autism. *Autism, 18*(5), 493–501. doi: 10.1177/1362361313485164.

McElhanon, B. O., McCracken, C., Karpen, S., and Sharp, W. G. (2014). Gastrointestinal symptoms in autism spectrum disorder: A meta-analysis. *Pediatrics, 133*(5), 872–883. doi: 10.1542/peds.2013-3995.

Melmed, R., Schneider, C., Fabes, R. A., Philips, J., and Reichelt, K. (2000). Metabolic markers and gastrointestinal symptoms in children with autism and related disorders. *Journal of Pediatric Gastroenterology and Nutrition, 31*, S31–S32.

Mikkelsen, K., Hallam, K., Stojanovska, L., and Apostolopoulos, V. (2018). Yeast based spreads improve anxiety and stress. *Journal of Functional Foods, 40*(1), 471–476. doi: 10.1016/j.jff.2017.11.034.

Muneer, A. (2016). Bipolar disorder: Role of inflammation and the development of disease biomarkers. *Psychiatry Investigations, 13*(1), 18–33. doi: 10.4306/pi.2016.13.1.18.

Nikolov, R. N., Bears, K. E., Lettinga, J., Erickson, C., Rodowski, M., Aman, M. G., ... Scahill, L. (2009). Gastrointestinal symptoms in a sample of children with pervasive developmental disorders. *Journal of Autism and Developmental Disorders, 39*(3), 405–413.

O'Neil, A., Quirk, S. E., Housden, S., Brennan, S. L., Williams, L. J., Pasco, J. A., ... Jacka, F. N. (2014). Relationship between and diet and mental health in children and adolescents: A systematic review. *American Journal of Public Health, 104*(10), 31–42. doi: 10.2105/AJPH.2014.302110.

Pirbaglou, M., Katz, J., de Souza, R. J., Stearns, J. C., Motamed, M., and Ritvo, P. (2016). Probiotic supplementation can positively affect anxiety and depressive symptoms: A systematic review of randomized controlled trials. *Nutrition Research, 36*(9), 889–898. doi: 10.1016/j.nutres.2016.06.009.

Pouteau, E., Kabir-Ahmadi, M., Noah, L., Mazur, A., Dye, L., Hellhammer, J., ... Dubray, C. (2018). Superiority of magnesium and vitamin B6 over magnesium alone on severe stress in healthy adults with low magnesemia: A randomized, single-blind clinical trial. *PLoS One, 13*(12), 1–17. doi: 10.1371/journal.pone.0208454.

Reis, D. J., Ilardi, S. S., and Punt, S. E. W. (2018). The anxiolytic effect of probiotics: A systematic review and meta-analysis of the clinical and preclinical literature. *PLoS ONE, 13*(6), 1–25. doi: 10.1371/journal.pone.0199041.

Robertson, R. C., Oriach, S. C., Murphy, K., Moloney, G. M., Cryan, J. F., Dinan, T. G., ... Stanton, C. (2017). Omega-3 polyunsaturated fatty acids critically regulate behaviour and gut microbiota development in adolescence and adulthood. *Brain, Behavior, and Immunity, 59*(1), 21–37. doi: 10.1016/j.bbi.2016.07.145.

Romijn, A. R., and Rucklidge, J. J. (2015). Systematic review of evidence to support the theory of psychobiotics. *Nutrition Reviews, 73*(10), 675–693. doi: 10.1093/nutrit/nuv025.

Sarris, J., Byrne, G. J., Cribb, L., Oliver, G., Murphy, J., Macdonald, P., ... Ng, C. H. (2019). L-theanine in the adjunctive treatment of generalized anxiety disorder: A double-blind, randomised, placebo-controlled trial. *Journal of Psychiatric Research, 110*(1), 31–37. doi: 10.1016/j.jpsychires.2018.12.014.

Schwalfenberg, G. K., and Genuis, S. J. (2017). The importance of magnesium in clinical healthcare. *Scientifica, 2017*(1), 1–14. doi: 10.1155/2017/4179326.

Slattery, J., MacFabe, D. F., and Frye, R. E. (2016). The significance of the enteric microbiome on the development of childhood disease: A review of prebiotic and probiotic therapies in disorders of childhood. *Clinical Medical Insights Pediatrics, 10*(1), 91–107. doi: 10.4137/CMPed.S38338.

Smith, D. G., Martinelli, R., Besra, G. S., Illarionov, P. A., Szatmari, I., Brazda, P., ... Lowry, C. A. (2019). Identification and characterization of a novel anti-inflammatory lipid isolated from Mycobacterium vaccae, a soil-derived bacterium with immunoregulatory and stress resilience properties. *Psychopharmacology (Berl), 236*(5), 1653–1670. doi: 10.1007/s00213-019-05253-9.

Su, K. P., Tseng, P. T., Lin, P. Y., Okubo, R., Chen, T. Y., Chen, Y. W., and Matsuoka, Y. J. (2018). Association of use of omega-3 polyunsaturated fatty acids with changes in severity of anxiety symptoms. *JAMA Network Open, 1*(5), 1–16. doi: 10.1001/jamanetworkopen.2018.2327.

Tahmasebi, K., Amani, R., Nazari, Z., Ahmadi, K., Moazzen, S., and Mostafavi, S. A. (2017). Association of mood disorders with serum zinc concentrations in adolescent female students. *Biological Trace Element Research, 178*(2), 180–188. doi: 10.1007/s12011-016-0917-7.

Tehrani, A. N., Salehpour, A., Beyzai, B., Farhadnejad, H., Molodi, R., Hekmatdoost, A., and Rashidkhani, B. (2018). Adherence to Mediterranean dietary pattern and depression, anxiety and stress among high-school female adolescents. *Mediterranean Journal of Nutrition and Metabolism, 11*(1), 73–83. doi: 10.3233/MNM-17192.

Valdes, A. M., Walter, J., Segal, E., and Spector, T. D. (2018). Role of the gut microbiota in nutrition and health. *BMJ, 361*(1), 36–44. doi: 10.1136/bmj.k2179.

Valicenti-McDermott, M., McVicar, K., Rapin, I., Wershil, B. K., Cohen, H., and Shinnar, S. (2006). Frequency of gastrointestinal symptoms in children with autism spectrum disorders and association with family history of autoimmune disease. *Journal of Developmental and Behavioral Pediatrics, 27*(2), 128–136.

Van Egmond-Fröhlich, A. W., Weghuber, D., and de Zwaan, M. (2012). Association of symptoms of attention-deficit/hyperactivity disorder with physical activity, media time, and food intake in children and adolescents. *PLoS One, 7*(11), 1–8. doi: 10.1371/journal.pone.0049781.

Wang, H., Lee, I. S., Braun, C., and Enck, P. (2016). Effect of probiotics on central nervous system functions in animals and humans: A systematic review. *Journal of Neurogastroenterology and Motility, 22*(4), 589–605. doi: 10.5056/jnm16018.

White, D. J., De Klerk, S., Woods, W., Gondalia, S., Noonan, C., Scholey, A. B. (2016). Anti-stress, behavioural and magnetoencephalography effects of an L-theanine-based nutrient drink: A randomised, double-blind, placebo-controlled, crossover trial. *Nutrients, 8*(53), 1–19. doi: 10.3390/nu8010053.

Wolraich, M. L., Lindgren, S. D., Stumbo, P. J., Stegink, L. D., Appelbaum, M. I., and Kirisy, M. C. (1994). Effects of diets high in sucrose or aspartame on the behavior and cognitive performance of children. *New England Journal of Medicine, 330*(1), 301–307. doi: 10.1056/NEJM199402033300501.

CHAPTER 6

Sensory Integration and Processing
Impact on Anxiety in Autism

Virginia Spielmann, M.S., O.T., Ph.D. candidate, and Lucy Jane Miller, Ph.D., OTR/L, Founder Emerita, STAR Institute for Sensory Processing Disorder, Colorado

Introduction

Sensory integration and processing refers to the neurobiological, sensory-perceptual, sensory-modulation, and sensory-motor mechanisms that underlie one's sense of safety, sense of self, body ownership, and function (Ayres, 1972a; Kilroy *et al.*, 2019; Mason, 2017b). In 2017, a Swedish study of 12,419 twin-pairs found that sensory over- and under-responsivity were strongly associated with autism at the genotype and phenotype levels (Taylor *et al.*, 2017). Multiple papers in recent years have suggested that atypical sensory processing and sensory-motor control may, in fact, be core to the autistic developmental process and experience (Bizzell *et al.*, 2019; Donnellan *et al.*, 2013; Hannant *et al.*, 2016; Hilton *et al.*, 2012; Mosconi and Sweeney, 2015; Robertson and Baron-Cohen, 2017; Whyatt and Craig, 2013). Furthermore, atypical sensory processing has been shown to be specifically associated with anxiety in autism (Glod *et al.*, 2015; Green and Ben-Sasson, 2010; South and Rodgers, 2017). How these dimensions of function interact and overlap warrants considerable thought and attention. Behaviors typically interpreted as "anxiety" might actually be a result of disordered sensory processing. Interruptions to an individual's interaction with the world, where everyday experiences are too intense, confusing, and/or disorganizing, can result in conditioned anxiety-related responses rather than causal scenarios.

The challenge in addressing these complex factors starts with the need for a thorough understanding of the topic. This book addresses numerous topics related to anxiety in autism; however, in this chapter the aim is to suggest the importance of disruptions in sensory processing (including sensory motor) as foundational to the autistic experience.

Overview of Sensory Processing

To engage in daily-life activities, all organisms must respond to stimuli from their own bodies and the external environment in a regulated manner (Miller *et al.*, 2017; Spitzer and Smith Roley, 2001). This process is complex and non-linear (Spitzer, 1999). It involves detection of stimuli; modulation of stimuli at the neuronal level; categorization of the sensory stimuli at the perceptual and cognitive levels; and prioritization, discrimination and response planning. Almost simultaneously, the execution of an affective, communicative, and/or motor response (or "behavior") takes place (Bundy and Murray, 2002; Guillery, 2017). This foundational process of producing responses to the environment and our internal sensations is rarely, if ever, uni-sensory, and usually involves integration of "combinatorial" sensory data from more than two sensory systems (Mason, 2017b). Each of the eight sensory systems will be briefly introduced below, with emphasis on its contribution to safety, mastery of one's own body, and sensory-affective combined effect. Implications for sensory mitigation or exacerbation of anxiety are discussed later in the chapter, from a developmental, dynamic systems perspective.

The terminology for categorization of sensory stimuli differs among disciplines. In this chapter, one categorization scheme used in the Occupational Therapy literature underlies the literature review. This nosology highlights eight sensory systems that influence one another multi-directionally (rather than being discrete self-contained constructs) (Miller *et al.*, 2019). Each system is comprised of neural hardware that detects stimuli and transmits the data through (often multiple) neural pathways to regions of the brain that prioritize and synthesize data from all sources to create the big picture. This ultimately produces an individual perception of the event in the context of the specific environment in which it happened.

Vestibular

The vestibular apparatus is located in the inner ear and detects the direction of gravity related to head and body position, speed of movement, direction of movement on multiple planes, and spatial orientation (Hain and Helminski, 2007; Lane, 2002; Mason, 2017b). Vestibular hardware is located in both ears and includes the utricle, saccule, and three semicircular canals that operate as halves of circles separated into the two sides of the body. The semicircular canals operate as a whole (right and left together) to provide more sophisticated and nuanced data about velocity, direction, and location of self (Baloh *et al.*, 2013; Hain and Helminski, 2007).

These peripheral receptors in the vestibular apparatus detect linear acceleration and head angular velocity. Processing of vestibular data primarily takes place in the vestibular nuclear complex (a multi-sensory processing locus) and the cerebellum. Output of the central vestibular system directly influences essential reflexes that keep the head and gaze stabilized, and keep our bodies secure, balanced, and upright. They are critical non-conscious mechanisms for safety, constantly monitored by the central nervous system (CNS), and supplemented by higher level (slower) cortical processes (Hain and Helminski, 2007).

The vestibular system is "extensively networked" (Rajagopalan *et al.*, 2017, p.13) within the limbic brain (Kilroy *et al.*, 2019) and many other regions of the brain, *and* it has a direct influence on emotional well-being and behavior (Rajagopalan *et al.*, 2017). Vestibular processing is also proposed to contribute to distinguishing self- versus non-self motion and sense of agency (Deroualle and Lopez, 2014).

Thus, it can be said that the vestibular system supports function from the most primitive of mechanisms through to affective experience and higher-level development of cognition, sense of self (Baloh *et al.*, 2013; Deroualle and Lopez, 2014; Rajagopalan *et al.*, 2017), and personality-trait development (C. Lopez, personal communication, February 4, 2019).

Visual

The visual system is the one most consciously relied upon during day-to-day functioning (Lane, 2002). It informs all levels of functioning, from low-level in the CNS, e.g., visual reflexes, to high level, e.g., frontal lobe decision making. The eyes house extremely complex and sophisticated photoreceptors and synaptic terminals that are hardwired via the optic nerve to structures at a wide variety of levels, e.g., the lateral geniculate nucleus (LGN) of the thalamus, superior colliculus, and primary visual cortex (Lane,

2002; Mason, 2017b). Visual processing also occurs in the inferotemporal and anterior temporal regions, where, as hypothesized by Rolls (2003), visual-affective integration occurs, including the assignment of emotional valence to otherwise neutral visual stimuli. Incoming information from the eyes far exceeds the replication of optical information, in the way a camera takes a photograph (Mason, 2017b). Visual data enables comprehension of the visual scene, depth perception, visual memory, and visual perception of motion (Anderson, 2011; Snowden and Freeman, 2004); the same data is also used for critical foundational functions such as entrainment of circadian rhythm, as well as pupillary reflexes and control of eye movements.

The vestibular and visual systems collaborate to provide information about where an organism is in relation to the ground, orientation of the body in space and time (Butterworth and Hicks, 1977), and velocity of movement (Gibson, 2009). Vision supports postural control and balance, although less so than the somatosensory and vestibular systems (Henderson *et al.*, 2002).

Previous research suggests that one's emotional state influences one's visual processing. For example, when fearful, visual orientation occurs only to certain cues at the expense of other visual data in the environment (Anderson *et al.*, 2011; Bruno and René, 2009).

Tactile

The tactile system refers to cutaneous sensors that register form, spatial, temporal, localization, pressure, and affective qualities of contact to the epidermis (McGlone and Reilly, 2010; Pawling *et al.*, 2017). It also refers to skin-based pain, pruritic, and thermal sensations (Haggard *et al.*, 2003; McGlone and Reilly, 2010). Tactile processing occurs predominantly in the primary somatosensory region, orbitofrontal cortex, and anterior cingulate cortex, as well as in the insula, which is currently considered the interoceptive "mainframe" (Björnsdotter *et al.*, 2010; Lane, 2002; McGlone and Reilly, 2010). Tactile experiences are the first bonding experiences between parent and child, and are neither solely sensory nor entirely affective. Rather, bonding is dually sensory and affective. Touch has a major influence on development of attachment (Beebe *et al.*, 2010). It is notable that recent literature on interoception (see below) indicates the importance of many of these tactile subsystems as contributors to the sense of internal well-being (Björnsdotter *et al.*, 2010).

Proprioceptive

The proprioceptive system includes the mechanoreceptors in the joints, muscle spindles, Golgi tendons, and certain tactile receptors in the skin (Proske and Gandevia, 2012; Tuthill and Azim, 2018). These receptors detect compression and traction on the joints, muscle-stretch, muscle-length, muscle-force, and muscle-tension, and when joints and muscles have been moved to their extreme (Lane, 2002; Proske and Gandevia, 2012). Proprioceptive receptors send feedback about body and limb position, detecting postural perturbations, heaviness of work, body and limb movement, sense of body shape, sense of physical self, and pre-reflective self-awareness (Arnfred *et al.*, 2015; Cole and Montero, 2010; Tuthill and Azim, 2018). Processing of proprioceptive data primarily takes place in the cerebellum, dorsal column nuclei, somatosensory cortex, motor cortex, multi-sensory regions in the parietal cortex, and notably also in the thalamus and insula (Lane, 2002; Tuthill and Azim, 2018). Thus it is apparent that proprioceptive processing occurs in and across multiple levels.

Proprioceptive sensory integration is proposed to be pivotal to the experience of pleasure in movement and the "harmony between intention, action, and sensory return" (Cole and Montero, 2010, p.313). In this way proprioception has an affective dimension that is considered to contribute to sense of agency, the embodied feeling/moving self, and also potentially the development of affective empathy (Cole and Montero, 2010). The partnership of tactile and proprioceptive sensory data is often labeled somatosensation (Bundy and Murray, 2002).

Vignette—Impact of Challenges in Sensory Discrimination on Stress and Anxiety

José is a 21-year-old man in the process of transitioning to university life on campus. He presents with stress headaches (all medical causes have been ruled out) and diagnoses of generalized anxiety disorder and autism. He is seeking help for social anxiety and difficulty transitioning to life on campus, especially making friends. An evaluation of sensory processing indicates that José has poor discrimination of all body-based senses (vestibular, proprioceptive, interoceptive, and tactile systems) and tends to over-rely on his other senses (vision, hearing, taste, and smell) for information about the world. His sensory discrimination challenges also contribute to postural difficulties, which puts further stress on his body and nervous system as he expends conscious energy on remaining upright and fatigues easily.

José also has difficulty managing personal space and appears clumsy, especially in more dynamic social situations. People have often commented that José gets too close when speaking to them, and he has a history of challenges at school, with classmates complaining he is invading their personal space. José can sometimes be difficult to understand and his challenges with self-perception have also impacted his ability to tune into his visceral and physiological experiences of emotional state. His affect usually appears flat and he finds it very effortful to identify emotions other than anxiety in himself, and also has difficulty reading the social cues of others.

The imbalances in José's sensory systems combined with his postural challenges likely contribute to his persistent and frequent headaches due to the cumulative stress of mental and physical strain.

Auditory

The auditory system codes and processes all acoustic stimuli, enabling spatial and temporal localization of sound, auditory discrimination, and pattern recognition, and contributing to awareness of self in space and time and interpersonal communication (Burleigh *et al.*, 2002; Mason, 2017a). The auditory apparatus consists of the outer, middle (ossicles and eardrum), and inner ear. The outer and middle ear and cochlea in the inner ear are critical for hearing (Kollmeier, 2008). The auditory software starts with the brainstem, runs up through the lateral lemniscus and the medial lemniscus into the inferior colliculus and the medial geniculate body, and ultimately reaches the primary auditory cortex (Kollmeier, 2008).

Affective reactions to sound have been well researched by sound designers in industries like film and automobile manufacturing (Tajadura-Jiménez and Västfjäll, 2008). These studies indicate that we may process and attend to the emotional timbre of sounds before we process the content.

All preceding sensory systems wire to the hemispheres, ensuring laterality and providing data that benefits spatial-temporal awareness and contributes to bi-lateral coordination.

Vignette—Impact of Sensory Over-Responsivity on Anxiety in the Workplace

Linda is a 34-year-old woman on the autism spectrum struggling with meltdowns, anxiety, anger, and needing earplugs. Although Linda displays only a few signs of sensory over-responsiveness during her day-to-day life, it is common for individuals her age to have well-developed "camouflaging" strategies. This may be due to cultural expectations of what is and is not socially acceptable behavior, and masking her reactions to diminish overt symptoms of sensory over responsiveness. Linda likely uses a considerable amount of mental energy to maintain self-control in distressing situations. At a certain point Linda no longer has capacity to tolerate bothersome inputs and she becomes overwhelmed and experiences a sensory shutdown or "meltdown." When this happens, Linda has limited abilities to communicate, and limited or no capacity for frustration tolerance and problem solving. At these times she is prone to outbursts, and/or withdrawal. Anticipation of these situations, and the strain of masking her sensory over-responsivity in day-to-day life, means that Linda experiences considerable anxiety as her baseline state.

Linda reports significant tactile, auditory, and visual sensitivities. Linda's nervous system experiences touch, auditory, and visual sensations more intensely than the neuromajority. Her intense experiences of sensation cause a spike in her natural stress response commonly known as fight or flight. As a result, she is often on edge despite her pleasant demeanor. Linda's ability to tolerate and discriminate auditory stimuli varies based on her arousal state. For example, Linda is able to distinguish words and tolerate background noise when in a calm state, but the same stimuli (air conditioners, refrigerators, ticking clocks) bombard her nervous system when she is over-aroused, and she loses the ability to distinguish words and process conversation.

Linda reports that she avoids certain public places or activities, and often wears headphones or earplugs to block out the constant noise. As the day progresses, the effort it requires to manage her sensory over-responsivity increases until at a certain point in the day, usually the late afternoon, Linda moves into hyperarousal and is no longer able to perform at work. Her window of functional arousal is very small, and one stressful experience can be enough to place her into the over-aroused zone, where she is easily startled and hypervigilant; at that point she is no longer able to manage her anxiety.

Gustatory and Olfactory

The olfactory (smell) and gustatory (taste) systems respond to chemical stimuli—thus they are key for ensuring safety by providing information about our environment and what we are ingesting. Both systems include peripheral sensors and a number of central pathways, and are considered functional by the second trimester in utero. Gustatory and olfactory sensations are processed separately in the olfactory bulb and gustatory cortex, as well as the hippocampus, amygdala, thalamus, insula, and orbitofrontal cortex; reciprocal connections have been found between olfactory and gustatory pathways (Sugai *et al.*, 2005). Interestingly, olfactory sensory processing does not need to pass through the thalamus to reach cortical areas (Mouly and Sullivan, 2010), and the more direct connection may explain the powerful phenomenon of odor-cued memories, which are generally considered to be more emotionally laden than memories evoked by other sensory systems (Mouly and Sullivan, 2010).

These systems are significant contributors to the development of attachment, and contribute not only to development of feeding behaviors, taste, and palate (Lipchock *et al.*, 2011), but also to sensory affective development (Schore, 2015). According to Mouly and Sullivan (2010), odor sensing contributes to selection of a mate and mother bonding to child.

Vignette—Impact of Olfactory, Gustatory, Tactile, and Visual Over-Responsivity on Development of Feeding Skills

Kiara is a 16-year-old girl on the autism spectrum; when regulated she uses an Augmentative and Alternative Communication (AAC) device for communication. She has a full-time caregiver with her at all times.

Kiara often communicates through behaviors, sometimes removing her clothing, sometimes pulling her hair and pinching her caregivers. She has a limited repertoire of food that she accepts, and recently the number of food items has dropped to just dinosaur-shaped chicken nuggets and goldfish crackers; she also accepts Pediasure (a nutritious supplement drink for children who are behind in growth). When these foods have not been available Kiara has had loud, aggressive outbursts, sometimes tipping furniture over and other times crying inconsolably.

Kiara has a history of gag responses when looking at soft and pureed foods, and in response to certain food smells (especially fish and broth smells). She also has aversions to tactile experiences like "messy play," lotions, and shaving foam. When presented with grits (a dish of ground cornmeal boiled with milk or water), porridge, and macaroni and cheese at a young age, Kiara would make a loud keening sound that was interpreted as humorous by her aide at school; she was still expected to eat the food. Kiara also had gag reactions to the texture and smell of green vegetables, particularly leafy vegetables, sometimes bringing these foods back up; it was common for her to be asked to put the food back in her mouth after these incidents. Kiara also finds the cafeteria environment challenging—especially the fluorescent lights, smells, and seeing other people eat. This meant that while Kiara obtained the calories she needed for physical growth, she developed anxiety around food and mealtimes, especially in school settings where she has very specific requirements around where she eats, which spoon and bowl she will use to eat from, and what foods are acceptable.

Kiara's care team were not reading her social cues or communication around food, and this added to her stress levels, increasing her anxiety and her need for control and predictability. This is likely why she dropped down to two foods and Pediasure for all her nutritional intake.

With support from a Feeding Therapist who understands sensory processing and integration, Kiara and her family were able to adopt a problem-solving, understanding-based approach to menu options. Using the AAC device to ensure she was comfortable and felt safe and listened to, she was able to discover a wider range of foods that she could tolerate and remain organized around. She continues to have rigid requirements around packaging, because food needs to be predictable for her.

Interoceptive

Interoception not only senses the physiological condition of the body and internal well-being, but also includes affective or sensual touch and tickle (Craig, 2008). The insula and the anterior cingulate cortex are the most recognized regions where interoceptive signals converge, although it is acknowledged that the story is richer, and thus the research continues (Murphy *et al.*, 2017).

Interoception encompasses sensing thirst, hunger, satiety, temperature, gut motility, heartrate, and blood-sugar levels, as well as the prediction of onset of illness (Fiene and Brownlow, 2015; Murphy *et al.*, 2017). Interoception is considered by many to be entirely sensoriaffective in nature, or, as coined by Schulz and Vögele (2015), "visceral affective"; e.g., butterflies in your stomach, being "hangry," and gut feelings are all physiological descriptors of primarily emotional states (Holzer, 2017). This kind of bodily intelligence is not cognitive, but is also not entirely subconscious. A separate but not entirely removed dimension of bodily knowing is neuroception, a phrase coined by Stephen Porges (2018) to describe a neural-level capacity to fluidly and rapidly distinguish environmental and visceral cues on threat and safety. As Ayres (1972a) and others (Brazelton and Greenspan, 2009; Sacks, 1990) stated so many years ago, the autonomic nervous system is connected to affect and to behavior (Kilroy *et al.*, 2019). The field's increased understanding of interoceptive and neuroceptive function and influence emphasizes the need for understanding and exploring the fully lived, embodied, sensoriaffective experience of each individual (Porges, 2015; Van Nest, 2018). "The neural substrates responsible for subjective awareness of your emotional state are based on the neural representation of your physiological state" (Craig, 2008, p.214). Interoception has been widely linked with emotional and psychological well-being, and a new wave of research into this concept is well under way (Khalsa *et al.*, 2018).

Nosology of Sensory Processing

Disordered sensory processing phenotypes were first identified by A. Jean Ayres (1972b) based primarily on factor analyses of her tests, the Southern CA Sensory Integration Test battery (1972a), and the Sensory Integration and Praxis Test (1989). Miller, Anzalone, Lane, Cermak and Osten (2007) proposed a nosology of sensory processing that demarcates subgroups.

Specificity in subtypes of disordered sensory processing provides clarity for intervention planning, as well as a way to homogenize sample inclusion criteria for research studies. Multiple diagnostic bodies have acknowledged Miller *et al.*'s classification system.[1] Miller and others have called for a revision of this nosology (Miller *et al.*, 2020). As research continues and new data becomes available from new standardized scales, it is expected that the nosology of sensory processing will be updated.[2] Figure 6.1 illustrates the 2007 nosology.

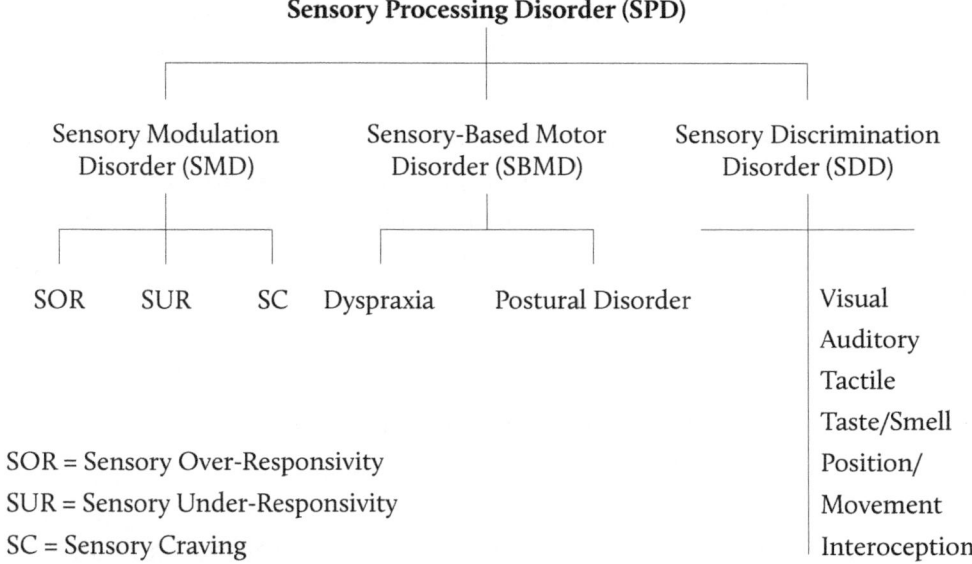

Figure 6.1 The 2007 Nosology for Sensory Processing Patterns
Source: Reproduced with permission from Miller *et al.*, 2007.

It is of critical significance to note that while the literature estimates that more than 90 percent of the autistic population experiences dysfunctional sensory processing (Robertson and Baron-Cohen, 2017), most of the focus for research has been in the areas of sensory over-responsivity (SOR) and sensory under-responsivity (SUR); there is a paucity of research into other

1 The Diagnostic Classification of Mental Health and Developmental Disorders of Infancy and Early Childhood, Revised (DC: 0-3R), Diagnostic Manual for Infancy and Early Childhood, Interdisciplinary Council on Development and Learning (ICDL-DMIC), Psychodynamic Diagnostic Manual—2nd Edition (PDM-2).

2 The Evaluation of Ayres Sensory Integration (EASI, to be published by CLASI), Structured Observations of Sensory Integration-Motor (SOSI-M, to be published by Academic Therapy Publishing), and the Sensory Processing 3-Dimensions Scale (SP3D, to be published by WPS).

presentations and phenotypes of disordered sensory processing. Therefore, the estimated number of individuals on the spectrum impacted by sensory processing dysfunction may be higher, which is consistent with testimonials from autistic self-advocates (Grandin, 2009; Robledo *et al.*, 2012; Schaber, 2014). Clinically more than one disordered sensory processing pattern is frequently observed within the same individual on the spectrum (Glod *et al.*, 2015). Co-occurring sensory processing patterns in autism need further empirical research.

In the following section each subtype in the 2007 nosology will be summarized, followed by discussion related to that subtype and its co-occurrence with anxiety. As seen in the outline of sensory system mechanisms above, sensory processing and anxiety exert bi-directional influence on one another. Note that patterns of sensory processing dysfunction are heterogeneous within this population, and no single template exists for disordered sensory processing in autistic people. Every individual deserves to explore and discover their own unique patterns of strengths and challenges in sensory processing.

Vignette—Impact of Anxiety on Sensory Over-Responsivity Symptoms

Ashley is a bright nine-year-old boy living in a wealthy downtown neighborhood of a densely populated city. Ashley was diagnosed on the autism spectrum at the age of four. His teacher reports that he is not coping in the classroom, is lazy, resists instructions, and interferes with his classmates' work. His parents report that he is exhausted when he comes home and preoccupied with school in conversations throughout the weekend.

At the point of evaluation, Ashley scored with profound differences in all areas of sensory processing and integration. Teacher report and classroom observations indicated that his biggest challenges were visual over-responsivity. He would orient and respond to every visual stimulus in his environment, including people walking past in the corridor through the classroom window, the branches of trees moving outside, or light and shadows; artwork that moved and art mobiles hanging from the ceiling would often grab his attention for extended periods of time.

The classroom observation revealed a considerable amount of anxiety-type behaviors; for example, during tidy-up time the class teacher put an animation of a ticking time bomb on the interactive whiteboard to cue the children on the transition. When this happened, Ashley would freeze in place with his eyes transfixed on the whiteboard; his teacher perceived his behavior as avoidant, but on observation it was apparent that he was in an immobilized fear state as he anticipated the explosion of the time bomb on the screen—and that both the visual and auditory aspects of that experience were overwhelming for his nervous system.

The occupational therapist and psychologist worked together with his parents to reduce stressors in Ashley's day-to-day life, and as they did so his symptoms of sensory over-responsivity diminished. His family eventually decided to move to the country with him; after nine months they had him reassessed for sensory-processing differences. He scored within normal range for all aspects of sensory processing and integration, with slightly higher scores for over-responsivity to visual, auditory, and tactile sensation (still within normal range). Ashley's sensory-processing differences were highly vulnerable to his stress levels and state of anxiety; in his situation it was treatment of anxiety that was the key factor in supporting psychological well-being and diminished sensory symptoms.

Sensory-Modulation Patterns

The most-researched presentation of disruptions in sensory processing (Glod *et al.*, 2015), sensory modulation disorders (SMD) are hypothesized to be the result of dysfunction of the neurological mechanisms related to habituation and sensitization (Miller *et al.*, 2001). SMD occur at the neurological level where pre- and post-synaptic signal modulation are either inhibited or propagated, affecting detection. Behavioral manifestations of disordered sensory modulation may include hyperresponsivity, hyporesponsivity, or fluctuating responses to sensory stimuli, and/or exhibition of unusual patterns of sensation seeking or avoiding (e.g., fight-or-flight reactions).

Sensory Over-Responsivity

Characterized as an exaggerated and disproportionate behavioral reaction (Glod *et al.*, 2015) to sensory stimuli (especially non-threatening stimuli), SOR is widely attributed to the autistic experience (Tavassoli *et al.*, 2014), as are elevated incidents of SOR and co-occurring anxiety in the autistic population (Green and Ben-Sasson, 2010). Correlations between SOR and anxiety were found to be significant in Glod *et al.*'s systematic review of 2015. SOR in autism is documented in the tactile, auditory, gustatory, and olfactory domains (Rogers *et al.*, 2003), as well as in the visual domain (Leekam *et al.*, 2007; Nyström *et al.*, 2015), and the vestibular domain (Ayres and Tickle, 1980; Kern *et al.*, 2007). SOR challenges cause considerable difficulty navigating day-to-day life and relationships (Green and Ben-Sasson, 2010; Kirby *et al.*, 2019). This over-responsivity to stimuli that would be considered non-noxious by a functional nervous system disrupts arousal modulation and often pushes a system into fight-or-flight mode. Clinical experience suggests that this continuous state of hypervigilance creates a loss of locus of control, interferes with development of self, and cultivates a state of chronic apprehension (Green and Ben-Sasson, 2010; Grillon, 2008). The converse is also true: increased arousal tends to impact threat detection in the environment, and in all likelihood the relationship is cyclical and somewhat bi-directional (Green and Ben-Sasson, 2010).

Sensory Under-Responsivity

At the behavioral level, SUR presents as diminished, insufficient, or delayed responses to sensory stimuli (Glod *et al.*, 2015). These individuals need more intense sensory stimulation in order to generate an adaptive response (Case-Smith and Ratliff-Schaub, 2009; Miller *et al.*, 2007). SUR often co-exists with SOR in autism across different sensory systems (Lane *et al.*, 2010). Individuals can exhibit SMD patterns differently based on times of day or location (Case-Smith and Ratliff-Schaub, 2009).

SUR in autism is proposed to be associated particularly with the proprioceptive system (Riquelme *et al.*, 2016) and in response to noise (Foss-Feig *et al.*, 2012). Functionally, SUR in autism has been associated with academic under-achievement (Ashburner *et al.*, 2008), slowness to adapt (Brock *et al.*, 2012), and lower adaptive functioning (Liss *et al.*, 2006).

Sensory Craving

Clinical experience strongly suggests that an individual experiencing insatiable desire for sensory experiences is more than seeking input. These individuals do not become regulated as a result of increased intense input, but rather arousal levels continue to remain elevated and dysregulation and challenges with response inhibition continue (Miller *et al.*, 2014). This phenomenon is yet to be empirically researched.

Sensory-Based Motor Patterns

Atypical sensory motor processing, lack of coordination, and slow motor learning are highly prevalent in autism (Torres and Whyatt, 2016; Hannant *et al.*, 2016; Robledo *et al.*, 2012; Torres and Donnellan, 2015). Specific motor challenges commonly identified in the literature include diminished fine and gross motor performance (Lloyd *et al.*, 2013; Riquelme *et al.*, 2016; Tomchek *et al.*, 2015) and atypical motor learning, which includes learning from mistakes and developing accurate and reliable sensory memories of movements (Marko *et al.*, 2015; Moraes *et al.*, 2017).

Posture-Based Patterns

"Postural control involves controlling the body's position in space for the dual purposes of stability and orientation" (Shumway-Cook and Wollacott, 2017, p.153). Functional posture involves sustaining steady-state balance (alignment, muscle and postural tone), being ready for action, and being able to react to events in the world (Shumway-Cook and Wollacott, 2017). To attain functional posture, continuous data from multiple sensory systems (visual, somatosensory, and vestibular) must be co-registered and interpreted by the individual (Miller *et al.*, 2007).

Autism-specific challenges related to difficulty with postural control include head lag in infancy (Hannant *et al.*, 2016), ocular motor control (Johnson *et al.*, 2016), hypotonia (Ming *et al.*, 2007), and the ability to adjust posture in anticipation of movement/action (Schmitz *et al.*, 2003; Trevarthen and Delafield-Butt, 2013); these all have an impact on the performance of gross motor skills (Mache and Todd, 2016). Researchers hypothesize that challenges with postural control in autistic people across the lifespan are due to poor multi-channel sensory integration (Doumas *et al.*, 2016; Lim *et al.*, 2017; Molloy *et al.*, 2003).

Difficulties with sustaining resistance against gravity, balance, hypotonia, and ocular motor control often demand development of compensatory strategies for minimal function in day-to-day life. This increases likelihood of fatigue and irritability, and sets a poor foundation for development of coordination of the two sides of the body, and more refined and demanding gross motor control. Posture also reflects a bodily expression of affective state, and as such has been shown to have a bi-directional influence on how one feels—posture can make mood worse or better and vice versa (Hainaut *et al.*, 2018; Riskind and Gotay, 1982).

Dyspraxia

Praxis is the ability to conceptualize, plan, sequence, and execute novel purposeful movements. "In order to carry out volitional activities, our cognitive skills need to interact with a range of performance skills, namely sensation and perception, memory and learning concepts, high-level executive functions, emotions, and motor skills" (Tempest, 2017, p.149). There are two main categories of purposeful movement: those involving objects, for example interacting with the environment and/or manipulating tools, and those that are sociocultural in nature, for example gestural communication (Tempest, 2017); it is also, of course, common for an action to simultaneously represent both types of purposeful movement.

Well-developed praxis is also necessary for the ability to sense time with reasonable accuracy and anticipate, plan for, and form expectations. These skills are necessary for the ability to transition between activities, make cognitive shifts, and inhibit unwanted responses related to thwarted expectations (Amos, 2013).

First-hand accounts report challenges with controlling, executing, combining action or movements, and marrying intention with action (Robledo *et al.*, 2012). Research also demonstrates challenges with imitation praxis (Smith Roley *et al.*, 2015), the somatosensory aspects of praxis (Schaaf *et al.*, 2015), the generation of ideas, and the ability to participate in play and leisure (Bodison, 2015). It is recommended that all individuals with a diagnosis of autism also receive evaluation for dyspraxia (Caçola *et al.*, 2017).

The ability to "make meaning" from motor gestures, motor experiences, and facial expressions of self and other is impacted by sensory motor challenges in autism, and impedes ability to infer meaning and understand others (Trevarthen and Delafield-Butt, 2013). The psychosocial impacts of dyspraxia include anxiety and depression and are considered the most disabling aspect of these challenges (Zwicker *et al.*, 2013).

Vignette—Impact of Dyspraxia on Social Anxiety, Transitions, and Play

Yat Ming is a six-year-old boy with a new diagnosis of autism. He presents with anxiety behaviors around transitions at school and at home. He has not made friends in his classroom and avoids free play and playground time, preferring to play by himself with a toy he brought from home.

Yat Ming's challenges with interpreting sensation affect his ability to produce complex sequences of movement (praxis). He has difficulty therefore shifting between activities and engaging purposefully, with others, in play. His challenges with praxis manifest as poor understanding of object properties, challenges understanding time, difficulty generating ideas for play, problems anticipating what will happen, and trouble organizing and sequencing his actions. Yat Ming enjoys imaginative play and is able to act out some elements of familiar TV shows, but has trouble following suggested actions and using novel objects. When presented with novel play objects, his play repertoire includes throwing, kicking, and hitting. These challenges with praxis mean that he has not yet developed purposeful play schemes beyond basic cause and effect or sensory motor play. This results in poor task completion and scattered play schemes, because there is no clear beginning, middle, or end to the activity.

These skill deficits mean that Yat Ming's arousal increases when he is provided a warning that it is time, or almost time, to stop an activity. This heightened arousal often results in a fight-or-flight response that looks like refusal of help and assistance. He often resorts to behavioral communicative strategies around his distress—these include hitting, kicking, and refusing to be moved or picked up.

These challenges also mean that Yat Ming is unable to successfully engage with his peers in age-appropriate play schemes, and is not invited to participate in playground games; this means he is missing out on important opportunities to develop social confidence and social pragmatic skills.

Sensory Discrimination Dysfunction

This pattern represents difficulty with discerning, differentiating, and interpreting specific details concerning sensory stimuli. The details, timing, and nuances of sensory stimuli must all be discriminated in order for refined and efficient adaptive responses to be formulated and executed. Sensory discrimination challenges can be present with or without modulation and motor-based challenges, and can be present in a combination of sensory systems. Clinical experience suggests that challenges with sensory discrimination manifest as disorganization, poor awareness of self and others, misinterpretation of real-time events, risk taking, or disproportionate risk aversion and constricted development of sense of self and mastery. Empirically identified discrimination challenges were outlined in the sections on sensory systems above.

Anxiety and Sensory Processing
The Autism Constellation

Both autism and anxiety are diagnosed based on a cluster of behaviors; underneath observable behaviors, there are multiple factors to consider. Sensory features such as sensory modulation capacity, sensory motor efficacy, postural maturity, and ability to discriminate accurately must be considered in tandem with the development of mental health features such as sense of self, relationships to others, and relationship with the world. Disordered sensory processing profoundly impacts interaction with environmental factors, and may therefore predispose an individual to anxiety behaviors such as fear, withdrawal, rigidity, separation anxiety, social anxiety, panic attacks, specific phobias, and rigidity (Green and Ben-Sasson, 2010; Mazurek et al., 2013; Neil et al., 2016). In addition, presentation of disordered sensory processing across multiple subtypes or patterns in one individual, which is quite common, is associated with increased withdrawal, negative mood, and stress behaviors (Brock et al., 2012; South and Rodgers, 2017).

A helpful conceptualization of the complexity of co-occurring conditions in autism comes from Caroline Hearst (n.d.) and is presented by Fletcher-Watson and Happé (2019). Rather than illustrating autism as a spectrum from high- to low-functioning, the constellation analogy takes into account how specific features of autism/associated diagnoses might be plotted on a three-dimensional chart. "Autistic people, with a diagnosis, may locate themselves anywhere in the resulting three-dimensional space. Their exact location would further vary with context and across the lifespan" (Fletcher-Watson and Happé, 2019, p.34). Figure 6.2 displays the conceptualization of the autistic constellation.

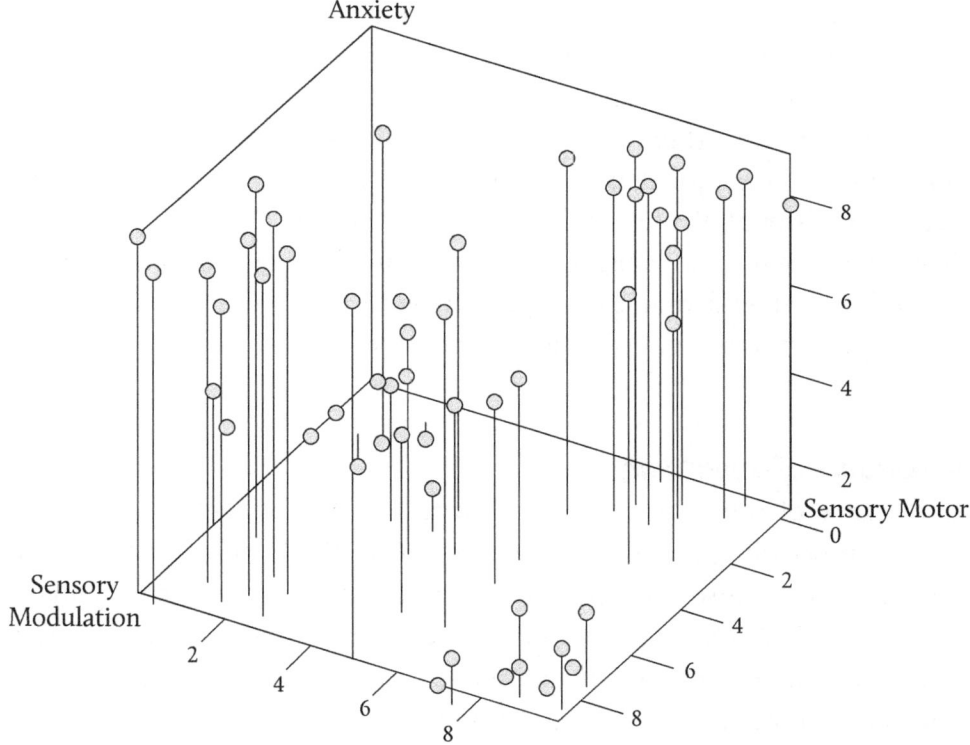

Figure 6.2 The Autism Constellation

Source: Reproduced from *Autism*, 2nd Edition by Sue Fletcher-Watson and Francesca Happé, published by Routledge. © 2019 Sue Fletcher-Watson and Francesca Happé. Reproduced by arrangement with Taylor & Francis Books UK.

In the autistic constellation, the interaction between patterns of sensory modulation, sensory-based motor, and sensory discrimination challenges with anxiety are cyclically causative.

Restricted and Repetitive Behaviors and Interests (RRBIs)

Identified sensory processing contributors to RRBIs include postural control (Radonovich *et al.*, 2013) and sensory hypersensitivity (Schulz and Stevenson, 2018). More profound sensory processing challenges seem to have a causative relationship with the intensity of RRBIs (Gabriels *et al.*, 2008). SOR has been shown to be associated with insistence on sameness behaviors, while SUR appears to relate to repetitive motor behaviors *and* insistence on sameness (Wigham *et al.*, 2015).

RRBs (repetitive motor movements) might be a manifestation of sensory- and/or social-anxiety, and are reported to be soothing to some people on the autistic spectrum. Conversely, some individuals may not engage in RRBs volitionally, but rather because of deficient motor control, and therefore RRBs contribute to their anxiety (Fletcher-Watson and Happé, 2019).

It is likely that there are multiple "causes" of RRBs. While they are sometimes dysfunctional, or harmful to self or others, they often support regulation through the joy of the movement (Fletcher-Watson and Happé, 2019). This means that RRBIs can impact well-being for the better, and the general recommendation is to respect the individual's wishes and leave the RRBI alone if it is not interfering with function.

Intolerance of Uncertainty

Intolerance of uncertainty strongly correlates with anxiety and atypical sensory processing in autism (Neil *et al.*, 2016; Wigham *et al.*, 2015). It is proposed as a transdiagnostic psychological vulnerability factor by many (Ouellet *et al.*, 2019)—even potentially a core component of anxiety itself. Intolerance of uncertainty manifests as "an excessive tendency to find uncertain situations stressful and upsetting, to believe that unexpected events are negative and should be avoided, and to think that being uncertain about the future is unfair" (Dugas *et al.*, 2005, p.58).

Indeed, clinical experience suggests that individuals with sensory processing differences are often highly invested in controlling the outcome of social interactions and activities. One possible explanation of this is that when our sensory systems are disordered, our experience of the world is generally out of our control—therefore controlling other dynamic and unpredictable situations becomes necessary for self-regulation and management of energy expenditure. It is logical that a lived experience of the world as fundamentally disorganizing and confusing, due to dysfunctional sensory processing, would lead to a strong drive to control the daily agenda and avoid uncertainty at all costs. Current best practice recommendations for support include multi-faceted approaches to support that consider the interplay of sensation, emotion regulation, and cognition (South and Rodgers, 2017).

Developmental Perspective

The importance of positive early experiences is generally agreed upon across disciplines for the development of a social brain, self-regulation, and a strong sense of self (Fogel, 1993; Gerhardt, 2009; Lurie-Hurvitz, 2009; Shonkoff and Phillips, 2000). Although concepts of emotional development have historically been separated out from sensory perceptual and sensory motor development, the more that is learned about functional neuroanatomy, the more apparent it becomes that these are two intersecting ways of feeling, impossible to parse out from each other. The concept of sensoriaffective development can be traced back to the 1940s (Alvarado, 2017), and in 1966 it was proposed as a developmental stage that ought to supersede the Piagetian sensory motor phase by Stechler and Latz (cited in Alvarado, 2017). Consideration must be given to the developmental implications of disordered sensory processing on arousal and regulation, mitigation or exacerbation of anxiety, and especially the ability of the child to access soothing relational overtures from caregivers (Garfinkel *et al.*, 2016).

Sensory processing is necessary for successful infant–caregiver interactions. For example, in order for the child to mold to the caregiver's body, proprioceptive awareness must be online and functioning well; to exchange gestural and affective communication, head control and postural control against gravity must be developed (Spitzer and Smith Roley, 2001). Mastery of movement through space, feelings of control over the environment, and well-developed body schema are multi-sensory developmental domains (Spitzer and Smith Roley, 2001).

Inhibited development of bodily/environment precept (Kilroy *et al.*, 2019) naturally limits development of differentiation of self and non-self and pre-reflective sense of self. Furthermore, difficulties with "sense making" has clear implications for development of self-perception and self-efficacy (De Jaegher, 2013), as well as development of social capacity and relationships (Tronick, 2007). This may be easily related to concepts of embodied cognition—in other words, how the brain and body are able to produce meaningful action in real time within context (De Jaegher *et al.*, 2016; Gjelsvik *et al.*, 2015; Wellsby and Pexman, 2014).

Evaluation and Treatment Considerations

Evaluation and treatment for anxiety and sensory processing challenges in autism should be holistic, interdisciplinary, and relationship based. Treatment of co-occurring conditions like anxiety and disordered sensory processing must move beyond siloed, domain-specific interventions into dynamic, collaborative support for the entire profile of the individual, as evident in this multi-disciplinary book. Without an interdisciplinary perspective, symptom overlap and professional perspective may obscure the ability to distinguish/differentiate between these clinical conditions, as well as establish priorities for intervention.

The dimensions of function that contribute to the autistic constellation are dynamic and influence each other, as open systems, anxiety, and other challenging aspects of the autistic experience must be addressed accordingly. Relationships are considered the most dynamic and effective way to support and strengthen dynamic systems (Johnston, 2008). The STAR Frame of Reference (Miller *et al.*, 2019), developed by Dr. Lucy Jane Miller and team, stipulates that treatment for sensory processing should intentionally and skillfully address the domains of sensory processing equally with regulation and relationships.

Alongside the mental health team (i.e., psychologist and/or psychiatrist), an evaluation of an individual with sensory-related anxiety must include a licensed occupational therapist trained in Ayres Sensory Integration® (ASI) (Smith Roley *et al.*, 2019), and ideally in DIR/Floortime™—a Developmental, Relationship and Individual Differences-based approach (Greenspan and Wieder, 2006).

Although it would be preferable to include a comprehensive guide to treatment in this chapter, any adequate discussion of treatment would be at least 20 pages long. We refer you instead to a recent discussion of both ASI and the STAR Frame of Reference in Kramer, Hinojosa, and Howe (2019).

Conclusion

From conception through the lifespan, senses provide fundamental information about self and environment, and inform development globally. Every domain of health is impacted by sensory processing function or dysfunction. Sensory-perception *is* affect-perception. Sense of agency and sense of self must start with pre-reflective sense of self, body schema, body map, and the ability to create and execute intentional affective-motor responses, or behaviors.

Sensory processing can mitigate or exacerbate challenges with emotional regulation and anxiety, and conversely anxiety can impact sensory processing function and efficacy. There is overwhelming evidence that sensory processing, which in this discussion includes sensory modulation, sensory-based motor capacities, and sensory discriminative abilities, is a pivotal part of the autistic experience. Atypical sensory processing and anxiety are strongly associated in autism, and these two influencing dimensions present with incredible diversity and nuance from individual to individual. Additionally, greater sensory dysfunction is associated with increased stress and likelihood of co-occurring mental health challenges.

References

Alvarado, C. (2017). *The Sensoriaffective Interactional Attunement Scale: Development and Preliminary Validation of a Measure Geared Toward Interactional Enhancement Between Primary Caregivers and their Young Children with Autism Spectrum Disorders (dissertation).* Fielding Graduate University, School of Leadership Studies/Infant and Early Child Development Program.

Amos, P. (2013). Rhythm and timing in autism: Learning to dance. *Frontiers in Integrative Neuroscience, 7*(April), 1–15. https://doi.org/10.3389/fnint.2013.00027.

Anderson, B. L. (2011). Visual perception of materials and surfaces. *Current Biology, 21*(24), R978–R983. https://doi.org/10.1016/j.cub.2011.11.022.

Anderson, E., Siegel, E. H., and Barrett, L. F. (2011). What you feel influences what you see: The role of affective feelings in resolving binocular rivalry. *Journal of Experimental Social Psychology, 47*(4), 856–860. https://doi.org/10.1016/j.jesp.2011.02.009.

Arnfred, S. M., Raballo, A., Morup, M., and Parnas, J. (2015). Self-disorder and brain processing of proprioception in schizophrenia spectrum patients: A re-analysis. *Psychopathology, 48*(1), 60–64. https://doi.org/10.1159/000366081.

Ashburner, J., Ziviani, J., and Rodger, S. (2008). Sensory processing and classroom emotional, behavioral, and educational outcomes in children with autism spectrum disorder. *American Journal of Occupational Therapy, 62*(5), 564–573. Retrieved from http://ajot.aota.org.

Ayres, A. J. (1972a). *Sensory Integration and Learning Disorders.* Los Angeles, CA: Western Psychological Services.

Ayres, A. J. (1972b). *Southern California Sensory Integration Tests.* Los Angeles, CA: Western Psychological Services.

Ayres, A. J. (1989). *Sensory Integration and Praxis Test: SIPT Manual*. Los Angeles, CA: Western Psychological Services.

Ayres, A. J., and Tickle, L. S. (1980). Hyper-responsivity to touch and vestibular stimuli as a predictor of positive response to sensory integration procedures by autistic children. *American Journal of Occupational Therapy, 34*(6), 375–381. https://doi.org/10.5014/ajot.34.6.375.

Baloh, R. W., Honrubia, V., and Kerber, K. A. (2013). *Baloh and Honrubia's Clinical Neurophysiology of the Vestibular System* (4th ed.). https://doi.org/10.1093/med/9780195387834.001.0001.

Beebe, B., Jaffe, J., Markese, S., Buck, K., Chen, H., Cohen, P., ... Feldstein, S. (2010). The origins of 12-month attachment: A microanalysis of 4-month mother–infant interaction. *Attachment and Human Development, 12*(1–2), 3–141. https://doi.org/10.1080/14616730903338985

Bizzell, E., Ross, J., Rosenthal, C., Dumont, R., and Schaaf, R. (2019). Sensory features as a marker of autism spectrum disorders. *Journal of Autism and Developmental Disorders*. https://doi.org/10.1007/s10803-019-03948-8.

Björnsdotter, M., Morrison, I., and Olausson, H. (2010). Feeling good: On the role of C fiber mediated touch in interoception. *Experimental Brain Research, 207*(3–4), 149–155. https://doi.org/10.1007/s00221-010-2408-y.

Bodison, S. C. (2015). Developmental dyspraxia and the play skills of children with autism. *American Journal of Occupational Therapy, 69*(5), 6905185060p1. https://doi.org/10.5014/ajot.2015.017954.

Brazelton, T. B., and Greenspan, S. I. (2009). *The Irreducible Needs of Children: What Every Child Must Have to Grow, Learn, and Flourish*. Da Capo Lifelong Books.

Brock, M. E., Freuler, A., Baranek, G. T., Watson, L. R., Poe, M. D., and Sabatino, A. (2012). Temperament and sensory features of children with autism. *Journal of Autism and Developmental Disorders, 42*(11), 2271–2284. https://doi.org/10.1007/s10803-012-1472-5.

Bruno, R. B., and René, Z. (2009). Emotion improves and impairs early vision. *Psychological Science, 20*(6), 707–713. Retrieved from http://dx.doi.org/10.1111/j.1467-9280.2009.02354.x.

Bundy, A. C., and Murray, E. A. (2002). Sensory integration: A. Jean Ayres' theory revisited. In A. C. Bundy, S. J. Lane, and E. A. Murray (Eds.), *Sensory Integration Theory and Practice*. Philadelphia, PA: F.A. Davis Company.

Burleigh, J. M., McIntosh, K. W., and Thompson, M. W. (2002). Central auditory processing disorders. In A. C. Bundy, S. J. Lane, and E. A. Murray (Eds.), *Sensory Integration Theory and Practice*. Philadelphia, PA: F.A. Davis Company.

Butterworth, G., and Hicks, L. (1977). Visual proprioception and postural stability in infancy. A developmental study. *Perception, 6*, 255–262.

Caçola, P., Miller, H. L., and Williamson, P. O. (2017). Behavioral comparisons in Autism Spectrum Disorder and Developmental Coordination Disorder: A systematic literature review. *Research in Autism Spectrum Disorders, 38*, 6–18. https://doi.org/10.1016/j.rasd.2017.03.004.

Case-Smith, J., and Ratliff-Schaub, K. (2009). Other sensory problems. In W. B. Carey, A. C. Crocker, E. R. Elias, H. M. Feldman, and W. L. Coleman (Eds.), *Developmental-Behavioral Pediatrics*. Philadelphia, PA: Elsevier. https://doi.org/10.1016/B978-1-4160-3370-7.00073-0.

Cole, J., and Montero, B. (2010). Affective proprioception. *Janus Head, 9*(2), 299–317. Retrieved from http://eprints.bournemouth.ac.uk/6356.

Craig, A. D. (2008). Interoception and emotion: A neuroanatomical perspective. *Handbook of Emotions, 3*(602), 272–288.

De Jaegher, H. (2013). Embodiment and sense-making in autism. *Frontiers in Integrative Neuroscience, 7*. https://doi.org/10.3389/fnint.2013.00015.

De Jaegher, H., Peräkylä, A., and Stevanovic, M. (2016). The co-creation of meaningful action: Bridging enaction and interactional sociology. *Philosophical Transactions of the Royal Society*, 1–22. https://doi.org/10.1098/not.

Deroualle, D., and Lopez, C. (2014). Toward a vestibular contribution to social cognition. *Frontiers in Integrative Neuroscience, 8*. https://doi.org/10.3389/fnint.2014.00016.

Donnellan, A. M., Hill, D. A., and Leary, M. R. (2013). Rethinking autism: Implications of sensory and movement differences for understanding and support. *Frontiers in Integrative Neuroscience, 6*. https://doi.org/10.3389/fnint.2012.00124.

Doumas, M., McKenna, R., and Murphy, B. (2016). Postural control deficits in autism spectrum disorder: The role of sensory integration. *Journal of Autism and Developmental Disorders, 46*(3), 853–861. https://doi.org/10.1007/s10803-015-2621-4.

Dugas, M. J., Hedayati, M., Karavidas, A., Buhr, K., Francis, K., and Phillips, N. A. (2005). Intolerance of uncertainty and information processing: Evidence of biased recall and interpretations. *Cognitive Therapy and Research, 29*(1), 57–70. https://doi.org/10.1007/s10608-005-1648-9.

Fiene, L., and Brownlow, C. (2015). Investigating interoception and body awareness in adults with and without autism spectrum disorder. *Autism Research, 8*(6), 709–716. https://doi.org/10.1002/aur.1486.

Fletcher-Watson, S. and Happé, F. (2019). *Autism: A New Introduction to Psychological Theory and Current Debate*. London: Routledge.

Fogel, A. (1993). *Developing Through Relationships*. Chicago, IL: University of Chicago Press.

Foss-Feig, J. H., Stone, W. L., and Wallace, M. T. (2012). Processing of non-speech auditory stimuli in individuals with autism spectrum disorders: The impact of stimulus characteristics. *International Review of Research in Developmental Disabilities, 43*, 87–145). https://doi.org/10.1016/B978-0-12-398261-2.00003-9.

Gabriels, R. L., Agnew, J. A., Miller, L. J., Gralla, J., Pan, Z., Goldson, E., ... Hooks, E. (2008). Is there a relationship between restricted, repetitive, stereotyped behaviors and interests and abnormal sensory response in children with autism spectrum disorders? *Research in Autism Spectrum Disorders, 2*(4), 660–670. https://doi.org/10.1016/j.rasd.2008.02.002.

Garfinkel, S. N., Tiley, C., O'Keeffe, S., Harrison, N. A., Seth, A. K., and Critchley, H. D. (2016). Discrepancies between dimensions of interoception in autism: Implications for emotion and anxiety. *Biological Psychology, 114*, 117–126. https://doi.org/10.1016/j.biopsycho.2015.12.003.

Gerhardt, S. (2009). Why Love Matters: How Affection Shapes a Baby's Brain. In *Quality of Childhood Group* (pp. 81–96). European Parliament. https://doi.org/10.1177/089033440602200422.

Gibson, J. J. (2009). Visually controlled locomotion and visual orientation in animals. *British Journal of Psychology, 100*(S1), 259–271. https://doi.org/10.1348/000712608X336077.

Gjelsvik, B., Lovric, D., and Williams, M. (2015). Embodied cognition and emotional disorders: Embodiment and abstraction in understanding depression. *Psychopathology Review*. https://doi.org/10.5127/pr.035714.

Glod, M., Riby, D. M., Honey, E., and Rodgers, J. (2015). Psychological correlates of sensory processing patterns in individuals with autism spectrum disorder: A systematic review. *Review Journal of Autism and Developmental Disorders, 2*(2), 199–221. https://doi.org/10.1007/s40489-015-0047-8.

Grandin, T. (2009). Visual abilities and sensory differences in a person with autism. *Biological Psychiatry, 65*(1), 15–16. https://doi.org/10.1016/j.biopsych.2008.11.005.

Green, S. A., and Ben-Sasson, A. (2010). Anxiety disorders and sensory over-responsivity in children with autism spectrum disorders: Is there a causal relationship? *Journal of Autism and Developmental Disorders, 40*(12), 1495–1504. https://doi.org/10.1007/s10803-010-1007-x.

Greenspan, S. I., and Wieder, S. (2006). *Engaging Autism: Using the Floortime Approach to Help Children, Relate, Communicate, and Think*. Philadelphia, PA: Da Capo/Lifelong Books.

Grillon, C. (2008). Models and mechanisms of anxiety: Evidence from startle studies. *Psychopharmacology, 199*(3), 421–437. https://doi.org/10.1007/s00213-007-1019-1.

Guillery, R. (2017). *The Brain as a Tool: A Neuroscientist's Account*. Oxford: Oxford University Press.

Haggard, P., Taylor-Clarke, M., and Kennett, S. (2003). Tactile perception, cortical representation and the bodily self. *Current Biology, 13*(5), R170–R173.

Hain, T. C., and Helminski, J. O. (2007). Anatomy and physiology of the normal vestibular system. In T. C. Hain and J. O. Helminski (Eds.), *Vestibular Rehabilitation* (Vol. 3). Philadelphia, PA: F.A. Davis Company.

Hainaut, J.-P., Caillet, G., Lestienne, F. G., and Bolmont, B. (2018). The role of trait anxiety on static balance performance in control and anxiogenic situations. *Gait and Posture, 33*(4), 604–608. https://doi.org/10.1016/j.gaitpost.2011.01.017.

Hannant, P., Tavassoli, T., and Cassidy, S. (2016). The role of sensorimotor difficulties in autism spectrum conditions. *Frontiers in Neurology, 7*(Aug), 1–11. https://doi.org/10.3389/fneur.2016.00124.

Henderson, A., Pehoski, C., and Murray, E. (2002). Visual spatial abilities. In A. C. Bundy, S. J. Lane, and E. A. Murray (Eds.), *Sensory Integration Theory and Practice*. Philadelphia, PA: F.A. Davis Company.

Hilton, C. L., Zhang, Y., Whilte, M. R., Klohr, C. L., and Constantino, J. (2012). Motor impairment in sibling pairs concordant and discordant for autism spectrum disorders. *Autism, 16*(4), 430–441. https://doi.org/10.1177/1362361311423018.

Holzer, P. (2017). Interoception and gut feelings: Unconscious body signals' impact on brain function, behavior and belief processes. In H. F. Angel, L. Oviedo, R. F. Paloutzian, A. L. C. Runehov, and R. J. Seitz (Eds.), *Processes of Believing: The Acquisition, Maintenance, and Change in Creditions* (Vol. 1). Cham, Switzerland: Springer. https://doi.org/10.1007/978-3-319-50924-2.

Johnson, B. P., Lum, J. A. G., Rinehart, N. J., and Fielding, J. (2016). Ocular motor disturbances in autism spectrum disorders: Systematic review and comprehensive meta-analysis. *Neuroscience and Biobehavioral Reviews, 69*, 260–279. https://doi.org/10.1016/j.neubiorev.2016.08.007.

Johnston, T. D. (2008). Genes, experience, and behavior. In S. Shanker, A. Fogel, and B. J. King (Eds.), *Human Development in the Twenty-First Century*. New York, NY: Cambridge University Press.

Kern, J. K., Garver, C. R., Grannemann, B. D., Trivedi, M. H., Carmody, T., Andrews, A. A., and Mehta, J. A. (2007). Response to vestibular sensory events in autism. *Research in Autism Spectrum Disorders, 1*(1), 67–74. https://doi.org/10.1016/j.rasd.2006.07.006.

Khalsa, S. S., Adolphs, R., Cameron, O. G., Critchley, H. D., Davenport, P. W., Feinstein, J. S., ... Zucker, N. (2018). Interoception and mental health: A roadmap. *Biological Psychiatry: Cognitive Neuroscience and Neuroimaging, 3*(6), 501–513. https://doi.org/10.1016/j.bpsc.2017.12.004.

Kilroy, E., Aziz-Zadeh, L., Cermak, S., Kilroy, E., Aziz-Zadeh, L., and Cermak, S. (2019). Ayres theories of autism and sensory integration revisited: What contemporary neuroscience has to say. *Brain Sciences, 9*(3), 68. https://doi.org/10.3390/brainsci9030068.

Kirby, A. V., Williams, K. L., Watson, L. R., Sideris, J., Bulluck, J., and Baranek, G. T. (2019). Sensory features and family functioning in families of children with autism and developmental disabilities: Longitudinal associations. *The American Journal of Occupational Therapy: Official Publication of the American Occupational Therapy Association, 73*(2), 7302205040p1-7302205040p14. https://doi.org/10.5014/ajot.2018.027391.

Kollmeier, B. (2008). Anatomy, physiology and function of the auditory system. *Handbook of Signal Processing in Acoustics*, 147–158. https://doi.org/10.1007/978-0-387-30441-0_10.

Kramer, P., Hinojosa, J., and Howe, T.-H. (Eds.) (2019), *Frames of Reference for Pediatric Occupational Therapy*. Mexico: Wolters Kluwer.

Lane, A. E., Young, R. L., Baker, A. E. Z., and Angley, M. T. (2010). Sensory processing subtypes in autism: Association with adaptive behavior. *Journal of Autism and Developmental Disorders, 40*(1), 112–122. https://doi.org/10.1007/s10803-009-0840-2.

Lane, S. J. (2002). Structure and function of the sensory systems. In A. C. Bundy, S. J. Lane, and E. A. Murray (Eds.), *Sensory Integration Theory and Practice*. Philadelphia, PA: F.A. Davis Company.

Leekam, S. R., Nieto, C., Libby, S. J., Wing, L., and Gould, J. (2007). Describing the sensory abnormalities of children and adults with autism. *Journal of Autism and Developmental Disorders, 37*(5), 894–910. https://doi.org/10.1007/s10803-006-0218-7.

Lim, Y. H., Partridge, K., Girdler, S., and Morris, S. L. (2017). Standing postural control in individuals with autism spectrum disorder: Systematic review and meta-analysis. *Journal of Autism and Developmental Disorders, 47*(7), 2238–2253. https://doi.org/10.1007/s10803-017-3144-y.

Lipchock, S. V., Reed, D. R., and Mennella, J. A. (2011). The gustatory and olfactory systems during infancy: Implications for development of feeding behaviors in the high-risk neonate. *Clinics in Perinatology, 38*(4), 627–641. https://doi.org/10.1016/j.clp.2011.08.008.

Liss, M., Saulnier, C., Fein, D., and Kinsbourne, M. (2006). Sensory and attention abnormalities in autistic spectrum disorders. *Autism, 10*(2), 155–172. https://doi.org/10.1177/1362361306062021.

Lloyd, M., MacDonald, M., and Lord, C. (2013). Motor skills of toddlers with autism spectrum disorders. *Autism, 17*(2), 133–146. https://doi.org/10.1177/1362361311402230.

Lurie-Hurvitz, E. (2009). Early experiences matter: Making the case for a comprehensive infant and toddler policy agenda. Zero to Three Policy Center. Retrieved from www.zerotothree.org/resources/1025-making-the-case-for-a-comprehensive-infant-and-toddler-policy-agenda.

Mache, M. A., and Todd, T. A. (2016). Gross motor skills are related to postural stability and age in children with autism spectrum disorder. *Research in Autism Spectrum Disorders, 23*, 179–187. https://doi.org/10.1016/j.rasd.2016.01.001.

Marko, M. K., Crocetti, D., Hulst, T., Donchin, O., Shadmehr, R., and Mostofsky, S. H. (2015). Behavioural and neural basis of anomalous motor learning in children with autism. *Brain, 138*(3), 784–797. https://doi.org/10.1093/brain/awu394.

Mason, P. (2017a). Audition. In *Medical Neurobiology*. New York, NY: Oxford University Press.

Mason, P. (2017b). *Medical Neurobiology*. New York, NY: Oxford University Press.

Mazurek, M. O., Vasa, R. A., Kalb, L. G., Kanne, S. M., Rosenberg, D., Keefer, A., ... Lowery, L. A. (2013). Anxiety, sensory over-responsivity, and gastrointestinal problems in children with autism spectrum disorders. *Journal of Abnormal Child Psychology, 41*(1), 165–176. https://doi.org/10.1007/s10802-012-9668-x.

McGlone, F., and Reilly, D. (2010). The cutaneous sensory system. *Neuroscience and Biobehavioral Reviews, 34*(2), 148–159. https://doi.org/10.1016/j.neubiorev.2009.08.004.

Miller, L. J., Reisman, J. E., McIntosh, D. N., and Simon, J. (2001). An ecological model of sensory modulation. In *Understanding the Nature of Sensory Integration with Diverse Populations*. Austin, TX: Pro-ed.

Miller, L. J., Anzalone, M. E., Lane, S. J., Cermak, S. A., and Osten, E. T. (2007). Concept evolution in sensory integration: A proposed nosology for diagnosis. *American Journal of Occupational Therapy, 61*(2), 135–142. https://doi.org/10.5014/ajot.61.2.135.

Miller, L. J., Fuller, D. A., and Roetenberg, J. (2014). *Sensational Kids Revised Edition: Hope and Help for Children with Sensory Processing Disorder (SPD)*. Harmondsworth: Penguin.

Miller, L. J., Schoen, S. A., Mulligan, S., and Sullivan, J. (2017). Identification of sensory processing and integration symptom clusters: A preliminary study. *Occupational Therapy International, 2017*, 1–10. https://doi.org/10.1155/2017/2876080.

Miller, L. J., Schoen, S. A., and Spielmann, V. (2019). A frame of reference for sensory processing difficulties: Sensory therapies and research (STAR). In Paula Kramer, J. Hinojosa, and T.-H. Howe (Eds.), *Frames of Reference for Pediatric Occupational Therapy*. Philadelphia, PA: Wolters Kluwer.

Miller, L. J., Witten, M., Ahn, R. R., and Schoen, S. A. (2020). Assessment of Sensory Processing Disorder. *The Oxford Handbook of Infant, Toddler, and Preschool Mental Health Assessment* (2nd Ed.), 286–314. doi: 10.1093/oxfordhb/9780199837182.013.12.

Ming, X., Brimacombe, M., and Wagner, G. C. (2007). Prevalence of motor impairment in autism spectrum disorders. *Brain and Development, 29*(9), 565–570. https://doi.org/10.1016/j.braindev.2007.03.002.

Molloy, C. A., Dietrich, K. N., and Bhattacharya, A. (2003). Postural stability in children with autism spectrum disorder. *Journal of Autism and Developmental Disorders, 33*(6), 643–652. https://doi.org/10.1023/B:JADD.0000006001.00667.4c.

Moraes, Í. A. P. de, Massetti, T., Crocetta, T. B., Silva, T. D. da, Menezes, L. D. C. de, Monteiro, C. B. de M., and Magalhães, F. H. (2017). Motor learning characterization in people with autism spectrum disorder: A systematic review. *Dementia and Neuropsychologia, 11*(3), 276–286. https://doi.org/10.1590/1980-57642016dn11-030010.

Mosconi, M. W., and Sweeney, J. A. (2015). Sensorimotor dysfunctions as primary features of autism spectrum disorders. *Science China Life Sciences, 58*(10), 1016–1023. https://doi.org/10.1007/s11427-015-4894-4.

Mouly, A. M., and Sullivan, R. (2010). Memory and plasticity in the olfactory system: From infancy to adulthood. In A. Menini (Ed.), *The Neurobiology of Olfaction*. Boca Raton, FL: Taylor & Francis.

Murphy, J., Brewer, R., and Bird, G. (2017). Interoception and psychopathology: A developmental neuroscience perspective. *Developmental Cognitive Neuroscience, 23*, 45–56. https://doi.org/10.1016/j.dcn.2016.12.006.

Neil, L., Olsson, N. C., and Pellicano, E. (2016). The relationship between intolerance of uncertainty, sensory sensitivities, and anxiety in autistic and typically developing children. *Journal of Autism and Developmental Disorders, 46*(6), 1962–1973. https://doi.org/10.1007/s10803-016-2721-9.

Nyström, P., Gredebäck, G., Bölte, S., and Falck-Ytter, T. (2015). Hypersensitive pupillary light reflex in infants at risk for autism. *Molecular Autism, 6*(1), 6–11. https://doi.org/10.1186/s13229-015-0011-6.

Ouellet, C., Langlois, F., Provencher, M. D., and Gosselin, P. (2019). Intolerance of uncertainty and difficulties in emotion regulation: Proposal for an integrative model of generalized anxiety disorder. *Revue Européenne de Psychologie Appliquée, 69*(1), 9–18. https://doi.org/10.1016/j.erap.2019.01.001.

Pawling, R., Cannon, P. R., McGlone, F. P., and Walker, S. C. (2017). C-tactile afferent stimulating touch carries a positive affective value. *PLoS ONE, 12*(3), 1–15. https://doi.org/10.1371/journal.pone.0173457.

Porges, S. W. (2015). Making the world safe for our children: Down-regulating defence and up-regulating social engagement to "optimise" the human experience. *Children Australia, 40*(2), 114–123. https://doi.org/10.1017/cha.2015.12.

Porges, S. W. (2018). Ployvagal theory: A primer. In S. W. Porges and D. Dana (Eds.), *Clinical Applications of the Polyvagal Theory: The Emergence of Polyvagal-Informed Therapies*. New York, NY: Norton.

Proske, U., and Gandevia, S. C. (2012). The proprioceptive senses: Their roles in signaling body shape, body position and movement, and muscle force. *Physiological Reviews, 92*(4), 1651–1697. https://doi.org/10.1152/physrev.00048.2011.

Radonovich, K. J., Fournier, K. A., and Hass, C. J. (2013). Relationship between postural control and restricted, repetitive behaviors in autism spectrum disorders. *Frontiers in Integrative Neuroscience, 7*. https://doi.org/10.3389/fnint.2013.00028.

Rajagopalan, A., Jinu, K., Sailesh, K. S., Mishra, S., Reddy, U. K., and Mukkadan, J. K. (2017). Understanding the links between vestibular and limbic systems regulating emotions. *Journal of Natural Science, Biology and Medicine, 8*(1), 11. https://doi.org/10.4103/0976-9668.198350.

Riquelme, I., Hatem, S. M., and Montoya, P. (2016). Abnormal pressure pain, touch sensitivity, proprioception, and manual dexterity in children with autism spectrum disorders. *Neural Plasticity, 2016*, 1–9. https://doi.org/10.1155/2016/1723401.

Riskind, J. H., and Gotay, C. C. (1982). Physical posture: Could it have regulatory or feedback effects on motivation and emotion? *Motivation and Emotion, 6*(3), 273–298. https://doi.org/10.1007/BF00992249.

Robertson, C. E., and Baron-Cohen, S. (2017). Sensory perception in autism. *Nature Reviews Neuroscience, 18*(11), 671–684. https://doi.org/10.1038/nrn.2017.112.

Robledo, J., Donnellan, A. M., and Strandt-Conroy, K. (2012). An exploration of sensory and movement differences from the perspective of individuals with autism. *Frontiers in Integrative Neuroscience, 6*. https://doi.org/10.3389/fnint.2012.00107.

Rogers, S. J., Hepburn, S., and Wehner, E. (2003). Parent reports of sensory symptoms in toddlers with autism and those with other developmental disorders. *Journal of Autism and Developmental Disorders, 33*(6), 631–642. https://doi.org/10.1023/B:JADD.0000006000.38991.a7.

Rolls, E. T. (2003). Vision, emotion and memory: From neurophysiology to computation. *International Congress Series, 1250*(C), 547–573. https://doi.org/10.1016/S0531-5131(03)00981-6.

Sacks, O. (1990). *Neurology and the Soul*. Fidia.

Schaaf, R. C., Cohn, E. S., Burke, J., Dumont, R., Miller, A., and Mailloux, Z. (2015). Linking sensory factors to participation: Establishing intervention goals with parents for children with autism spectrum disorder. *American Journal of Occupational Therapy, 69*(5). https://doi.org/10.5014/ajot.2015.018036.

Schaber, A. (2014). Ask an Autistic #9 – What is Sensory Processing Disorder? Neurowonderful. Retrieved from www.youtube.com/watch?v=upU-dc19Taw.

Schmitz, C., Martineau, J., Barthélémy, C., and Assaiante, C. (2003). Motor control and children with autism: Deficit of anticipatory function? *Neuroscience Letters, 348*(1), 17–20. https://doi.org/10.1016/S0304-3940(03)00644-X.

Schore, A. N. (2015). *Affect Regulation and the Origin of the Self: The Neurobiology of Emotional Development* (Classic). New York, NY: Routledge.

Schulz, A., and Vögele, C. (2015). Interoception and stress. *Frontiers in Psychology, 6*(July), 1–23. https://doi.org/10.3389/fpsyg.2015.00993.

Schulz, S. E., and Stevenson, R. A. (2018). Sensory hypersensitivity predicts repetitive behaviours in autistic and typically-developing children. *Autism*. https://doi.org/10.1177/1362361318774559.

Shonkoff, J. P., and Phillips, D. (Eds.) (2000). *From Neurons to Neighborhoods: The Science of Early Childhood Development*. Washington, DC: Committee on Integrating the Science of Early Childhood Development, Board on Children, Youth, and Families.

Shumway-Cook, A., and Wollacott, M. H. (2017). *Motor Control: Translating Research into Clinical Practice*. Philadelphia, PA: Wolters Kluwer.

Smith Roley, S., Mailloux, Z., Parham, L. D., Schaaf, R. C., Lane, C. J., and Cermak, S. (2015). Sensory integration and praxis patterns in children with autism. *American Journal of Occupational Therapy, 69*(1). https://doi.org/10.5014/ajot.2015.012476.

Smith Roley, S., Schaaf, R. C., and Baltazar Mori, A. (2019). Ayres Sensory Integration® Frame of Reference. In Paul Kramer, J. Hinojosa, and T.-H. Howe (Eds.), *Frames of Reference for Pediatric Occupational Therapy*. Mexico: Wolters Kluwer.

Snowden, R. J., and Freeman, T. C. (2004). The perception of visual motion. *Current Opinion in Neurobiology, 2*(2), R828–R831. https://doi.org/10.1016/j.cub.2004.09.033.

South, M., and Rodgers, J. (2017). Sensory, emotional and cognitive contributions to anxiety in autism spectrum disorders. *Frontiers in Human Neuroscience, 11*(January), 1–7. https://doi.org/10.3389/fnhum.2017.00020.

Spitzer, S. L. (1999). Dynamic systems theory: Relevance to the theory of sensory integration and the study of occupation. *Sensory Integration Special Interest Section Quarterly AOTA, 22*(2), 1–4.

Spitzer, S. L., and Smith Roley, S. (2001). Sensory integration revisited: A philosophy of practice. In S. Smith Roley, E. I. Blanche, and R. C. Schaaf (Eds.), *Understanding the Nature of Sensory Integration with Diverse Populations*. Austin, TX: Pro-ed.

Sugai, T., Yoshimura, H., and Onoda, N. (2005). Functional reciprocal connections between olfactory and gustatory pathways. *Chemical Senses, 30*(Supplement 1), i166–i167. https://doi.org/10.1093/chemse/bjh166.

Tajadura-Jiménez, A., and Västfjäll, D. (2008). Auditory-induced emotion: A neglected channel for communication in human-computer interaction. In *Affect and Emotion in Human-Computer Interaction*. New York, NY: Springer.

Tavassoli, T., Miller, L. J., Schoen, S. A., Nielsen, D. M., and Baron-Cohen, S. (2014). Sensory over-responsivity in adults with autism spectrum conditions. *Autism, 18*(4), 428–432.

Taylor, M. J., Gustafsson, P., Larsson, H., Gillberg, C., Lundström, S., and Lichstenstein, P. (2017). Examining the association between autistic traits and atypical sensory reactivity: A twin study. *Journal of the American Academy of Child and Adolescent Psychiatry*. https://doi.org/10.1016/j.jaac.2017.11.019

Tempest, S. (2017). Purposeful Movement and Apraxia. In L. Maskill and S. Tempest (Eds.), *Neuropsychology for Occupational Therapists: Cognition in Occupational Performance*. Oxford: Wiley-Blackwell.

Tomchek, S. D., Little, L. M., and Dunn, W. (2015). Sensory pattern contributions to developmental performance in children with autism spectrum disorder. *American Journal of Occupational Therapy, 69*(5), 1–10. https://doi.org/10.5014/ajot.2015.018044.

Torres, E. B., and Donnellan, A. M. (2015). Editorial for research topic "Autism: the movement perspective." *Frontiers in Integrative Neuroscience, 9*. https://doi.org/10.3389/fnint.2015.00012.

Torres, E. B. and Whyatt, C. (2016). *Autism: The Movement-Sensing Perspective*. Taylor & Francis.

Trevarthen, C., and Delafield-Butt, J. T. (2013). Autism as a developmental disorder in intentional movement and affective engagement. *Frontiers in Integrative Neuroscience, 7*(July), 1–16. https://doi.org/10.3389/fnint.2013.00049.

Tronick, E. Z. (2007). The neurobehavioral and social-emotional development of infants and children. *The Neurobehavioral and Social-Emotional Development of Infants and Children*. Retrieved from http://ovidsp.ovid.com/ovidweb.cgi?T=JS&PAGE=reference&D=psyc5&NEWS=N&AN=2006-13259-000.

Tuthill, J. C., and Azim, E. (2018). Proprioception. *Current Biology, 28*(5), R194–R203. https://doi.org/10.1016/j.cub.2018.01.064.

Van Nest, S. (2018). Sensory integration theory in psychotherapy: A case study. *Clinical Social Work Journal, 47*(2), 167–175. https://doi.org/10.1007/s10615-018-0685-2.

Wellsby, M., and Pexman, P. M. (2014). Developing embodied cognition: Insights from children's concepts and language processing. *Frontiers in Psychology, 5*(May), 1–10. https://doi.org/10.3389/fpsyg.2014.00506.

Whyatt, C., and Craig, C. (2013). Sensory-motor problems in autism. *Frontiers in Integrative Neuroscience, 7*(51), 12. https://doi.org/10.3389/fnint.2013.00051.

Wigham, S., Rodgers, J., South, M., McConachie, H., and Freeston, M. (2015). The interplay between sensory processing abnormalities, intolerance of uncertainty, anxiety and restricted and repetitive behaviours in autism spectrum disorder. *Journal of Autism and Developmental Disorders, 45*(4), 943–952. https://doi.org/10.1007/s10803-014-2248-x.

Zwicker, J. G., Harris, S. R., and Klassen, A. F. (2013). Quality of life domains affected in children with developmental coordination disorder: A systematic review. *Child: Care, Health and Development, 39*(4), 562–580. https://doi.org/10.1111/j.1365-2214.2012.01379.x.

CHAPTER 7

Anxiety and Autism Spectrum Disorders

Causes, Clinical Presentations, and Interventions

Margaret L. Bauman, M.D., Boston University School of Medicine, with a personal commentary by Temple Grandin, Ph.D. Animal Science at Colorado State University

Anxiety disorders have been reported to be some of the most common psychiatric conditions in the western world (Simpson *et al.*, 2010). These disorders often include symptoms of excessive worry, fear, and hyper-arousal—symptoms that can be both debilitating and counter-productive to the individual affected. It has been estimated that the prevalence of anxiety disorders in the United States is approximately 18 percent of the general population (Kessler *et al.*, 2005).

Autism spectrum disorder (ASD) has been defined as a neurodevelopmental disorder characterized by delayed and disordered language/communication, impaired social interaction, restricted areas of interest, and the presence of repetitive and stereotypic behaviors (American Psychiatric Association, 2013). Although the diagnostic features of ASD have been fairly well established, there is a growing appreciation that the disorder is heterogeneous in its etiology and neurobiology as well as in the severity and complexity of its clinical presentation. In addition, there is an increasing awareness that many of the clinical features of the disorder can be significantly impacted by medical and psychiatric co-morbidities, and that these conditions often have a negative impact on the developmental trajectory of the individual, frequently causing stress and increased behavioral dysfunction.

Among the medical and psychiatric conditions reported to be associated with ASD, anxiety disorders have been one of the most common. The reported prevalence rates among the ASD population have varied widely, ranging from 11 percent to 84 percent in some studies; this variability is potentially related to the heterogeneity of the disorder, in which there are significant differences in intellectual and verbal abilities. There is also some evidence that the differing assessment tools used to diagnose anxiety disorders in ASD may impact estimated outcomes, with higher rates of generalized anxiety disorders being reported in studies using questionnaires compared with studies using interviews. Additional confounding factors may include overlapping symptoms and unconventional presentations of anxiety in ASD, combined with the fact that most diagnostic measures used to assess anxiety disorders have not been designed for individuals on the spectrum (Postorino *et al.*, 2018).

Symptomatically, anxiety disorders within the ASD population can vary widely. Much of this variability may relate to differing clinical presentations of the disorder itself, but it may also be related to how anxiety is expressed by those with intellectual disabilities and by those who are non-verbal and cannot adequately express their fears and discomfort (Magiati *et al.*, 2017). Further, some of the symptoms associated with anxiety, including social withdrawal and stereotypic behaviors, may overlap with and therefore be difficult to separate from ASD-related behaviors. Anxiety-related symptoms, especially in non-verbal persons, have been reported to include screaming, avoidance, disruptive behaviors, disturbed sleep patterns, and/or unexplained changes in behavior.

The underlying neurobiological mechanisms related to anxiety in ASD remain poorly defined and controversial. There has been some suggestion that both ASD and anxiety share the same structural and functional brain abnormalities. Imaging studies, using fMRI, have found abnormalities in the amygdala, hippocampus, ventromedial prefrontal cortex, and insula in the brains of ASD individuals, as well as in those with generalized anxiety disorders (Goossen *et al.*, 2019; Mikita *et al.*, 2016). However, not all individuals with ASD demonstrate a co-occurring anxiety disorder. Thus, whether ASD and anxiety disorders share the same or similar neurobiological connections remains as yet unclear and will require further research.

Potential Causes of Anxiety in ASD

The etiology of anxiety disorders in ASD may be related to a number of different factors. Research has suggested that one of the potential causes may be an intolerance of uncertainty (IU). This hypothesis has been supported by the fact that some of the core features of ASD, including the insistence on sameness, restricted and repetitive behaviors, inflexible adherence to routines, and difficulty tolerating change (Kanner, 1943), symptoms that overlap with anxiety, would be consistent with this hypothesis (Rodgers *et al.*, 2012; Joyce *et al.*, 2017). Thus, the avoidance of the unexpected and a desire to make life as predictable as possible appears to support the concept of IU.

In 2014, Boulter *et al.* reported on a study of anxiety in a group of ASD children and noted a significant relationship between IU and anxiety among the research subjects. Further, the investigators noted that IU accounted for a substantial increase in anxiety in ASD children as compared with neurotypical controls. These observations have been further supported by more recent studies that have suggested that fears of uncertainty may be a significant factor in the development and maintenance of anxiety in ASD (Kerns *et al.*, 2016).

Relatively little research has explored treatment approaches for anxiety within the autism population, much of the work having been pursued in typically developing subjects. This research has suggested that a reduction of IU in neurotypical individuals can result in a reduction in anxiety and improvements in everyday functioning (Boswell *et al.*, 2013). The use of cognitive behavioral therapy (CBT) has been found to be effective in neurotypical patients, with a focus on increasing their tolerance of uncertainty and reducing their anxiety. Research has confirmed that the use of cognitive behavioral treatments that help neurotypical patients increase their tolerance of uncertainty and reduce their anxiety results in significant and sustainable changes long term (Payne *et al.*, 2011). Intervention using similar protocols is now being piloted in children with ASD. One such project that is currently under way involves an eight-week parent intervention approach (CUES: Coping with Uncertainty in Everyday Situations) that provides parents of ASD children with strategies to increase their tolerance of uncertainty in daily life and to improve everyday functioning (Rodgers *et al.*, 2019). It is anticipated that this project will assess the acceptability and feasibility of this approach as well as its effectiveness and clinical outcome.

While intolerance of the unexpected may be a significant factor in the etiology and exacerbation of anxiety among those on the spectrum, it has become increasingly apparent that medical and physiologic co-morbidities may be playing a contributing role.

Anxiety Associated with Gastrointestinal Dysfunction

There is a growing body of evidence that ASD is frequently associated with a variety of co-morbid gastrointestinal disorders, including gastroesophageal reflux disease (GERD), constipation, diarrhea, celiac disease, Crohn's disease, eosinophilic esophagitis, and irritable bowel syndrome (Buie *et al.*, 2010). In the general population, a strong relationship has been demonstrated between psychological and physical stress and gastrointestinal disorders (Lyte *et al.*, 2011). Recent data suggests that there is a bidirectional communication between the brain and the gut through a number of pathways including the autonomic, central, and enteric nervous systems (Collins *et al.*, 2012). However, despite literature describing alterations in both the autonomic nervous system and gastrointestinal function in ASD, little is known about the relationship of the two systems in this disorder.

In 2017, Ferguson *et al.* published a study focused on the potential connection between the sympathetic and parasympathetic nervous systems and gastrointestinal dysfunction by measuring heart rate variability and skin conductance in a large cohort of ASD children and adolescents with a variety of gastrointestinal disorders. The results suggested that individuals with ASD and anxiety disorders may be at increased risk for lower bowel/gastrointestinal disorders, and that the mechanism by which this relationship occurs is through an enhanced stress response. These findings are consistent with previously published research that found anxiety to be associated with a range of gastrointestinal disorders, including constipation, in individuals on the autism spectrum (Mazurek *et al.*, 2013).

Sleep Disorders and Anxiety

Disordered sleep patterns have also been associated with anxiety in ASD subjects. Sleep problems are defined as difficulties related to falling asleep, interrupted sleep, sleep maintenance, night terrors, enuresis, sleep walking, and other parasomnias (Lehmkuhl *et al.*, 2008). Sleep problems are common in typically developing children with anxiety and approximately 80–90 percent of clinically anxious children have at least one sleep problem

(Alfano *et al.*, 2006, 2007; Chase and Pincus, 2011). Elevated sleep problems and anxiety are also common in children with ASD, with the prevalence rate of sleep problems in this population ranging from 50 percent to 80 percent (Krakowiak *et al.*, 2008; Polimeni *et al.*, 2005). The frequency of anxiety disorders in ASD has been reported to be 40 percent as compared with 10–20 percent in typically developing children (Alfano *et al.*, 2009; Van Steensel *et al.*, 2011). While it is recognized that a relationship exists between poor sleep and anxiety, the direction of this relationship and whether one precedes the other remains unclear.

In 2019, Uren *et al.* published the results of a longitudinal study in which they investigated the possible association between sleep and anxiety at two years of age and at age eight years, as well as the additional influence of autistic traits at age two years on sleep and anxiety at eight years. The outcome of this research found that anxiety at age eight was the best predictor of sleep problems at eight years, supporting previous studies showing that sleep and anxiety problems are interrelated and occur contemporaneously in eight-year-olds. Further, it was found that anxiety's contribution to poor sleep at age eight years was entirely accounted for by autistic traits and sleep at two years, highlighting the interrelationship between sleep problems, anxiety symptoms, and autistic traits in young children.

The Role of Sensory Processing Disorders

Since the publication of the *Diagnostic and Statistical Manual—V* in 2013, disorders of sensory processing have been included as a core clinical feature of ASD. Sensory features have been conceptualized as a response to sensory events and are associated with four profiles, including (a) low registration, (b) sensation seeking, (c) sensory sensitivity, and (d) sensation avoiding (Dunn, 1999). These responses can involve the processing of sensory information across differing domains including auditory, visual, vestibular, touch, multisensory, and oral. Sensory sensitivities—both hyper- and hypo-sensitivity—have been considered to be contributors to anxiety. In 2012, Trembath *et al.* published a study of anxiety in young ASD adults and found that sound and light sensitivities were key sources of anxiety among the subjects sampled. More recently, quantitative studies have shown a greater degree of severe sensory sensitivities in ASD subjects with high levels of anxiety (Gillott and Standen, 2007; Uljarevic *et al.*, 2016).

In 2019, Hwang *et al.* published the results of a study of 292 ASD adults, ages 25 years and older, analyzed in comparison with 116 non-autistic adults, ages 25–78 years, with regard to IU, measures of sensory sensitivities (using the Glasgow Sensory Questionnaire—GSQ), anxiety as defined by the Severity Measure for Generalized Anxiety Disorder (American Psychiatric Association, 2013), and the presence of restricted and repetitive behaviors using the Repetitive Behaviors Questionnaire-2 for adults (RBQ-2A) (Leekam *et al.*, 2007). The results of this study found a strong correlation between repetitive behaviors and sensory sensitivities. In addition, there was a strong association between anxiety and the insistence on sameness, with a weaker association between hypo-sensitivity and repetitive sensory-motor behaviors. The findings from this study suggest that IU is an important mechanism underlying the relationship between anxiety and sensory sensitivities (both hyper- and hypo-sensitivity), as well as between anxiety and insistence on sameness.

Evaluation and Management of Anxiety in ASD

Given emerging evidence for the presence of medical co-morbidities in ASD, it is important to consider potential healthcare conditions that could be the cause of or a contributor to symptoms of anxiety. This can be a challenging process in the ASD patient, especially in those who are non-verbal. Further, it has been recognized that the ASD individual may not present with symptoms that are easily recognized by the average practitioner, since the presenting features often appear as atypical or disruptive behaviors. Every effort should be made to rule out any underlying medically related disorders that could be contributing to the presenting anxiety symptoms.

Other possible contributing factors should include school-related issues, including the lack of appropriate support services and interventions in the school environment and the potential presence and impact of bullying. The presence of sensory processing symptoms should be fully evaluated by a qualified occupational therapist skilled in working with ASD patients and knowledgeable about appropriate therapies and accommodations. Sleep management may require a referral to a sleep specialist, and gastrointestinal dysfunction may require a referral to a gastroenterologist.

Assuming that medical conditions have been treated and ruled out, a referral to a psychiatrist/psychopharmacologist skilled in working with individuals on the spectrum should be considered, and medication management and monitoring should be under the care of this provider. Counseling for both the person with ASD and their parent/caretaker should also be sought and implemented.

Medication Management

A review of anxiety studies in ASD children and adolescents has found that 11–84 percent have experienced anxiety. Symptoms have included stereotypies including repetitive noises, body movements, shaking, and hand movements (White *et al.*, 2009). Evidence of effective treatment of anxiety disorders in typically developing children has included a combination of CBT and the administration of selective serotonin reuptake inhibitors (SSRIs) (Walkup *et al.*, 2008). In 2018, Delli *et al.* reported on a review of published studies of interventions used in ASD children and adolescents, based primarily on pharmacotherapy, CBT, and social recreational therapy, provided individually or in combination. Many of the earlier studies regarding the treatment of anxiety in ASD were medication-related and generally involved drugs used to treat anxiety in typically developing children and adults. Research directed toward the treatment of anxiety in ASD individuals has suggested that the SSRIs have a positive response rate in approximately two-thirds of the subjects studied (Couturier and Nicolson, 2002). Of the SSRIs investigated, citalopram was the most commonly studied medication in ASD and appeared to be well tolerated. The authors noted that, for all anxiety disorders associated with ASD, medications should be started at low doses since many ASD individuals appear to be particularly sensitive to the effect of medications in general. Gradual increases to therapeutic levels as tolerated should be carefully monitored in order to avoid worsening of the anxiety symptoms (Delli *et al.*, 2018).

Benzodiazepines have also been useful in the treatment of anxiety disorders, particularly for short-term management, but are considered limited by their potential for dependence long term. Short-acting medications such as alprazolam (Xanax) may be associated with symptoms of withdrawal, whereas longer-acting benzodiazepines such as clonazepam (Klonipin) are considered preferable (Delli *et al.*, 2018).

A recent retrospective review of the effectiveness of buspirone in the treatment of anxiety in youth with high-functioning ASD has suggested improvement in the severity of anxiety symptoms using this medication. Significant improvement was observed in 58 percent of the participants, with mild improvement in 29 percent. The medication appeared to be well tolerated with no adverse side effects reported in the majority of the patients studied (Ceranoglu *et al.*, 2019).

Some children with anxiety may exhibit acute symptoms of elevated blood pressure and heart rate, sweating, and muscle tension. Despite the lack of research evidence, many of these symptoms have been successfully managed with the use of α-agonists such as clonidine or guanfacine, as well as propranolol, a β-blocker (Kolevzon *et al.*, 2006). Presently, there is no data on the management of situational anxiety. However, short-acting benzodiazepines such as lorazepam or the beta-blocker propranolol have been utilized as short-term measures, with careful monitoring of behavioral activation, sedation, and cognitive impairments.

Based on the research to date, there appears to be a consensus that, while most anxiety disorders will require long-term treatment, improvement in symptoms can be achieved with appropriate intervention (Owen *et al.*, 2009). Lifelong management with medication and/or CBT is not uncommon. Further, there is growing evidence that positive outcomes are most likely to depend on a combination of medication management and non-pharmacological interventions, most especially the use of CBT.

Cognitive Behavioral Therapy

Many of the original studies of CBT as an intervention for anxiety disorders in ASD have been performed in academic clinical environments, rather than in real-life settings such as schools and/or community situations; as a result, the generalization of these research findings has been limited. It has been noted, however, that the efficacy of CBT depends heavily on the experience of the therapist, the connection between the patient and the therapist, and supervision and treatment reliability (Clarke *et al.*, 2016). CBT generally involves a focus on both behavioral and cognitive approaches, designed to support the patient's understanding of anxiety-provoking situations and to teach behavioral strategies to help the individual to reflect on their thoughts, feelings, and reactions to stressful situations.

Research data indicates that ASD children respond well to CBT treatment, with intervention lasting from six weeks to 16 weeks. Parental involvement has been found to be an important component in achieving positive outcomes, with parents playing the role of supporter, trainer, and friend (Derguy *et al.*, 2018). CBT programs may vary depending upon the age and cognitive ability of the patient as well as their cultural background. Participants are taught to recognize what triggers their anxiety and to learn techniques to defuse their stress levels, including specific relaxation skills, recruiting help from others, and developing positive ways of thinking. Typically, those undergoing therapy should be able to practice these skills under the supervision of the therapist and should be provided with strategies to generalize these skills outside of the therapy sessions.

For many children with ASD, CBT adaptations are needed to facilitate understanding of emotional and cognitive concepts. These include the use of visual supports and concrete language as well as the use of written materials and lists, opportunities for repetition and practice, incorporating special interests, video modeling, and active parent engagement in the therapy. Behavioral therapy may be particularly helpful, especially for those ASD children who have cognitive and language challenges (Vasa *et al.*, 2018).

Other Psychosocial Interventions

A number of additional interventions have been used to reduce anxiety in ASD youth, including improving social skills and participating in recreational programs and group activities. It has been found that group activities can provide opportunities to learn and practice pre-social skills through participation in collaborative exercises such as board games and team-based activities. A number of programs have been developed to build self-confidence, develop coping skills, and expand friendship skills. Many of these programs focus on the child's relationships and his or her interactions in school and in the community (McConachie *et al.*, 2014) as well as in the home.

Temple Grandin, Ph.D.

M.B.: Temple Grandin is an iconic figure in our society. She has shared her experiences living with autism in her writings and lectures, and this has provided invaluable insights to all shareholders in the autism community. In fact, Temple was named one of the 100 "most influential people" by Time *magazine in 2010.*

I have known Temple for over 30 years, and we have often talked about anxiety. She has shared her thoughts on this subject matter below. The following excerpt is reprinted with permission from Thinking in Pictures *by Temple Grandin.*

Puberty arrived when I was fourteen, and nerve attacks accompanied it. I started living in a constant state of stage fright, the way you feel before your first big job interview or public speaking engagement. But in my case, the anxiety seized me for no good reason. Many people with autism find that the symptoms worsen at puberty. When my anxiety went away, it was replaced with bouts of colitis or terrible headaches. My nervous system was constantly under stress. I was like a frightened animal, and every little thing triggered a fear reaction.

For the next twenty years, I tried to find psychological reasons for the panic attacks. I now realize that because of the autism, my nervous system was in a state of hypervigilance. Any minor disturbance could cause an intense reaction. I was like a high-strung cow or horse that goes into instant antipredator mode when it is surprised by an unexpected disturbance. As I got older, my anxiety attacks got worse, and even minor stresses triggered colitis or panic. By the time I was thirty, these attacks were destroying me and causing serious stress-related health problems. The intensification of my symptoms over time was similar to the well-documented worsening of symptoms that occurs in people with manic-depression and is common in other people with autism.

Reaction After Taking 50 mg/day of Tofranil: My body was no longer in a state of hyperarousal. Before taking the drug, I had been in a constant state of physiological alertness, as if ready to flee from nonexistent predators. Many non-autistic people who are depressed and anxious also have a nervous system that is biologically prepared for flight. Small stresses of daily life that are insignificant to most people trigger anxiety attacks.

Taking the medication is like adjusting the ideal adjustment screw on an old-fashioned automobile engine. Before I took Tofranil, my "engine" was racing all the time, doing so many revolutions per minute that it was tearing itself up. Now my nervous system is running at 55 mph instead of 200 mph, as it used to. Note: SSRI drugs such as Prozac were not on the market when I started taking tricyclics.

Summary

For individuals on the autism spectrum, anxiety and anxiety-provoking experiences are common in day-to-day life as the result of a wide range of factors. In adults, contributors may include problems in navigating the healthcare system, where lack of clinician training may be a factor, as well as negative experiences with employment, including underemployment and employment instability (Hwang *et al.*, 2019). Research in both ASD children and adults has suggested that interventions aimed at reducing anxiety should target IU, using interventions that have successfully reduced anxiety severity in non-autistic individuals. Studies in ASD adults suggest that such interventions may have a positive effect on insistence on sameness behaviors and may have additional benefits for those with sensory sensitivities (Hwang *et al.*, 2019).

It is important to acknowledge the heterogeneity of ASD and the precipitators and presentation of medical co-morbidities, sensory sensitivities, repetitive behaviors, and anxiety in people on the spectrum. As such, a one-size-fits-all approach to intervention may be limited in its effectiveness, and each person with ASD and their presenting symptoms should be considered individually. Until research can provide more definitive guidelines and approaches to anxiety in this population, each client and their symptomatic profile must be evaluated and treated on a case-by-case basis in order to achieve the best outcomes.

References

Alfano, C. A., Beidel, D. C., Turner, S. M., and Lewin, D. S. (2006). Preliminary evidence for sleep complaints among children referred for anxiety. *Sleep Medicine, 7*, 467–473.

Alfano, C. A., Ginsburg, G. S., and Kingery, J. N. (2007). Sleep-related problems among children and adolescents with anxiety disorders. *Journal of the American Academy of Child and Adolescent Psychiatry, 46*, 224–232.

Alfano, C. A., Zakem, A. H., Costa, N. M., Taylor, L. K., and Weems, C. F. (2009). Sleep problems and their relationship to cognitive factors, anxiety and depressive symptoms in children and adolescents. *Depression and Anxiety, 26*, 503–512.

American Psychiatric Association (2013). *Diagnostic and Statistical Manual of Mental Disorders* (5th ed.). Washington, DC: American Psychiatric Association.

Boswell, J. F., Thompson-Hollands, J., Farchione, T. J., and Barlow, D. H. (2013). Intolerance of uncertainty: A common factor in the treatment of emotional disorders. *Journal of Clinical Psychology 69*(6), 630–645.

Boulter, C., Freeman, M., South, M., and Rodgers, J. (2014). Intolerance of uncertainty as a framework for understanding anxiety in children and adolescents with autism spectrum disorder. *Journal of Autism and Developmental Disorders, 44*(6), 391–402.

Buie, T., Campbell, D. B., Fuchs III, G. J., Furuta, G. T., Levy, J., Van de Water, J., ... Winter, H. (2010). Evaluation, diagnosis, and treatment of gastrointestinal disorders in individuals with ASDs: A consensus report. *Pediatrics, 125*(Supplement 1), S1–S18.

Ceranoglu, T. A., Wozniak, J., Fried, R., Galdo, M., Hoskova, B., DeLeon Fong, M., Biederman, J., and Joshi, G. A. (2019). Retrospective chart review of buspirone for treatment of anxiety in psychiatrically referred youth with high-functioning autism spectrum spectrum disorder. *Journal of Child and Adolescent Psychopharmacology, 29*, 28–33.

Chase, R. M., and Pincus, D. B. (2011). Sleep-related problems in children and adolescents with anxiety disorders. *Behavioral Sleep Medicine, 9*, 224–236.

Clarke, C., Hill, V., and Charman, T. (2016). School based cognitive behavioural therapy targeting anxiety in children with autistic spectrum disorder: A quasi-experimental randomized controlled trial incorporating a mixed methods approach. *Journal of Autism and Developmental Disorders, 47*(12), 3883–3895.

Collins, S. M., Surette, M., and Bercik, P. (2012). The interplay between the intestinal microbiota and the brain. *Nature Reviews Microbiology, 10*, 735–742.

Couturier, J. L., and Nicolson, R. A (2002). Retrospective assessment of citalopram in children and adolescents with pervasive developmental disorders. *Journal of Child and Adolescent Psychopharmacology, 12*(3), 243–248.

Delli, C. K. S., Polychronopoulou, S. A., Kolaitis, A., and Antoniou, A. S. G. (2018). Review of interventions for the management of anxiety symptoms in children with ASD. *Neuroscience and Biobehavioral Reviews, 95*, 449–463.

Derguy, C., Poumeyreau, M., Pingault, S., and M'bailara, K. (2018). A therapeutic education program for parents of children with ASD: Preliminary results about the effectiveness of the ETAP program. *L'Encephale, 44*(5), 421–428.

Dunn, W. (1999). *Sensory Profile.* San Antonio, TX: Psychological Corporation.

Ferguson, B. J., Marler, S., Altstein, L. L., Lee, E. B., Akers, K., Sohl, K., McLaughlin A., Kartnett, K., Kille, B., Mazurek, M., Macklin, E. A., McDonnell, E., Barstow, M., Bauman, M. L., Margolis, K. G., Veenstra-VanderWeele, J., and Beversdorf, D. Q. (2017). Psychophysiological associations with gastrointestinal symptomatology in autism spectrum disorder. *Autism Research 10*(2), 276–288.

Gillott, A. and Standen, P. J. (2007). Levels of anxiety and sources of stress in adults with autism. *Journal of Intellectual Disabilities, 11*, 359–370.

Goossen, B., van der Starre, J., and van der Heiden, C. (2019). A review of neuroimaging studies in generalized anxiety disorder: "So where do we stand?" *Journal of Neural Transmission, 126*(7), 1203–1216.

Hwang, Y. I., Arnold, S., Srasuebkul, P., and Trollor, J. (2019). Understanding anxiety in adults on the autism spectrum: An investigation of its relationship with intolerance of uncertainty, sensory sensitivities and repetitive behaviours. *Autism, 24*(2), 411–422.

Joyce, C., Honey, E., Leekam, S. R., Barrett, S. L., Rodgers, J. and Joyce, C. (2017). Anxiety and intolerance of uncertainty and restricted and repetitive behavior: Insights directly from young people with ASD. *Journal of Autism and Developmental Disorders, 47*, 3789–3802.

Kanner, L. (1943). Autistic disturbances of affective contact. *Nervous Child, 2*, 212–250.

Kerns, C. M., Rump, K., Worley, J., Kratz, H., McVey, A., Herrington, J., and Miller, J. (2016). The differential diagnosis of anxiety disorders in cognitively able youth with autism. *Cognitive and Behavioral Practice, 23*(4), 530–547.

Kessler, R. C., Berglund, P., Demler, O., Jin, R., Merikangas, K. R., and Walters, E. E. (2005). Life-time prevalence and age-of-onset distributions of DSM-IV disorders in the National Comorbidity Survey Replication. *Archives of General Psychiatry, 62*, 593–602.

Kolevzon, A., Mathewson, K. A., and Hollander, E. (2006). Selective serotonin reuptake inhibitors in autism: A review of efficacy and tolerability. *Journal of Clinical Psychiatry, 67*(3), 407–414.

Krakowiak, P., Goodlin-Jones, B., Hertz-Picoiotto, I., Croen, L. A., and Hansen, R. I. (2008). Sleep problems in children with autism spectrum disorders, developmental delays, and typical development: A population-based study. *Journal of Sleep Research, 17*, 197–206.

Leekam, S., Tandos, J., McConachie, J., Meins, E., Parkinson, K., and Wright, C. (2007). Repetitive behaviours in typically developing 2-year-olds. *Journal of Child Psychology and Psychiatry, 48*, 1131–1138.

Lehmkuhl, G., Waiter, A., Mitschke, A., and Fricke-Oerkermann, L. (2008). Sleep disorders in children beginning school: Their causes and effects. *Deutsches Ärzteblatt International, 105*, 809–814.

Lyte, M., Vulchanova, L., and Brown, D. R. (2011). Stress at the intestinal surface: Catecholamines and mucosa-bacteria interactions. *Cell Tissue Research, 343*, 23–32.

Magiati, I., Ozsivadjian, A., and Kerns, C. (2017). Phenomenology and presentation of anxiety in autism spectrum disorder. In C. M. Kerns, P. Renno, E. A. Storch, P. C. Kendall, and J. J. Wood (Eds.), *Anxiety in Children and Adolescents with Autism Spectrum Disorder: Evidence-Based Assessment and Treatment.* San Diego, CA: Elsevier Academic Press.

Mazurek, N., Vasa, R. A., Kalb, S. M., Rosenberg, D., Keefer, A., Murray, D. S., Freedman, B., and Lowery, L. A. (2013). Anxiety, sensory over-responsivity and gastrointestinal problems in children with autism spectrum disorder. *Journal of Abnormal Child Psychology, 41,* 165–176.

McConachie, H., McLaughlin, E., Grahame, V., Taylor, H., Honey, E., Tavernor, L., Rodgers, J., Freeston, M., Hamm, C., Steen, N., and Le Couteur, A. (2014). Group therapy for anxiety in children with autism spectrum disorder. *Autism, 18*(6), 723–732.

Mikita, N., Siminoff, E., Pine, D. S., Goodman, R., Artiges, E., Banaschewski, T., ... Stringaris, A. (2016). Disentangling the autism-anxiety overlap: fMRI of reward processing in a community-based longitudinal study. *Translational Psychiatry, 6*(6), e845.

Owen, H., Sikich, L., Marcus, R. N., Corey-Lisle, P., Manos, G., McQuade, R. D., Carson, W. H., and Findling, R. L. (2009). Aripiprazole in the treatment of irritability in children and adolescents with autistic disorder. *Pediatrics, 124*(6), 1533–1540.

Payne, S., Bolton, D., and Perrin, S. (2011). A pilot investigation of cognitive therapy for generalized anxiety disorder in children aged 7–17 years. *Cognitive Therapy and Research, 35*(2), 71–80.

Polimeni, M. A., Richdale, A. L., and Francis, A. J. P. (2005). A survey of sleep problems in autism, Asperger's disorder and typically developing children. *Journal of Intellectual Disability Research, 49,* 260–268.

Postorino, V., Kerns, C. M., Vivanti, G., Bradshaw, J., Siracusano, M., and Mazzone, L. (2018). Anxiety disorders and Obsessive-Compulsive Disorder in individuals with Autism Spectrum Disorder. *Current Psychiatry Reports, 19*(12), 92.

Rodgers, J., Glod, M., Connolly, B., and McConachie, H. (2012). The relationship between anxiety and repetitive behaviours in autism spectrum disorder. *Journal of Autism and Developmental Disorders, 42*(11), 2404–2409.

Rodgers, J., Goodwin, J., Parr, J., Grahame, V., Wright, C., Padget, J., Garland, D., Osborne, M., Labus, M., Kernohan, A., and Freeston, M. (2019). Coping with Uncertainty in Everyday Situations (CUES) to address intolerance of uncertainty in autistic children: Study protocol for intervention feasibility trial. *Nature, 20,* 385.

Simpson, H. B., Neria, Y., Lewis-Fernandez, R., and Shneier, F. (2010). *Anxiety Disorders – Theory, Research and Clinical Perspectives.* Cambridge: Cambridge University Press.

Trembath, D., Germano, C., Johanson, G., and Dissanayake, C. (2012). The evidence of anxiety in young adults with autism spectrum disorders. *Focus of Autism and Other Developmental Disabilities, 27,* 213–224.

Uljarevic, M., Lane, A., Kelly, A., and Leekam, S. (2016). Sensory subtypes and anxiety in older children and adolescents with autism spectrum disorder. *Autism Research, 9,* 1073–1078.

Uren, J., Richdale, A. L., Cotton, S. M., and Whitehouse, A. J. O. (2019). Sleep problems and anxiety from 2 to 8 years and the influence of autistic traits: A longitudinal study. *European Child and Adolescent Psychiatry, 28,* 1117–1127.

Van Steensel, F. J., Bogel, S. M., and Perrin, S. (2011). Anxiety disorders in children and adolescents with autistic spectrum disorders: A meta-analysis. *Clinical Child and Family Psychology Review, 14,* 302–317.

Vasa, R. A., Keefer, A., Reaven, J., South, M., and White, S. W. (2018). Priorities for advancing research in youth with autism spectrum disorder and co-existing anxiety. *Journal of Autism and Developmental Disorders, 137* (Supplement 2), 115–123.

Walkup, J. T., Albano, A. M., Piacentini, J., Birmaher, B., Compton, S. N., Sherrill, J. T., ... Kendall, P.C. (2008). Cognitive behavioral therapy, sertraline, or a combination in childhood anxiety. *New England Journal of Medicine, 359*(26), 2753–2766.

White, S. W., Oswald, D., Ollendick, T., and Scahill, L. (2009). Anxiety in children and adolescents with autism spectrum disorders. *Clinical Psychology Review, 29*(3), 216–229.

CHAPTER 8

Pharmacotherapy for Anxiety in Individuals with Autism Spectrum Disorder

Tomoya Hirtoa, M.D., University of California San Francisco, Department of Psychiatry, Jordan Brooks, B.S., University of California San Francisco, School of Pharmacy, and Robert L. Hendren, D.O., University of California San Francisco, Department of Psychiatry

When Should Pharmacological Treatment Be Considered for Anxiety in ASD?

Currently available medications are not effective for treatment of core symptoms of autism spectrum disorder (ASD), including social communication and speech difficulties as well as repetitive and restricted behaviors or interests (Howes *et al.*, 2018; King *et al.*, 2009). However, a growing number of research studies suggest the effectiveness of pharmacotherapy for other symptoms that occur more often in individuals with ASD compared with those without ASD (defined as "ASD-associated symptoms"). These symptoms include inattention, hyperactivity-impulsivity, aggression and irritability, self-injurious behavior, depression, anxiety, obsessive compulsive disorder (OCD), and sleep difficulties (Simonoff *et al.*, 2008). As these symptoms affect the severity of core ASD symptoms (for example, more social communication challenges in the context of co-occurring anxiety) and negatively contribute to psychosocial functioning (Joshi *et al.*, 2013), addressing ASD-associated symptoms is of clinical importance.

Although there are currently no practice guidelines in pharmacological treatment in ASD (Murray *et al.*, 2014), psychotropic medication use is sometimes recommended by clinicians based on the severity of ASD-associated symptoms (including anxiety), the level of functional impairment due to these ASD-associated symptoms, and treatment response to non-medication treatment, such as psychoeducation and psychotherapy. For example, if someone with ASD experiences heightened generalized anxiety multiple times within a single day and frequent panic attacks, the severity of the anxiety symptoms, defined by their intensity and frequency, would lead practitioners to consider medication treatment as these individuals may not be able to fully engage in psychotherapy due to their anxiety symptoms. Another important factor that can come into play in making a decision for pharmacotherapy is the individual's level of speech. Although psychotherapy such as cognitive behavioral therapy (CBT) is recommended for anxiety both in individuals with and without ASD, CBT requires an individual's engagement, which is highly affected by the level of their receptive and expressive speech. In such cases, medication treatment may be prioritized then combined with other types of therapy, such as behavior therapy.

How Should Prescribers Present Medication Treatment to Patients and Their Families?

Before discussing pharmacological treatment with caregivers, clinicians need to acknowledge their reservations and concern about the use of medication. They may feel that medication is a last resort and may have a concern that there will be no other treatment if there is no response to pharmacotherapy. Some may be discouraged by multiple failures with other treatment modalities before they arrive at the clinic.

In discussing a trial of psychotropic medication, there are several factors, well summarized in the *Parents' Medication Guide* published by the American Academy of Child and Adolescent Psychiatry Work Group (AACAP Autism Parents' Medication Guide Work Group, 2016) that should be covered: informed consent, risks and benefits of pharmacotherapy, treatment options, dosage of medication, side effects, duration of treatment, and off-label use of medication (for example, in the treatment for anxiety in ASD, no medications are approved by the Food and Drug Administration: FDA).

In obtaining informed consent from caregivers of children or adults with ASD, the potential prescriber should discuss diagnosis and target symptoms for pharmacotherapy, other treatment options, including complementary and integrative medicine and non-pharmacological approaches, recommended medication options and evidence level supporting those options, estimated duration of pharmacotherapy, specific outcomes determining continuation or termination of pharmacotherapy, and benefits and risks of not pursuing pharmacotherapy. As stated in the *Parents' Medication Guide*, these discussions need to be repeated whenever a different medication is considered. Although it can be challenging depending on the child's cognitive ability, obtaining the child's assent is ideal and can lead to therapeutic alliance.

Physicians also need to explain to caregivers that side effects of psychotropics can aggravate pre-existing conditions in individuals with ASD. For example, some selective serotonin reuptake inhibitors (SSRIs) may lead to upset stomach, which may exacerbate pre-existing eating problems (for example, picky eating). Also, SSRIs can lead to changes in bowel movements (for example, sertraline is more likely to cause diarrhea compared with other SSRIs, and paroxetine is more likely to cause constipation compared with other SSRIs), which often co-occur in individuals with ASD. Although not explicitly reported in drug trials, some medications used for anxiety potentially cause insomnia that may negatively impact behaviors and attention.

Pathophysiology of Anxiety to Justify Medication Treatment: Serotonergic, GABAnergic, and Noradrenergic Systems

Pharmacotherapy of anxiety disorders is guided by the current understanding of their underlying pathophysiology. The serotonergic, GABAnergic, and noradrenergic systems have each been implicated in the pathophysiology of anxiety disorders; thus, many of the most effective current anxiety medications target these systems. While no theorized models to describe the pathophysiology of anxiety perfectly unifies these systems, the nature of each system's individual association with anxiety disorders is elucidated in both animal and human studies.

Within the serotonergic system, 5-HT1A receptors, 5-HT2 receptors, and the 5-HT transporter (5-HTT) have each displayed an association with anxiety. 5-HT1A receptors are present as autoreceptors on 5-HT neurons, where they modify 5-HT signaling via feedback inhibition. Human imaging and genetic studies of 5-HT1A receptors show both their density and regulation are associated with both anxiety and response to antidepressant medications. In addition to 5-HT1A receptors, 5-HT2 receptors are implicated in the pathophysiology of anxiety. 5-HTT has been associated with the regulation of mood and anxiety, given it is the target of SSRIs. SSRIs are currently the preferred class of medication for the long-term treatment of anxiety and are thought to decrease anxiety by raising 5-HT output. In studying 5-HTT in humans, the complex relationship between genotype, developmental, environmental, and epigenetic factors is still being elucidated (Olivier *et al.*, 2013).

Along with the serotonergic system, both the GABAnergic and noradrenergic systems also are associated with the pathophysiology of anxiety disorders. While many GABAnergic single nucleotide polymorphisms are individually correlated with anxiety disorders, a limited number of genome-wide association studies have described specific culprit mutations unequivocally. While the genetic and environmental relationships between the GABAnergic system and anxiety are still being investigated, the fact that benzodiazepines (BZPs) derive their anxiolytic activity by modulating the GABAnergic system is well described. Specifically, BZs enhance GABA-A receptor chloride channel opening in the presence of GABA, and overall increase inhibitory signaling throughout the brain (Olivier *et al.*, 2013).

Complex dysregulation of the noradrenergic system is also implicated in the pathophysiology of anxiety disorders. Abnormal norepinephrine turnover, decreased norepinephrine transporter (NET) and α2 receptor density, and possibly changed norepinephrine neuronal density in the locus coeruleus, are all correlated with the presence of anxiety disorders. Anxiolytic drugs that modify the noradrenergic system include serotonin noradrenaline reuptake inhibitors (SNRIs), which inhibit NET, and guanfacine, an α2 agonist (Ressler and Nemeroff, 2000).

Overview of Pharmacotherapy for Anxiety in Individuals without ASD

Before we discuss the efficacy and safety of pharmacotherapy in people with ASD, we first summarize the updated evidence of pharmacotherapy in individuals without ASD, as prescribers generally utilize the findings of pharmacological studies conducted in a general population (where the majority of study participants are non-ASD) in providing pharmacotherapy for those with ASD.

Pharmacotherapy for Anxiety Disorders in Adults Without ASD

For anxiety disorders in adults, including generalized anxiety disorder (GAD), social anxiety disorder (SAD), and panic disorder, several medications are approved by the FDA in the United States: SSRIs, including escitalopram, fluoxetine, fluvoxamine, paroxetine, and sertraline, and SNRIs, including duloxetine and venlafaxine, buspirone, and BZPs. In controlled trials conducted in adult patients with GAD, SSRIs and SNRIs were more efficacious than placebo; however, placebo response was relatively high (40%) in a recent systematic review, where response rate to SSRIs was 60–70 percent (Kapczinski *et al.*, 2003). BZPs have also been found to be efficacious in the treatment of GAD, generally leading to a reduction of emotional and somatic symptoms within minutes to hours (Offidani *et al.*, 2013). BZPs can be used in GAD for acute management of anxiety during the period before SSRIs or SNRIs take effect. Use of BZPs should be short term and be tapered off gradually, mainly due to concerns about the risks of dependence and tolerance. For the treatment of SAD, a beta-blocker (propranolol) and as-needed use of BZP are historically used mostly to reduce performance-related anxiety; however, there is no evidence sufficient to support their efficacy. For general anxiety in SAD, the efficacy of SSRIs, SNRIs, BZPs, and gabapentin has been shown in controlled trials.

Pharmacotherapy for Anxiety Disorders in Children and Adolescents Without ASD

Compared with the adult population, fewer controlled studies have been conducted to assess the efficacy and safety of psychotropic medications for anxiety in children and adolescents. At this time, there are no medications approved by the FDA for the treatment of anxiety disorders in youth. However, there are some FDA-approved medications for other disorders that often co-occur with anxiety, including fluoxetine (depression and OCD), escitalopram (depression alone), fluvoxamine (OCD alone), and sertraline (OCD alone).

Although fewer in number than the adult studies, several randomized controlled studies show that the efficacy of serotonin reuptake inhibitors, including SSRIs and SNRIs, outperformed that of placebo in pediatric patients with anxiety disorders. A meta-analysis of nine randomized controlled trials of SSRIs and SNRIs vs. placebo for pediatric anxiety revealed the superiority of these agents to placebo (Strawn *et al.*, 2015). Use of serotonergic agents, including SSRIs and SNRIs, may be counterbalanced by a possible increased risk of suicidality (suicidal thinking and behavior)—a black-box warning was issued by the FDA in 2004—from these agents. A meta-analysis of 39 medication trials conducted in children and adolescents treated with SSRIs, SNRIs, nefazodone, venlafaxine, or mirtazapine for an anxiety disorder showed a small increase in the risk of suicidal ideation and suicide attempts compared with those assigned to placebo (0.5% for OCD; 0.7% for anxiety disorders other than OCD) (Bridge *et al.*, 2007); however, whether SSRIs have a direct effect on an increase in suicide remains unclear and controversial.

Other medications for pediatric anxiety include buspirone and guanfacine (alpha agonist), neither of which is superior to placebo in reducing anxiety symptoms in controlled trials. An anticonvulsant, tiagabine, which is a selective GABA reuptake inhibitor, also failed to show superiority to placebo in reducing symptoms of generalized anxiety disorder in randomized controlled trials. BZPs, propranolol, and gabapentin are considered treatment options in clinical practice; however, there is no published evidence supporting the use of these agents for pediatric anxiety in children and adolescents with ASD.

Literature Review and Current Evidence of Pharmacotherapy for Anxiety in ASD: Effectiveness and Safety
Pharmacotherapy for Anxiety in Adults with ASD

A statistically significant decrease in anxiety as measured by the Hamilton Rating Scales for Anxiety was reported in a 16-week placebo-controlled crossover study with six adults diagnosed with ASD with fluoxetine at 40 mg/day. The mean age of the group was 30.5 ± 8.6 years, five of the individuals were men, and the mean IQ was 95. One of the individuals studied experienced frontal headaches and received a dose reduction to 20 mg/day, while the other five reported experiencing no adverse effects from fluoxetine (Buchsbaum *et al.*, 2001).

Pharmacotherapy for Pediatric Anxiety in Children and Adolescents With ASD

Serotonergic medications are often used for the treatment of anxiety in children with ASD, and several of these medications have been investigated clinically, including citalopram, fluvoxamine, sertraline, and buspirone. Other serotonergic medications (fluoxetine, for example) are also commonly used in clinical practice. Citalopram's efficacy in treating anxiety in ASD has been studied in two retrospective chart reviews containing both children and adolescents. Couturier and Nicolson (2002) reviewed the charts of 17 individuals aged 4–15 years. Of the 17 included in the study, 14 were male and eight were previously diagnosed with intellectual disability. Similarly, Namerow *et al.* (2003) reviewed the charts of 15 individuals aged 5–16 years with 13 males; four were previously diagnosed with intellectual disability. Both studies found that citalopram dosed 5–40 mg/day improved anxiety symptoms as measured by the Clinical Global Impression (CGI) scale. Overall, citalopram was well tolerated, but side effects were noted in both studies, including agitation, headaches, and aggressiveness. A total of six of the 32 individuals studied discontinued citalopram due to its side effects.

A ten-week open-label study in children and adolescents with ASD conducted by Martin *et al.* (2003) found that fluvoxamine dosed at 1.5 mg/kg/day was not significantly associated with a decrease in anxiety as measured by the Screen for Childhood Anxiety Related Emotional Disorders. This study of 18 individuals aged 7–18 years included 14 males, and five had been diagnosed with comorbid intellectual disability. Notably, an intention-to-treat analysis found that eight individuals were at least partial responders, and this group included all four female participants. Adverse effects were experienced by 13 of the 18 participants and included behavioral activation (50%), difficulties sleeping (50%), headaches (33%), changes in appetite (22%), abdominal discomfort (17%), and rhinitis (11%). Though most of the adverse effects above were noted as tolerable, severe behavioral activation resulted in three participants discontinuing fluvoxamine prematurely.

Sertraline for transition-associated anxiety and agitation in nine children with ASD aged 6–12 years (Steingard *et al.*, 1997) found sertraline given at 25–50 mg/day resulted in improvement of anxiety symptoms in eight of the nine cases. Minimal adverse effects were experienced, including stomachaches in one case and behavioral activation in two cases when sertraline was increased to 75 mg/day. Additionally, in three of the cases, initial anxiety improvement declined after 3–7 months of treatment.

Two studies have investigated the use of buspirone in children with ASD. Chugani *et al.* (2016) conducted a randomized placebo-controlled trial and examined the efficacy of low-dose buspirone for restricted and repetitive behaviors in children with ASD. The 166 participants (aged 2–6 years) in the study were divided into placebo, 2.5 mg buspirone, and 5 mg buspirone treatment groups. In this study, anxiety was a secondary outcome measured as a composite score based on the Aberrant Behavior Checklist subscale and Leiter Emotion regulation score. The reduction of anxiety composite score from baseline to the study endpoint (24 weeks) was significant at 2.5 mg buspirone but not at 5 mg buspirone. Although the lower dose of buspirone showed efficacy in anxiety in children with ASD, this effect was not significant when compared with that of placebo, which also showed a significant reduction in anxiety composite score in this study. Therefore, it is unclear if buspirone is superior to placebo in reducing anxiety in this population. An open-label study conducted by Buitelaar *et al.* (1998) containing 22 individuals with ASD age 6–17 years found 15–45 mg of buspirone daily resulted in maintained therapeutic responses in 16 of the participants as measured by the CGI scale. Overall, adverse effects of buspirone were minimal in the two studies above. Chugani *et al.* found no differences in adverse effects between the three study groups, and Buitelaar *et al.* found only one participant displayed an adverse effect of abnormal involuntary movements.

Non-serotonergic medications are also used for anxiety treatment in individuals with ASD in clinical practice. The efficacy of single-dose propranolol on conversational reciprocity in 20 adults with ASD (mean age 21.4 years), in which study anxiety was measured as a secondary outcome, was not significant (Zamzow *et al.*, 2016). In the study, participants were given either propranolol 40 mg or placebo while they were engaging in tasks evaluating their conversational reciprocity. Changes in anxiety measured by self-report anxiety questionnaire using the Spence Children's Anxiety Scale and the Beck Anxiety Inventory were comparable between the two intervention groups. Although not published, there is one study presented at an international meeting in which the efficacy of propranolol for anxiety and aggression in children with ASD treated at a clinic in the U.K. was observed in a naturalistic fashion (Sagar-Ouriaghli *et al.*, 2017). The symptoms were quantitatively measured using the CGI scale and Therapeutic Efficacy Index. The reduction of symptoms in children who were treated with propranolol (24.0 +/- 12.7 mg) suggested good efficacy. Other than the studies above, no published studies pertaining to propranolol use for anxiety in ASD were identified in electronic databases, suggesting a lack of evidence despite the fact that this medication has been historically used for anxiety both in ASD and in non-ASD populations.

Similar to propranolol, the evidence regarding the use of alpha agonists for anxiety in ASD is limited. Children and adolescents aged 5–14 years with ASD and attention deficit hyperactivity disorder (ADHD) symptoms were assigned to either guanfacine extended-release or placebo in an eight-week placebo-controlled randomized trial, in which anxiety was measured as a secondary outcome (Politte *et al.*, 2018). In the study, the anxiety subscale of the Child and Adolescent Symptom Inventory (CASI) was used as a secondary outcome measure. Guanfacine did not significantly change the anxiety subscale of the CASI from baseline to Week 8 compared with placebo.

Use of BZPs in ASD is mostly reported in cases with catatonia. Catatonia is a condition defined by a group of symptoms that usually involve a lack of movement and communication, and sometimes also agitation, confusion, and restlessness. In clinical practice, short-term use of BZPs can be beneficial for some individuals (particularly children and adolescents) to ease their fear and anxiety before procedures (for example, dental procedures). Use of BZPs requires some caution, particularly in individuals with ASD and other neurodevelopmental disorders, given that it is anecdotally reported that these individuals are more likely to have paradoxical reactions to GABA-enforcing agents, including BZPs, compared with typically developing individuals. Paradoxical reactions are characterized by increased talkativeness, emotional release, excitement, and excessive movement (Mancuso *et al.*, 2004).

Anticonvulsants, such as valproic acid, are used for emotional and behavioral problems in ASD; however, no evidence supports their efficacy for anxiety in this population. There are no studies reported using these agents (valproic acid, gabapentin, tiagabine, for example) for anxiety in ASD. However, these agents can be beneficial for individuals with comorbid ASD, seizure disorder, and anxiety, as the stabilization of seizure symptoms may lead to the reduction of emotional symptoms, including anxiety.

Biomedical, Complementary, and Integrative Treatments for Anxiety in ASD

Families commonly use nutritional supplements in an effort to improve outcomes for their children with ASD. These supplements are often referred to as complementary and integrative medicine (CIM), and are found attractive by families who wish to avoid the side effects of psychotropic medications, preferring a more "health-promoting" approach. CIM treatments suggested for the treatment of anxiety in people with ASD include omega-3 fatty acids, oxytocin, N-acetylcysteine (NAC), GABA, l-theanine, magnesium, 5-HTP, inositol, kava probiotics, and butyric acid. While there are anecdotal reports and online testimonies,[1] there are no published positive clinical trials with blinded raters for people with autism and anxiety. This does not mean that the lack of scientific evidence proves a lack of efficacy. It is possible that effective CIM therapies have not been adequately studied, and parental reports of efficacy along with review articles suggest that some CIM therapies may be effective.

Cannabidiol/tetrahydrocannabinol (CBD/THC) and Anxiety Treatment in ASD

The endocannabinoid system is involved in autism pathophysiology, particularly in energy metabolism and immune system control, suggesting it may be a target for pharmacologic intervention (Brigida *et al.*, 2017). In addition, cannabidiol (CBD) modulates brain excitatory glutamate and inhibitory GABA, as measured by magnetic resonance spectroscopy—both play a strong role in anxiety associated with ASD (Pretzsch *et al.*, 2019a).

Published studies of CBD for the treatment of anxiety are few in number, but a controlled anxiety treatment study of simulated public speaking in subjects with social phobia found CBD significantly reduced anxiety in the CBD group (Bergamaschi *et al.*, 2011). A separate study from the same group but using subjects with social anxiety disorder also noted significant improvement, related to its effects on activity in the limbic and paralimbic brain areas (Crippa *et al.*, 2011).

---

1 www.healthline.com/health/anxiety/supplements-for-anxiety; www.webmd.com/vitamins/condition-1001/anxiety.aspx; www.foundationalmedicinereview.com/blog/autism-and-gut-health-butyric-acid-could-provide-multidimensional-symptom-relief.

In ASD, an fMRI study of low-frequency activity and functional connectivity found CBD altered the cerebellar vermis and the right fusiform gyrus, areas frequently implicated in ASD (Pretzsch *et al.*, 2019b).

A two-year study of CBD oil containing 30 percent CBD and 1.5 percent THC reported improvement without blind raters in the majority of subjects with ASD, with restlessness being the most common side effect. A preliminary report of CBD and THC 20:1 reported 60 children showed improved anxiety and behavior problems, with no standardized or blinded raters (Aran *et al.*, 2019). In another study, 53 children aged 4–22 years received CBD for a median duration of 66 days (range: 30–588). Sleep problems (n = 21) improved in 71.4 percent and worsened in 4.7 percent. Anxiety (n = 17) improved in 47.1 percent and worsened in 23.5 percent. Adverse effects, mostly somnolence and change in appetite, were mild (Barchel *et al.*, 2018).

Of concern, however, is that there is moderate evidence for a statistical association between CBD and impairment in cognitive functioning, and limited evidence for an association between CBD and impaired social functioning.[2]

Overall, the published evidence for the effects of CBD/THC on anxiety and ASD is very small and anecdotal. There are no studies of dosing, outcome measures, effect sizes, or side effects that can be used to guide treatment. Much more study, especially randomized controlled trials, is needed to recommend or discourage CBD/THC use in ASD with confidence.

Conclusion

Pharmacologic treatment for anxiety associated with ASD should be considered when other non-pharmacologic treatments have not been successful, or when anxiety is severe and interferes with the functioning of the individual with ASD and his or her family or close environment. A strong rationale for treatment with pharmacologic agents is based on the pathophysiology of anxiety and ASD and on studies of the pharmacological treatments of anxiety in adults and children without ASD. Published studies of pharmacologic and complementary and integrative treatments for ASD are few, but suggest variable benefits and generally good tolerance and safety. There is a growing literature of anecdotal reports and small studies

---

2 www.nationalacademies.org/hmd/Reports/2017/health-effects-of-cannabis-and-cannabinoids.aspx.

of the benefits (or lack of benefits) from SSRIs, buspirone, propranolol, benzodiazepines, and anticonvulsants for people with anxiety and ASD. Further case reports and series with clear outcome measures over time and controlled trials and comparative trials for subgroups of anxiety symptoms in ASD with meaningful outcome measures are needed.

References

AACAP Autism Parents' Medication Guide Work Group (2016). *Autism Spectrum Disorder: Parents' Medication Guide*. Washington, DC: American Academy of Child and Adolescent Psychiatry.

Aran, A., Cassuto, H., Lubotzky, A., Wattad, N., and Hazan, E. (2019). Brief report: Cannabidiol-rich cannabis in children with autism spectrum disorder and severe behavioral problems – a retrospective feasibility study. *Journal of Autism and Developmental Disorders, 49*(3), 1284–1288. https://doi.org/10.1007/s10803-018-3808-2.

Barchel, D., Stolar, O., De-Haan, T., Ziv-Baran, T., Saban, N., Fuchs, D. O., ... Berkovitch, M. (2018). Oral cannabidiol use in children with autism spectrum disorder to treat related symptoms and co-morbidities. *Frontiers in Pharmacology, 9*, 1521. https://doi.org/10.3389/fphar.2018.01521.

Bergamaschi, M. M., Queiroz, R. H. C., Chagas, M. H. N., de Oliveira, D. C. G., De Martinis, B. S., Kapczinski, F., ... Crippa, J. A. S. (2011). Cannabidiol reduces the anxiety induced by simulated public speaking in treatment-naïve social phobia patients. *Neuropsychopharmacology: Official Publication of the American College of Neuropsychopharmacology, 36*(6), 1219–1226. https://doi.org/10.1038/npp.2011.6.

Bridge, J. A., Iyengar, S., Salary, C. B., Barbe, R. P., Birmaher, B., Pincus, H. A., ... Brent, D. A. (2007). Clinical response and risk for reported suicidal ideation and suicide attempts in pediatric antidepressant treatment: A meta-analysis of randomized controlled trials. *JAMA, 297*(15), 1683–1696. https://doi.org/10.1001/jama.297.15.1683.

Brigida, A. L., Schultz, S., Cascone, M., Antonucci, N., and Siniscalco, D. (2017). Endocannabinod signal dysregulation in autism spectrum disorders: A correlation link between inflammatory state and neuro-immune alterations. *International Journal of Molecular Sciences, 18*(7). https://doi.org/10.3390/ijms18071425.

Buchsbaum, M. S., Hollander, E., Haznedar, M. M., Tang, C., Spiegel-Cohen, J., Wei, T. C., ... Mosovich, S. (2001). Effect of fluoxetine on regional cerebral metabolism in autistic spectrum disorders: A pilot study. *The International Journal of Neuropsychopharmacology, 4*(2), 119–125. https://doi.org/10.1017/S1461145701002280.

Buitelaar, J. K., van der Gaag, R. J., and van der Hoeven, J. (1998). Buspirone in the management of anxiety and irritability in children with pervasive developmental disorders: Results of an open-label study. *The Journal of Clinical Psychiatry, 59*(2), 56–59.

Chugani, D. C., Chugani, H. T., Wiznitzer, M., Parikh, S., Evans, P. A., Hansen, R. L., ... Autism Center of Excellence Network (2016). Efficacy of low-dose buspirone for restricted and repetitive behavior in young children with autism spectrum disorder: A randomized trial. *The Journal of Pediatrics, 170*, 45–53, e1–4. https://doi.org/10.1016/j.jpeds.2015.11.033.

Couturier, J. L., and Nicolson, R. (2002). A retrospective assessment of citalopram in children and adolescents with pervasive developmental disorders. *Journal of Child and Adolescent Psychopharmacology, 12*(3), 243–248. https://doi.org/10.1089/104454602760386932.

Crippa, J. A. S., Derenusson, G. N., Ferrari, T. B., Wichert-Ana, L., Duran, F. L. S., Martin-Santos, R., ... Hallak, J. E. C. (2011). Neural basis of anxiolytic effects of cannabidiol (CBD) in generalized social anxiety disorder: A preliminary report. *Journal of Psychopharmacology, 25*(1), 121–130. https://doi.org/10.1177/0269881110379283.

Howes, O. D., Rogdaki, M., Findon, J. L., Wichers, R. H., Charman, T., King, B. H., … Murphy, D. G. (2018). Autism spectrum disorder: Consensus guidelines on assessment, treatment and research from the British Association for Psychopharmacology. *Journal of Psychopharmacology, 32*(1), 3–29. https://doi.org/10.1177/0269881117741766.

Joshi, G., Wozniak, J., Petty, C., Martelon, M. K., Fried, R., Bolfek, A., … Biederman, J. (2013). Psychiatric comorbidity and functioning in a clinically referred population of adults with autism spectrum disorders: A comparative study. *Journal of Autism and Developmental Disorders, 43*(6), 1314–1325. https://doi.org/10.1007/s10803-012-1679-5.

Kapczinski, F., Lima, M. S., Souza, J. S., and Schmitt, R. (2003). Antidepressants for generalized anxiety disorder. *The Cochrane Database of Systematic Reviews* (2), CD003592. https://doi.org/10.1002/14651858.CD003592.

King, B. H., Hollander, E., Sikich, L., McCracken, J. T., Scahill, L., Bregman, J. D., … STAART Psychopharmacology Network (2009). Lack of efficacy of citalopram in children with autism spectrum disorders and high levels of repetitive behavior: Citalopram ineffective in children with autism. *Archives of General Psychiatry, 66*(6), 583–590. https://doi.org/10.1001/archgenpsychiatry.2009.30.

Mancuso, C. E., Tanzi, M. G., and Gabay, M. (2004). Paradoxical reactions to benzodiazepines: Literature review and treatment options. *Pharmacotherapy, 24*(9), 1177–1185.

Martin, A., Koenig, K., Anderson, G. M., and Scahill, L. (2003). Low-dose fluvoxamine treatment of children and adolescents with pervasive developmental disorders: A prospective, open-label study. *Journal of Autism and Developmental Disorders, 33*(1), 77–85.

Murray, M. L., Hsia, Y., Glaser, K., Simonoff, E., Murphy, D. G. M., Asherson, P. J., … Wong, I. C. K. (2014). Pharmacological treatments prescribed to people with autism spectrum disorder (ASD) in primary health care. *Psychopharmacology, 231*(6), 1011–1021. https://doi.org/10.1007/s00213-013-3140-7.

Namerow, L. B., Thomas, P., Bostic, J. Q., Prince, J., and Monuteaux, M. C. (2003). Use of citalopram in pervasive developmental disorders. *Journal of Developmental and Behavioral Pediatrics: JDBP, 24*(2), 104–108.

Offidani, E., Guidi, J., Tomba, E., and Fava, G. A. (2013). Efficacy and tolerability of benzodiazepines versus antidepressants in anxiety disorders: A systematic review and meta-analysis. *Psychotherapy and Psychosomatics, 82*(6), 355–362. https://doi.org/10.1159/000353198.

Olivier, J. D. A., Vinkers, C. H., and Olivier, B. (2013). The role of the serotonergic and GABA system in translational approaches in drug discovery for anxiety disorders. *Frontiers in Pharmacology, 4.* https://doi.org/10.3389/fphar.2013.00074.

Politte, L. C., Scahill, L., Figueroa, J., McCracken, J. T., King, B., and McDougle, C. J. (2018). A randomized, placebo-controlled trial of extended-release guanfacine in children with autism spectrum disorder and ADHD symptoms: An analysis of secondary outcome measures. *Neuropsychopharmacology: Official Publication of the American College of Neuropsychopharmacology, 43*(8), 1772–1778. https://doi.org/10.1038/s41386-018-0039-3.

Pretzsch, C. M., Freyberg, J., Voinescu, B., Lythgoe, D., Horder, J., Mendez, M. A., … McAlonan, G. M. (2019a). Effects of cannabidiol on brain excitation and inhibition systems: A randomised placebo-controlled single dose trial during magnetic resonance spectroscopy in adults with and without autism spectrum disorder. *Neuropsychopharmacology: Official Publication of the American College of Neuropsychopharmacology, 44*(8), 1398–1405. https://doi.org/10.1038/s41386-019-0333-8.

Pretzsch, C. M., Voinescu, B., Mendez, M. A., Wichers, R., Ajram, L., Ivin, G., … McAlonan, G. M. (2019b). The effect of cannabidiol (CBD) on low-frequency activity and functional connectivity in the brain of adults with and without autism spectrum disorder (ASD). *Journal of Psychopharmacology,* 269881119858306. https://doi.org/10.1177/0269881119858306.

Ressler, K. J., and Nemeroff, C. B. (2000). Role of serotonergic and noradrenergic systems in the pathophysiology of depression and anxiety disorders. *Depression and Anxiety, 12 Suppl 1,* 2–19. https://doi.org/10.1002/1520-6394(2000)12:1+<2::AID-DA2>3.0.CO;2-4.

Sagar-Ouriaghli, I., Lievesley, K., and Tarver, J. (2017). *Effectiveness of propranolol for treating anxiety and aggression in children and adolescents with autism spectrum disorder.* Presented at the Annual meeting for the International Society for Autism Research (INSAR), San Francisco, CA, USA.

Simonoff, E., Pickles, A., Charman, T., Chandler, S., Loucas, T., and Baird, G. (2008). Psychiatric disorders in children with autism spectrum disorders: Prevalence, comorbidity, and associated factors in a population-derived sample. *Journal of the American Academy of Child and Adolescent Psychiatry, 47*(8), 921–929. https://doi.org/10.1097/CHI.0b013e318179964f.

Steingard, R. J., Zimnitzky, B., DeMaso, D. R., Bauman, M. L., and Bucci, J. P. (1997). Sertraline treatment of transition-associated anxiety and agitation in children with autistic disorder. *Journal of Child and Adolescent Psychopharmacology, 7*(1), 9–15. https://doi.org/10.1089/cap.1997.7.9.

Strawn, J. R., Welge, J. A., Wehry, A. M., Keeshin, B., and Rynn, M. A. (2015). Efficacy and tolerability of antidepressants in pediatric anxiety disorders: A systematic review and meta-analysis. *Depression and Anxiety, 32*(3), 149–157. https://doi.org/10.1002/da.22329.

Zamzow, R. M., Ferguson, B. J., Stichter, J. P., Porges, E. C., Ragsdale, A. S., Lewis, M. L., and Beversdorf, D. Q. (2016). Effects of propranolol on conversational reciprocity in autism spectrum disorder: A pilot, double-blind, single-dose psychopharmacological challenge study. *Psychopharmacology, 233*(7), 1171–1178. https://doi.org/10.1007/s00213-015-4199-0.

CHAPTER 9

Stress and Autism
Adapted Coping Interventions for Everyone on the Spectrum

June Groden, Ph.D., Leslie Weidenman, Ph.D., and
Cooper R. Woodard, Ph.D., The Groden Center, Rhode Island

Introduction

At first glance a discussion of stress and autism seems like a fairly straightforward endeavor; however, due to the complexity of these terms it quickly becomes a challenging undertaking. Subsequently, considering one term in light of the other only compounds this complexity. Stress, for example, is a somewhat vague and nebulous concept that has a variety of definitions, a variety of causes that can be both common to certain groups as well as unique to the person (Hirvikoski and Blomqvist, 2015), and a variety of outcomes, both advantageous and detrimental. It is a term that is often used interchangeably with anxiety, even though anxiety is one of many possible responses to a stressful event. Autism can be equally intricate, with its sometimes difficult to identify diagnostic features and array of presentations and associated challenges (behavioral, medical, sensory, etc.), along with the differing explanations as to its etiology, best treatment practices, and relation to other diagnoses such as obsessive-compulsive disorder and attention-deficit disorder.

In this chapter we will begin by addressing these two areas both individually and in relation to each other, and then reviewing some of the main concerns and challenges that arise from such a discussion. Special attention will be paid to our concern that despite the fact that nearly two-thirds of persons with autism have intellectual disabilities (ID), the bulk of research in the stress and anxiety area is conducted with individuals for whom intellectual functioning is at or above the borderline range. In a similar vein, we will discuss how behavior problems for persons who have ID (more so than persons without ID) may result not only from anxiety or fear-based (distress) responses to stressors, but also as a result of hopeful, positive, active, or exciting (eustress) responses to stressors. We will then turn to the challenge of assessing stress levels in the person with autism, and how these issues indicate the need for specialized and targeted assessment procedures. Finally, we will discuss how current topics of interest in psychology and innovative intervention strategies might be adapted to address non-desired stress responses in persons with autism, ID, and challenging behaviors.

What is stress? And is there an optimal conceptualization of stress in light of autism? Stress has been defined differently by different people, and in layperson's terms is typically thought of somewhat narrowly as a fight or flight (and sometimes also fright and/or freeze) response to certain stimuli that are threatening in some way. When one of these responses occurs, those stimuli or antecedents are then considered to be stressors. There are many helpful definitions of the term "stress." Hufnagel *et al.* (2017) defined it as "adaptive behavioral or mental responses willing to address the common life consequences of stressors" (p.1), whereas Rance *et al.* (2017) described it as "a state in which an individual's homeostasis is interrupted" (p.2011). However, we have found a broader definition more useful when considering stress in relation to the full array of persons with autism, proposed by Hans Selye. He defined stress as the "non-specific response of the body to any demand for change" (1956), and he not only identified the term "stressor," but also contrasted the concepts of eustress and distress. Both eustress and distress are stress responses, with eustress being a hopeful, active, positive, or invigorating/meaningful response that leads to personal growth, and distress being the less adaptive, anxiety-ridden, "shutting down," and somehow damaging response to a stressor. Hence, both are potential adaptations to environmental demands, and both are the result of how the organism conceptualizes the demand. We have chosen this definition of stress because for persons with autism there is a higher likelihood that ID is also present. In contrast to a person with autism without ID, a person with autism with ID may be more likely to display problem behavior associated with both eustress and distress. For example, the stress of going on a field trip for ice cream could lead to problem behavior such as jumping, stereotypy, or screaming, even though the event is a desired one. We would suggest that a person with autism without ID is more likely to have the cognitive skills or aptitude to support a less problematic expression of eustress.

Stress and anxiety are related concepts and, as such, are frequently discussed together. Typical or common examples of anxiety-inducing events include: public speaking, threat of physical pain, flying on an airplane, or perhaps anticipated exposure to non-desired situations such as being in the dark or near snakes or spiders. This commonly held conceptualization of stress is likely the result of the well-known and non-desired stress response of anxiety, which is a reported emotional experience of worry, nervousness, and/or unease. Behaviorally, anxiety can be demonstrated with symptoms such as sweating, shaking/tremors, "high-alert" appearance, phobias, avoidance, or stuttering. Physiological responses to anxiety are found in cortisol levels, galvanic skin responses, and heart rate variability. An early and widely accepted conceptualization of anxiety was developed by Wolpe (1958). He wrote that anxiety included three components: a subjective state inferred from verbal reports from the individual experiencing anxiety; the extent of the avoidance of anxiety-provoking stimuli or situations; and sympathetic nervous system arousal. A fourth component of nonverbal behaviors such as crying, visible muscle tension, and shaking has been considered by clinicians to be important in determining the presence of anxiety.

A more succinct description is offered by Hollocks *et al.* (2014). The authors state: "Anxiety is described with respect to three elements: cognitions, behaviors, and physiological changes. When people are anxious they experience changes in one or more of these elements" (p.33). In their chapter titled "Autism and the Physiology of Stress and Anxiety," Romanczyk and Gillis (2006) address the complexity of the term "anxiety" and state that "it is a multifaceted event that is highly interactive not only with our current biological state, but also with our learning history, current emotional status, and the physical and social environment" (p.186). In considering the term "stress," the authors observe that it is often used indiscriminately to mean either a stressor or the stress response. They define the two terms as follows:

- Stressor: an individual response to an environmental event that produces, or results in, a stress response.

- Stress response: the individual's reaction to the real or imagined aversive situation.

Hufnagel *et al.* (2017) discuss the overlap between stress and anxiety and note that one of the negative effects of stress is anxiety. The authors use the term "stress" to mean the negative physiological and psychological impact of stressors. Groden *et al.* (1994) comment that the presence of anxiety always indicates that the individual is experiencing stress.

As with stress, autism needs to be conceived of in an expanded way. Autism is a defined diagnostic category, marked by impaired social engagement and communication, and repetitive or restricted patterns of behavior. Yet, people who work with persons with autism often note that if you know one person with autism, you know one person with autism. The unique cognitive, intellectual, and behavioral presentations can vary widely from person to person, making it less likely that a single stressor or stress response can be identified that will apply to all. However, there are some stressors that are prevalent in the ASD population, such as making transitions and tolerating changes. Researchers have attempted to minimize the issue of heterogeneity by, for example, excluding participants whose intellectual functioning is below the borderline range of intelligence, but this excludes nearly two-thirds of persons with this diagnosis. Further, this is only one dimension of what makes autism a truly complex and unusual disorder. When cognitive, social, and communicative development are altered, as they are in autism, the impact is significant and can include: altered verbal skills, impaired ability to appreciate the thinking of another person, difficulty understanding humor, impaired insight or self-awareness, altered social skills, altered experience of empathy, rigidity in thinking, preference for predictability, specific fears or unique responses to certain events, limited array of coping skills, the presence or absence of sensory sensitivity, and many other effects.

Recent research has demonstrated that the responses of typically developing children to items on the Stress Survey Schedule are dramatically different from the responses of children with autism (Harmony *et al.*, 2019, under review). Typically developing children did not find the autism-related stressors relevant to their own experience. Other research has demonstrated that individuals with autism often have inconsistent and unexpected responses to stressors (Hollocks *et al.*, 2014; Lanni *et al.*, 2012; Spratt *et al.*, 2012). These results support the notion that stressors and stress responses are unpredictable and unique to each person. As an example, a person with autism may have low average intelligence, no sensory issues, some understanding of the thinking of others, and some insight into his or her own behavior and thinking. This person may report stressors similar to those described by typically developing people, and some that are unique to the diagnosis of autism. The expression of stress may likewise have some similarities to typically developing individuals, but also be comparatively blunted or difficult to identify. Or, he or she may lash out suddenly, unexpectedly (as affect is blunted), and impulsively. In contrast, a person with a more severe presentation of autism who also has ID may not have a good understanding of the concepts of others and their thinking, and may have very limited social skills, sensory sensitivity, and limited insight. He or she may have a very different set of stressors from a typically developing person and a higher functioning person with autism, although there would likely be some overlap with the latter. Stressors for this person may include any social contact, changes in schedules or plans, sensory aversions to foods, noises, or other stimuli, or new experiences—even when these experiences are desired and rewarding. For this person, the stress response may be as unique as the stressors. It could present as anything from complete non-responsiveness and sweating, to severe problem behavior that is marked by dangerous aggression, self-injury, or excessive motor behavior. Therefore, we are proposing that to understand stress in relation to autism, both a wide definition of stress and an in-depth and multi-dimensional conceptualization of the many presentations of autism are needed. Only by approaching these topics in this manner can we more fully and completely conceive of their relation to each other, and design assessments and interventions that serve and support the full array of persons with autism.

Our discussion suggests that stressors for persons with autism may overlap with those of a typically developing person, and that there may also be groups of stressors that are unique to persons with autism as a function of the diagnosis. In the early 1990s, Groden *et al.* (1994) addressed this topic, suggesting that the core symptoms of autism had the potential to create significant negative and stress-inducing effects on functioning. The heightened presence of anxiety in persons with autism as compared with typically developing persons is commonly accepted and repeatedly cited in the literature (e.g., Bellini, 2004; Hirvikoski and Blomqvist, 2015). However, as noted above, this literature focuses predominantly on individuals with autism without intellectual impairment. Stressors proposed in Groden *et al.* (1994) to be unique to persons with autism included the inability to effectively express wants and needs, the inability to make use of common coping strategies available to many typically developing persons, difficulty engaging in effective and positive social interactions with others, difficulty interpreting the emotions and thinking of others, heightened sensory sensitivities, difficulty with change, and many others. These authors suggested that high stress resulted automatically for the person with autism, even prior to experiencing potential stressors: autism itself was stress-inducing.

In addition to this baseline of comparatively heightened stress and possibly anxiety, a person with autism may be further stressed once specific environmental stressors present themselves. For example, simple awareness or anticipation of having to engage with a social world is compounded by actual social interactions that subsequently take place. Further, the characteristics of autism may impair or deplete resources such as social buffers or adaptive skills that would otherwise be available to a typically developing person. For example, as social functioning improves, stress levels tend to decrease (Bishop-Fitzpatrick *et al.*, 2014). In short, having autism has the stress- and anxiety-inducing potential to impact a person's entire experience of engagement with a social-communicative, ever-changing, and sensory-laden world.

We have discussed how stress and autism require broad definitions and conceptualizations to be fully understood. This depth and breadth of understanding allows researchers and practitioners to better address the full range of common and unique stressors and stress responses in light of the many presentations of autism. This is particularly evident and true for persons with autism with intellectual impairments, who represent a group that is often overlooked or excluded from research and the products of that research. It is critical that researchers consider the intricacies of stress and autism when, for example, selecting stress assessment tools, identifying situations that may or may not induce stress in persons with autism, and/or drawing conclusions, creating interventions, or making recommendations based on data derived from research procedures designed for typically developing populations. We propose that stress assessment tools for persons with autism that are used in research, or for any purpose, need to be specifically designed for this population. Using tools that were designed for a typically developing population risks the introduction of test bias. These tools and the procedures used to implement them also need to be suitable for the full range of possible intellectual levels of persons with autism. Likewise, when one considers supports or intervention strategies, researchers and practitioners need to be sensitive to the characteristics of autism and the range of levels of intellectual functioning, even when appropriate tools are implemented. In the following sections, we will address these areas more specifically and offer assessment and intervention options based on these ideas.

Assessing Stress and Anxiety

Assessing stress and anxiety in individuals with ASD is not an easy matter given the complexities of the concepts and the recognition of the countless ways stress and anxiety can be expressed. As noted in the introduction, every individual with ASD is unique and has his or her own set of abilities and challenges. A review of available research supports the notion that individuals with ASD experience stress and anxiety at a higher rate than typically developing peers. A review article on anxiety in children and adolescents with ASD by MacNeil, Lopes, and Minnes (2008) found that youth with ASD experience greater levels of anxiety compared with community populations, and similarly high levels of anxiety compared with clinically anxious groups. Although the ASD group and clinically anxious typically developing individuals both had high levels of anxiety, they found that the patterns of anxiety in the ASD group were very different from those seen in other clinical groups. Rodgers *et al.* (2016) reported that between 22 and 84 percent of children with ASD experience impairing anxiety. In a paper on anxiety and stress in adults with autism, Gillot and Standon (2007) found that adults with ASD were three times more anxious than a comparison group comprised of individuals with intellectual disability. The authors reported that the autism group had higher scores on anxiety subscales of panic, agoraphobia, separation anxiety, obsessive-compulsive disorder, and generalized anxiety disorder. They also found that the sources of stress that correlated with high anxiety levels in the autism group included the ability to cope with change, anticipation, sensory stimuli, and unpleasant events. Kerns *et al.* (2014) studied the various presentations of anxiety in children with ASD. The authors were interested in whether the characteristics of autism, including sensory-processing abnormalities, restricted and repetitive behaviors, and impairments in social functioning, predisposed individuals to specific forms of anxiety. They found evidence that 15 percent of the ASD group studied presented with anxiety that was altered in its presentation by its interaction with ASD characteristics. Seventeen percent of the group presented with "traditional" anxiety and 31 percent had a combined profile.

In their discussion of the varied ways the term "stress" is used and how stressors and stress responses are so individualized, Romanczyk and Gillis (2006) concurred with Lazarus and Folkman (1984) that the measurement of stress should include "the measurement of stressors or antecedents (i.e., environmental variables appraised by the individual as a stressor), intervening variables (i.e., coping styles), and strains or outcomes (i.e., anxiety)" (p.187). The authors go on to say that anxiety is often measured by changes in body chemistry, the manifestations of which can be measured by self-report or physiological measures. Some of the characteristics of autism, for example communication challenges, desire for sameness, difficulty with social interactions, and sensory challenges, as well as the high incidence of intellectual disabilities in the ASD population, further complicate the challenge of assessing stress and anxiety. Individuals with autism may be particularly vulnerable to stress as a result of these challenges. For example, in the communication domain, Groden, Baron, and Groden (2006) point out that there are numerous communication stressors that individuals with ASD may experience. The authors cite the following examples:

1. Expressing feelings.

2. Processing verbal input that is spoken quickly.

3. Deciphering language when many people are talking at the same time.

4. Understanding words when they have no relevant concrete parallel.

5. Attending to verbal input that is too complex or too long to discriminate what the message is.

6. "Getting stuck" on a certain sound or combination of sounds.

They comment that even individuals with Asperger's or high functioning autism who have good verbal skills can feel frustrated by the requirements and social norms involved in holding a conversation, such as taking turns speaking, beginning and ending conversations appropriately, and maintaining a topic of interest to the listener. Each of the other areas of challenge for individuals with ASD has its own potential stressors and sources of anxiety, which supports the evidence that individuals on the spectrum are more likely to be experiencing stress and anxiety than the typical population.

Methods of Assessing Stress and Anxiety

A review of available literature on assessment of stress and anxiety in individuals with autism reveals a limited but growing body of research. The basic methods used to assess stress and anxiety are described below.

Interviews

One of the simplest ways to begin an assessment of stress and anxiety is to ask the individual. If the person is non-verbal or an unreliable reporter, interviewing significant others (e.g., parents, caretakers, and teachers) about the person's behavior and conditions under which he or she appears stressed or anxious can be very helpful. Information obtained from interviews and self-reports should be considered only as a starting point for further investigation, as such measures are often unreliable. Individuals may not be able to assess their skills or emotional states accurately, or to identify specific stressors. Research has documented that there is significant variability in how well individuals' self-reports of their sources of anxiety correspond with their parents' perceptions. For example, Bellini (2004) found that there was no correlation between parent reports of social skills and self-reports of social anxiety.

Direct Observation and Functional Assessment

Knowing the individual and observing his or her behavior in a variety of situations can be extremely helpful in identifying stressors and situations in which behaviors associated with anxiety and stress are observed. Problem or challenging behaviors are often the result of stressful antecedent events. Observing a person over time and recording details on the antecedent conditions and consequences of challenging behavior provides the information needed for a functional assessment. The analysis typically results in hypotheses about the function(s) of the behavior, as well as the antecedent stressors that are likely to trigger it. One of the methods used at the Groden Center in Providence, RI, a school and treatment program for young people with autism, is detailed in *Understanding Challenging Behavior: A Step-by-Step Behavior Analysis Guide* (Groden *et al.*, 1996). It structures the collection of relevant information surrounding a behavioral incident and provides a means of organizing the information—useful when assessing why events may be functionally related to the behavior. The ultimate goal of the functional assessment is to develop intervention strategies based on the analysis. The Detailed Behavior Report (DBR) is the tool used to systematically collect and organize relevant information, such as the target behavior, precursor behaviors, immediate antecedents, setting events, time of day, people present, activity, and consequences. In addition to determining the function of an individual's behavior, the functional assessment process often leads to the identification of an individual's unique stressors. For example, an analysis of DBRs may reveal that the maladaptive behavior always occurs when there is an unexpected change in the daily schedule. This pattern, often represented as an "escape" function, may suggest that unpredictable change is a stressor for the person. Once identified, antecedent, environmental, and consequent treatment strategies can be devised and implemented. Along with the functional analysis, an ecological assessment and discrepancy analysis can be very helpful in pinpointing skills that an individual will need in stressful situations. This is done by assessing the responses of typically developing individuals when they are faced with the identified stressor. Comparing the adaptive responses with the maladaptive ones can help pinpoint goals for program development and skills training.

Surveys and Assessment Instruments

Researchers and clinicians who want to develop methods to assess stress and anxiety in individuals with ASD often start with instruments that were designed for a typically developing population. Investigations into the usefulness of such instruments for the ASD population have shown them to have significant limitations. In Rodgers *et al.* (2016), the authors reviewed the suitability of measures of anxiety for the ASD population and found that a number of measures were less than satisfactory. They urged caution in using tools developed to assess anxiety in the typical population with the ASD population.

Anxiety Scale for Children with ASD (ASC-ASD)

This scale, developed by Rodgers *et al.* (2016), is an adaptation of the Revised Children's Anxiety and Depression Scale (RCADS), which was created by Chorpita *et al.* in 2000 and is designed specifically for persons with autism. The adaptation of the RCADS by Rodgers *et al.* included the addition of items that related to three ASD-specific anxiety constructs— sensory hypersensitivity, intolerance of uncertainty, and specific fears/ phobias. The authors proposed that the repetitive behaviors so commonly seen in individuals with ASD are an "attempt to impose predictability in the face of intolerable uncertainty" (p.1206). Specific fears were found to be one of the most common forms of anxiety. In their review of the literature, the authors found that the prevalence rates of fears and specific phobias in the ASD population ranged from 13 percent to 67 percent. In addition to the inclusion of items addressing the three ASD-related constructs, the revision of the RCADS included modifications of the wording of 37 of the original items. Two versions of the revised measure (child and parent) were evaluated with evidence of good reliability and validity. The resulting 24-item ASC-ASD measure has two versions, a self-report and a parent-report. Each version has four subscales: performance anxiety, uncertainty, anxious arousal, and separation anxiety. In the discussion of the development of the ASC-ASD and its evaluation, the authors note that their study only included children with ASD of average ability. Its usefulness in assessing anxiety and stress in individuals with ASD and intellectual disability was unknown, but it is a topic of future research.

Stress Survey Schedule for Persons with Autism and Other Developmental Disabilities (SSS)

Groden *et al.* (2001) developed an instrument for measuring stress in the lives of individuals with ASD, various levels of intellectual functioning, and other developmental disabilities. It consists of 49 statements of events that are rated on a five-point scale as to the intensity of stress each one would cause for the individual. A rating of "1" would indicate that the event or activity would result in no stress or only a mild degree. A rating of "5" would represent severe stress. In addition, there are sections to rate common fears and life stressors. Sample items include the following, which indicate both distress and eustress:

- Having personal objects or materials out of order.

- Receiving hugs and affection.

- Being prevented from carrying out a ritual.

- Transitioning from preferred to non-preferred activity.

- Having a conversation.

- Waiting for reinforcement.

Exploratory and confirmatory analyses resulted in the identification of eight dimensions of stress: Anticipation/Uncertainty, Changes and Threats, Unpleasant Events, Pleasant Events, Sensory/Personal Contact, Food-Related Activity, Social/Environmental Interactions, and Ritual-Related Stress. In validating the SSS, Goodwin *et al.* (2007) conducted a study in which it was completed for 180 individuals with autism who varied in age, intellectual ability, verbal ability, and gender. The results demonstrated high internal consistency for the stress scales, suggesting that it is a valid tool for assessing stressors for individuals across the autism spectrum.

Physiological Measures

For decades, researchers and clinicians have investigated the feasibility of using physiological measures to assess the stress and anxiety in their clients. For example, measures of cardiovascular activity (e.g., heart rate and heart rate variability), electrodermal responses (e.g., skin conductance or galvanic skin response), and hormonal levels (e.g., cortisol) have been explored as measures of stress and anxiety (Baron *et al.*, 2006). In choosing methods to use with individuals with autism, investigators have to consider the available technology, the invasiveness of the procedure, and the validity of the measure itself. Below is a brief description of some of the most frequently used methods of physiological assessment.

Heart Rate (HR)

HR has been demonstrated to be a robust measure of overall stress-based arousal in persons with autism (Groden *et al.* 2006). Increased arousal has been associated with stress. Investigators have been looking at how HR changes from a calm resting state when the individual is exposed to stressors. These changes in HR can help the clinician learn about the stress individuals are experiencing. Looking at patterns of heart rate variability (HRV) in a variety of situations can help identify individuals who respond with heightened arousal to stressors.

There continues to be debate about what (if any) differences in HR exist in the ASD population. Researchers have been interested in knowing if the ASD population differs from a typically developing population, as well as if there are differences within the ASD population depending on age, communication level, and intellectual ability. A study by Goodwin *et al.* (2006) compared the HR of five individuals with ASD with that of five typically developing age- and sex-matched peers when faced with a variety of stressors. One of the interesting findings was that the average HR of the ASD group was approximately 20 beats per minute higher than the typically developing group. A recent study by Zantinge *et al.* (2017) attempted to measure stress in children when faced with a difficult task. They compared heart rate patterns and behavioral regulation of emotion of children with ASD with those of typically developing children. HR was continually measured during a locked-box task designed to evoke frustration in preschool children by preventing them from playing with a desired toy. The task is part of the preschool Laboratory Temperament Assessment Battery by Goldsmith *et al.* (1999). Children select a desired toy to play with which is in a locked box. Frustration is induced by giving the children the wrong set of keys to open the box. Results showed that HR levels for both groups were identical during arousal and recovery stages of the test. However, the ASD group displayed less constructive methods of solving the problem and more venting and avoidance strategies. The authors concluded "that rather than abnormal levels of emotional arousal, a key impairment in young children with ASD may be difficulties in behaviorally regulating and expressing experienced emotions to others" (Zantinge *et al.*, 2017, p.2648).

HR can offer valuable information on how an individual responds to stressors, but more research is needed before it can be determined if it can be used as a reliable and valid measure of stress and anxiety in the ASD population. In an opinion article titled "The need for objective measures of stress in autism," Hufnagel *et al.* (2017) wrote that individuals with ASD would benefit from an objective, continuous measurement of stress. They posited that HRV, defined as the variation between two consecutive heart beats, could be such a measure. The rationale for the use of HRV is detailed in their paper. Briefly, the authors base their argument on the connection between HR and vagal tone, a measure of parasympathetic nervous system activity (the parasympathetic branch is associated with relaxation and a return to a calm state). The authors state:

> A high HRV reflects the fact that an individual can constantly adapt to micro-environmental changes. An overload of stress induces a decrease in HRV and the adaptation mechanisms are exceeded. Therefore, low HRV is both a marker of cardiovascular risk and a biomarker of stress. (Hufnagel *et al.*, 2017, p.2)

Measuring HRV can be done accurately and easily using small medical devices. They propose that such devices be used to measure stress during daily life activities instead of in the laboratory with simulated stressors. They note that recent development in device portability has made it possible to do continuous monitoring.

Hormonal Measures

Romanczyk and Gillis (2006) describe the basic physiological mechanisms of stress and note that it is a very complex system involving the ANS, endocrine system, hypothalamus, limbic system, pituitary gland, and thyroid gland, among others. Hormones and neurotransmitters released or activated during the stress response have been measured, including epinephrine, norepinephrine, and cortisol, which are controlled by the autonomic nervous system, and vasopressin, adrenocorticotrophic hormone (ACTH), and thyrotrophic hormone, released by the pituitary gland in the endocrine system. The thyroid gland is also involved in the stress response. It releases thyroxine, which is associated with increased perspiration and heart rate. The authors point out that cortisol and ACTH (a precursor to cortisol) are good indices of stress and negative emotions. Even though it can be a good indicator of stress, measuring cortisol has its challenges. There are two common ways of measuring cortisol levels—blood tests or saliva samples. Both methods may be stressful to an individual on the spectrum. For most, salivary cortisol is easier and less stressful to collect.

In 2009, Corbett *et al.* compared morning and evening cortisol levels in individuals with ASD with parent-report measures of stress. Parents of children with high functioning autism filled out the Stress Survey Schedule for Individuals with Autism and Other Developmental Disabilities (SSS) described above. The results demonstrated a positive relation between the SSS stress measure and cortisol levels. The higher the reported stress, the higher the cortisol levels were at the end of the day. In particular, the findings showed that higher levels of cortisol in the evening were associated with increased stress from changes in routines. It also was noteworthy that the parents' reports of higher stress and the measures of higher cortisol corresponded with the higher measures on the SSS.

Electrodermal Measures

Panju *et al.* (2015) reported that the existing literature suggests that there is quite a bit of variability in autonomic activity in the ASD population, and that it is often atypical or dysregulated. In their study, they compared electrodermal activity in individuals with ASD with low anxiety, individuals with ASD with high anxiety, and typically developing children. They found atypical autonomic function in the ASD groups compared with typically developing individuals. They also found distinct differences within the two ASD groups, indicating that anxiety had an impact on physiological responses. In addition, the authors reported behavioral differences in the ASD subgroups. The high anxiety subgroup showed more severe symptomatology on several measures, suggesting that the two subgroups present with different behavioral profiles. Overall, the authors state that "the results add to the body of literature supporting autonomic dysfunction in ASD and highlight the role of anxiety and autonomic features in explaining the variability in the autism spectrum" (p.2). The children involved in the study ranged in age from 7 to 18 across groups, with average IQs of 113.1 in the typical group and 94.3 in the ASD group.

Multimodal Approach

Each of the methods of assessing stress and anxiety has strengths and limitations. The experience of stress and anxiety is a very individual one, and can be affected by a host of variables such as age, intellectual ability, verbal and communication skills, personal experience, and behavioral repertoire and history. Given the challenges, clinicians and researchers alike support the use of multiple measures to investigate stress and anxiety. In their article on anxiety in children and adolescents with ASD, White *et al.* (2009) reviewed 40 papers on the topic. They found that anxiety, "whether measured categorically or dimensionally, is indeed common in children and adolescents with autism spectrum disorders and may be a source of additional morbidity" (p.216). They concluded that the assessment of anxiety disorders in ASD should be conducted using "multiple informants and modalities" (p.216).

Adapted Coping Interventions for Stress and Anxiety in Autism

We have discussed some of the challenges associated with addressing stress in persons with autism. Both stress and autism have been described separately as complex concepts, due to issues such as varied definitions, differing causes and etiologies, and a wide range of presentations. However, when stress is considered in light of an autism diagnosis, what is a stressor becomes even more challenging to identify because the entire cognitive and interactive experience of the person with autism is altered to varying degrees and often in unique ways. One of these variations has to do with the impact of an intellectual disability, which affects a person's ability to understand stressors when they are present, the ability to alter attributions related to that stressor, and/or otherwise cope with what is encountered. Even though nearly two-thirds of persons with autism have intellectual functioning below the average range, much of the recent coping-oriented trends in the field have been directed at persons with autism with average or higher levels of intellectual functioning.

We will discuss how a behavior therapy orientation has been used effectively at the Groden Center to develop stress-reducing relaxation therapy, cognitive picture rehearsal, changing attributions, and positive psychology. We will then briefly discuss two newer trends, mindfulness and Acceptance and Commitment Therapy (ACT), and consider how these are related to or can be integrated into existing intervention methods. This is done in an effort to make both existing and newer tools available to persons with autism who do not function at or above the average range of intelligence. This carries on a tradition of such adaptations begun many years ago at the

Groden Center. Persons in this program also typically present with significant developmental disabilities and severe behavior challenges. For many years, these behavior challenges have been treated from a behavioral perspective that includes innovative and adapted cognitive components. Treatment is also based on a belief that having autism is in and of itself stressful, and this stress is at the root of many of the behavioral manifestations. Because of this, learning and using coping strategies that target stress-reduction are considered essential to the successful functioning of a person with autism.

A Behavior Therapy Foundation

Behavior therapy is a psychological treatment that covers a wide range of procedures and has its roots in learning theory, and the work of B. F. Skinner, Joseph Wolpe, and many other learning theorists. It looks closely at how behaviors are acquired/learned, and emphasizes the effects of the environment and the use of data and empirical evidence. The use of behavior therapy to treat persons with developmental disabilities began in the late 1970s by psychologists Baer, Peterson, and Sherman (1967). These practitioners built upon the experimental work of Skinner and started to use what was then called behavior modification to teach imitative behavior and other basic skills. At the time, behavior modification relied primarily on the use of consequence-based interventions such as reinforcement and extinction. Ivar Lovaas *et al.* (1973) used these procedures with persons with autism and was able to show through data that this population was capable of significant learning that could lead to more independent and dignified lives. Previously, many of the children and adults with autism were living in institutions, both public and private, out of the mainstream of community life, and received little in the way of therapeutic interventions. The work of these early researchers began to open the door to new possibilities in the area of treatment.

In the late 1970s and throughout the 1980s, behavioral practitioners began using the term Applied Behavior Analysis (ABA) along with behavior modification to refer to the work being done in the field. ABA represents the larger systemic science designed to affect socially significant behaviors. It is now widely used in the field of autism, and focuses on identifying the variables that underlie behavior change. However, it is only one form of the application of the larger field of behavioral psychology, which also extends into cognitive psychology and more recently into the emergence of areas such as Acceptance and Commitment Therapy (ACT). ABA has many distinct tools or interventions, and can be particularly helpful in decreasing problem behaviors, as well as teaching discrimination skills, imitation, adaptive living skills, early reading, following instructions, social and play skills, writing, and many other lifelong adaptive skills. It is based on observing and assessing observable or "outer" behavior, and treating it with environmental alterations. For example, teaching a child to sit in his or her seat for a small period of time is observable, and it is usually treated with positive reinforcement once the child sits for a very short stipulated amount of time. Thus observable behavior (outer) is affected by altering environmental contingencies. This does not, however, negate the existence and importance of the "inner" behaviors of thinking and emotion that begin to emerge when behavioral psychology is considered in its fullest capacity.

Behavior Therapy at the Groden Center

The Groden Center is a non-profit education and treatment institute that was founded in Rhode Island in 1976. Drs. June and Gerry Groden formulated a model that combined a wide range of behavioral therapy procedures with a developmental and ecological perspective. In addition, they felt it was also critical to integrate the concept of "inner" behavior—or what Skinner termed private events—such as thoughts, feelings, emotions, and images into the treatment protocols for persons with autism. Taking the characteristics of autism into account, it was thought that persons with autism would have a great deal of stress (an inner behavior) dealing with everyday-life situations, and the need to develop treatments to reduce stress was paramount. At that time the feeling was prevalent that persons with autism did not experience stress or have imagery skills. This was evident in a critique of the book, *AUTISM, Strategies for Change* (1988), edited by Groden and Baron, which described stress reduction techniques such as relaxation and imagery that were used at the Groden Center. The reviewer felt that the procedures directed at inner-stress behavior described in the book could not be a benefit to this population—that persons with autism did not have the cognitive capacity to benefit from this method, and that these procedures were too sophisticated. However, a wide range of stress-reduction procedures to improve coping skills were adapted for use at the

Groden Center and have helped many students in the program. Coping strategies are behavioral and cognitive attempts to adjust to situational demands that are perceived to exceed a person's ability to adapt (Lazarus and Folkman, 1984). People who effectively use such strategies to deal with stress have been found to lead a healthier and better quality of life than people who do not (Turner and Roszell, 1994). These will be described in more detail later in the chapter.

Demand, Control, and Support

Three important variables to consider in focusing on strategies to reduce stress are demand, control, and support. Low demand, high control, and high support produce a low-stress condition. High demand, low control, and low support produce the opposite condition—that is, most stress is placed on the individual.

"Demand" is any force, pressure, or strain placed on the individual. "Support" refers to significant others, including family members, friends, and teachers, who help buffer the adverse mental and physical effects of stress-inducing situations. "Control" is the capacity to make active responses during stressful situations and is closely associated with a sense of mastery of the environment (Groden *et al.*, 2016b). Below are some of the ways to foster the optimal conditions of low demand, high control, and high support.

Fostering Low Demand

Demands may arise from the physical environment, social situations, or task requirements. Environmental accommodations, instructional strategies, and acquiring specific skills are ways to reduce the stress associated with high-demand situations.

Informed Choice Making

Giving a person the opportunity to make choices helps to obtain increased control over events in the environment. In order to learn to make choices, it is best to start with two simple items and advance to the use of choice-boards with or without pictures. It is important to make the type and the number of choices match the developmental level of the individual. The intrinsic reinforcement of obtaining the choices one has made can lead to personal satisfaction and a sense of well-being that may reduce stress.

Visual Supports

Visual supports are physical cues, environmental strategies, or specifically designed tools that help the learner receive, process, and act on information. Gestures and body language are often visual supports, as are furniture arrangements, object placements, and the common everyday signs and symbols we all use (Hodgdon, 1995). Visual supports used in many teaching programs for persons on the spectrum include schedules, calendars, reinforcement boards, rule cards, communication pictures, tablets, smartphones, and other technological tools. These strategies and devices are organizing tools that enhance the understanding of verbal input, provide predictability, and help make abstract concepts concrete, all of which help to improve the communication difficulties that can exacerbate stress in this population.

Building Skills

Although we have mentioned many strategies, treatments, and supports to reduce stress, it is critical to encompass these within a framework of building new skills. Many of these treatments and supports incorporate new skills in the procedures, but in addition, increasing a person's abilities in all areas leads to more opportunities to make choices and develop appropriate alternatives to stress responses. The proper schooling and curricula should include increasing academic knowledge (e.g., reading, writing, communicating), building physical fitness, knowing about good nutrition, and ongoing medical care, all to fit the development level of the individual. "The more abilities a person has, the more they are able to make choices and choose alternatives" (Groden *et al.*, 2016a, p.247).

Schedules and Routines

Schedules and routines are specific types of visual supports personalized to reflect the individual's need for structure, organization, and planning. Establishing routines to follow and having the visual support of a schedule can provide the assistance that is needed. Schedules also help to establish time and space relationships (what comes first and last, what was in the past, what is present, and what is in the future). This is often difficult for a person with autism. Schedules can be in picture form, written on paper, or on the latest technological device. Being able to predict what is happening next can reduce the stress of not knowing what to expect. Having a set routine can also provide this same structure. When a person participates in developing his/her own schedule or routine, it allows a feeling of control, which is another way to reduce stress.

Providing High Support

In this category a number of people are involved in the process of reducing stress—families, school personnel, peers, community friends, and fellow workers. Although the value of social support is commonly accepted in the general population, it is of particular importance with persons on the spectrum. Because of their communication difficulties and often inappropriate behaviors, their social lives can be greatly impaired or reduced. Often autistic persons are lonely, and do not make and keep friends easily. Some parents report that they cannot keep friends because of their child with autism, which also affects the social development of a child with autism.

Family

Children and adults with autism frequently develop an emotional closeness to family members. They learn that family members can help solve problems, clarify confusing situations, and provide comfort. In this way family members provide a high level of support that helps to maintain stability and counteract many of the inappropriate stress responses like tantrum, aggression, and property destruction.

Friends

Since it is often difficult for persons with autism to make friends, joining social groups and building support networks can be helpful. There is some controversy as to whether these groups should be restricted to persons on the spectrum or include typically developing peers. At the Groden Center there were many requests from teens in inclusive high school programs for opportunities to get together with others who share similar experiences. As a result, we offer several types of support groups: (1) groups that offer social-skill development and provide an opportunity for youth with high functioning autism to meet and make friends, (2) an after-school recreational group that allows youth with autism to share experiences and support each other, and (3) an adult recreational club that plans trips and other activities initiated by members. In these groups we have found that the members become friends, call each other, and offer support to each other. These groups offer the members meaningful and enjoyable experiences on weekends, vacations, and after school.

Teachers

Teachers are in a unique position to help students with disabilities to understand their problems, needs, and challenges associated with their disabilities. This extends to school personnel who monitor the cafeteria, library, and recess, where students with autism and other disabilities are often bullied or excluded from joining in on activities or sitting at particular lunch tables. Teacher training in these areas would help to facilitate the reduction of stress put upon those children who feel unwanted and uncomfortable. Teachers are also role models and can demonstrate positive character traits, foster desired values, and teach empathy, kindness, flexibility, self-confidence, and pride in accomplishment. All of the above would reduce the stress of children with autism and other disabilities.

Teaching High Control

A sense of personal control or mastery over life is one of the most frequently examined coping resources in the literature (Thoits, 1995). A number of studies show that a sense of control reduces psychological problems and physical illness, and buffers the negative effects of stressors (Turner and Roszell, 1994). The ultimate goal of high control is self-control. Self-control can be defined as learning a new, more appropriate response in the absence of external cues, prompts, or contingencies. Self-control is a personal quality that not only is possible for people of a higher cognitive range, but can also be learned by people with autism at all levels to reduce stress in their lives. It can help individuals be proactive in reducing stress by learning to act early, when first warning signs are evident (antecedents) (Hobfoil, 2001).

Because techniques to foster high control include so many opportunities, the next section includes examples of procedures to help promote high control through self-control. Special emphasis is given to the role and value of self-control to reduce the stress in the lives of individuals with autism and to increase the use of proactive, adaptive coping techniques.

Procedures to Promote High Control and Self-Control
Relaxation

Although there are many systems to teach relaxation, at the Groden Center we incorporate the use of relaxation into the students' day in two ways. We schedule daily relaxation practice sessions in which students refine their skills, and also teach them to use relaxation as a means of self-control when they encounter stressful situations. Practicing relaxation regularly and during times of stress greatly strengthens the effectiveness of the procedure. The relaxation response, when learned, can function as an adaptive behavior that is incompatible with stress and anxiety. Progressive muscle relaxation procedures (Jacobson, 1938) have been adapted to meet the needs of a population with autism (Groden *et al.*, 2016a). Although there are many techniques to promote relaxation, such as yoga, meditation, or Benson's relaxation response (1984), progressive relaxation was chosen because it adapted more easily to meet the needs of persons with autism. It involves building an awareness of muscle groups in the body, and learning to discriminate between the presence of tense muscles and then learning to relax the muscles. In addition, deep breathing is taught to facilitate relaxation of the whole body. One distinct advantage of relaxation is that it can be used in any setting and at any time a stressor occurs, whether in school, at home, or in the workplace.

Relaxation, as outlined in *Relaxation: A Comprehensive Manual for Children and Adults with Autism and Other Developmental Disabilities* (Groden *et al.*, 2016a), describes the adaptations made to the Jacobson progressive muscle relaxation procedure to accommodate the needs of persons with autism and other special needs. The manual includes an assessment/placement test to determine the step on which training should begin. Some people may need training on the fundamental skills needed before relaxation training begins. Fundamental skills include sitting in a chair, imitating basic motor actions, and following directions. Others may start with the basic relaxation procedure that focuses on tightening and relaxing major body parts, such as arms, hands, and legs, and learning to take deep breaths. More capable individuals may start training with the advanced relaxation procedures.

The advanced procedures follow the same sequence of tightening and relaxing muscles, but add more muscle groups, including: eyes, nose, mouth, face, shoulders, neck, stomach, and back. In both the basic and advanced procedures, the individual first learns to tighten and then relax each muscle group and take deep breaths. Immediately, the sequence is repeated, omitting the tightening aspect. The person practices just relaxing the muscles and taking deep breaths. The final steps of the process of learning the relaxation protocol are to practice relaxing the muscle groups and breathing deeply while standing and walking, and then generalizing the practice to other environments. The purpose of including the tightening of the muscle groups into the relaxation procedure is to help individuals discriminate a tight muscle from a relaxed one. Through this process, learners become more aware of what their muscles feel like when they are tight versus relaxed, and how to relax any muscles that feel tight or tense.

To become proficient in relaxation, it is recommended that the sequence be practiced for 20 minutes a day, and that a record of progress be maintained. This relaxation procedure, in its daily practice, focuses on directing attention to muscle groups, and deep breathing, and is complementary to mindfulness and related practices to be discussed later in this chapter.

Using the Relaxation Response

Using the relaxation response effectively requires that an individual's stressors be identified, thus allowing procedures to be personalized to match specific conditions or situations. As noted above, they can be identified via one or preferably multiple methods. Once they are identified, they should be prioritized according to intensity, frequency, and relevance to significant life situations. Since persons with autism often have many stressors, they can be addressed starting with the one considered to be the most substantial. Once the individual has mastered the relaxation process and is able to practice it on a regular basis, he or she can begin to use it in stressful situations. Depending on the person's functioning level, evoking relaxation may require some degree of prompting (or none at all). For lower functioning individuals, a caregiver, teacher, or parent would cue the relaxation response before the stressor occurs, again during the stress period, and then after the stressful situation. Once the participant is reliably able to relax when cued, the goal is to develop self-control. To begin the process of transferring control, when stressors occur, the participant is asked, "What do you do now?" The correct response is, "I relax." After this response is learned, the next step is for the participant to self-identify the stressor and then carry out the relaxation response, thus increasing self-control and self-management. For persons with autism and other developmental disabilities, it is not enough to learn self-controlling responses to reduce stress. Learning to *use* them in various life contexts is necessary for effective coping.

Vignette—An Example of the Use of Relaxation

Hailey is a ten-year-old girl with autism, with a moderate-to-severe level of intellectual disability. Hailey's grandmother takes care of her after school. The grandmother reports many occasions when Hailey becomes loud and noisy and exhibits stereotypic behavior such as rocking and flapping her hands. These behaviors occur most frequently on trips to the market. In working with Hailey's therapist, behavior programming addressing the possible escape function of her behavior has been put in place. This includes increasing levels of reinforcement for positive behavior, ignoring the problem behavior when it occurs, and starting with very short trips to the market. These interventions have had only a limited effect. Additionally, the grandmother is concerned that Hailey looks very distressed and alarmed during these incidents.

The behavior program is augmented with daily relaxation practice following Hailey's after-school snack. When she takes Hailey to the market, the grandmother cues her to practice relaxation while walking from the car to the market and upon entering the store. While shopping, if she notices Hailey becoming agitated or increasing her stereotypic behavior, she reminds her to use her relaxation. When Hailey responds to the cue to relax appropriately, the grandmother immediately praises her, and if the visit is successful, allows her to pick something she likes in the market. After she consistently responds to the instruction, she says, "Hailey, we have to go to the market, what can you do to make yourself feel calm?"

Hailey should respond by saying or showing relaxed arms, hands, and legs, and practicing deep breathing. After a few months, Hailey should begin to recognize when she is feeling anxious in the market and cue herself to relax by relaxing her arms, legs, and hands, and taking a deep breath. The grandmother is happy to see this self-controlling response and praises Hailey.

Cognitive Picture Rehearsal (CPR)

Cognitive picture rehearsal is a proactive instructional strategy, based on imagery techniques that use sequenced pictures and an accompanying script. The pictures and script create a scene or story that describes when, where, and how to use a particular behavioral sequence, and ends with a pleasant scene for successful performance (Groden and LeVasseur, 1995). It was developed in 1980 by June Groden and Joseph Cautela, and is the forerunner of programs that use scripts and pictures to address behavioral and stressful situations. Although there are many programs that use some form of scripts or scripting, the majority of them do not take advantage of information derived from the examination of outer behavior through formal identification of antecedent-based stressors. They also do not typically take advantage of integration of other therapies, including positive psychology concepts such as positive affirmations, messages of self-efficacy, or promoting positive traits such as optimism, all of which can be quickly and easily woven into scripts to maximize benefit. CPR also has the added benefit of incorporating pictures into the scripts to provide the visual support system that is important to persons with autism.

Creating CPR Scenes

The scripts developed for CPR scenes rely on information obtained by a thorough assessment process, as described earlier in the chapter. Once the stressors are identified and prioritized, the clinician creating the script identifies the desired, alternate, and appropriate behavior that should take place in the presence of the stressor. Based on the functioning level of the person for whom the script is designed, the format of the CPR scene and materials (real pictures, drawings, icons, words only, etc.) is selected. The scenes are developed and the scripts are written in a manner that typically presents the stressor, perhaps prompting the relaxation response or alternate attribution, and then incorporates the desired behavior. The scene ends with a real or imagined reinforcer. Typically, the CPR scenes and the relaxation procedure are used in conjunction with each other, as they are complementary. The length, order, and level of difficulty of the scenes can be altered depending on the needs of the individual and the particular stressful situation. More information on this is available in *Coping with Stress Through Picture Rehearsal* (Groden *et al.*, 2002).

The selection of a treatment procedure for each scene is based on the literature relevant to the problem, the individual's language level, and cognitive abilities. The steps in designing a CPR program are as follows:

- Step 1: Identify the antecedent events/stressor.

- Step 2: Identify the behavior to change and its appropriate replacement behavior.

- Step 3: Create the script and add a reinforcer from a menu of pleasurable events.

- Step 4: Develop a data system.

CPR scenes can be presented in a variety of formats, including index cards, small photo albums, computers, tablets, or smartphones, with pictures individually designed to match the child's or adult's interests, and developmental and cognitive levels. Pictures represent the image that the individual should form. The images can either be simple line drawings, Boardmaker symbols (icons), pictures, photographs, or, in some cases, actual objects. The number of images and the language used should match the individual's development level. A person who is functioning on an early level might only have three pictures or objects with a few words, whereas a higher functioning person may have many images and a more sophisticated script. Pictures are presented individually by the therapist or teacher. The teacher points to each card and reads the accompanying script. Then the scene is repeated by the participant. When the participant learns the script, she/he then reviews it independently. Daily practice of CPR scenes using this format is suggested.

In order to use the CPR scene as a means of self-control, it should be readily available to the participant. If the person is able, he or she should carry the scene and script with him or her. Before the identified stressor occurs, the caregiver can cue the response as delineated in the script. The system of cues is the same as described above for relaxation. When the individual begins to recognize the stressor or antecedent event, then he/she can self-cue and use the appropriate response. This is the ultimate aim of CPR: self-control. Note that CPR, as with relaxation and other treatment strategies, takes a long time to become effective, depending upon how long the inappropriate behavior has been in the person's repertoire, the individual's cognitive abilities and motivation, and the expertise of the therapist. However, the reward of a self-controlling response can be life changing and worth the effort.

An Example of the Use of CPR

The book *Coping with Stress Through Picture Rehearsal* (Groden *et al.*, 2002) is an excellent resource for CPR scenes on a variety of topics. It includes the Stress Survey Schedule and offers sample CPR scenes for each category of stress. The scene shown in Figure 9.1 from the book[AQ] incorporates the relaxation response (Card 4: "I take a deep breath and relax"), changing attributions (Card 5: "...soon it will be our turn to order"), practicing an appropriate and alternative behavior (Card 6: "I talk to Grandpa while we wait"), and positive reinforcement (Card 8: Eating hamburger and French fries in the restaurant).

What differentiates CPR from other strategies that use scripting is that CPR is specific, individualized, and incorporates positive coping mechanisms designed to address unique stressors. It is informed by evidence-based procedures such as functional behavioral assessment, and also builds in positive reinforcement that is specific to the person.

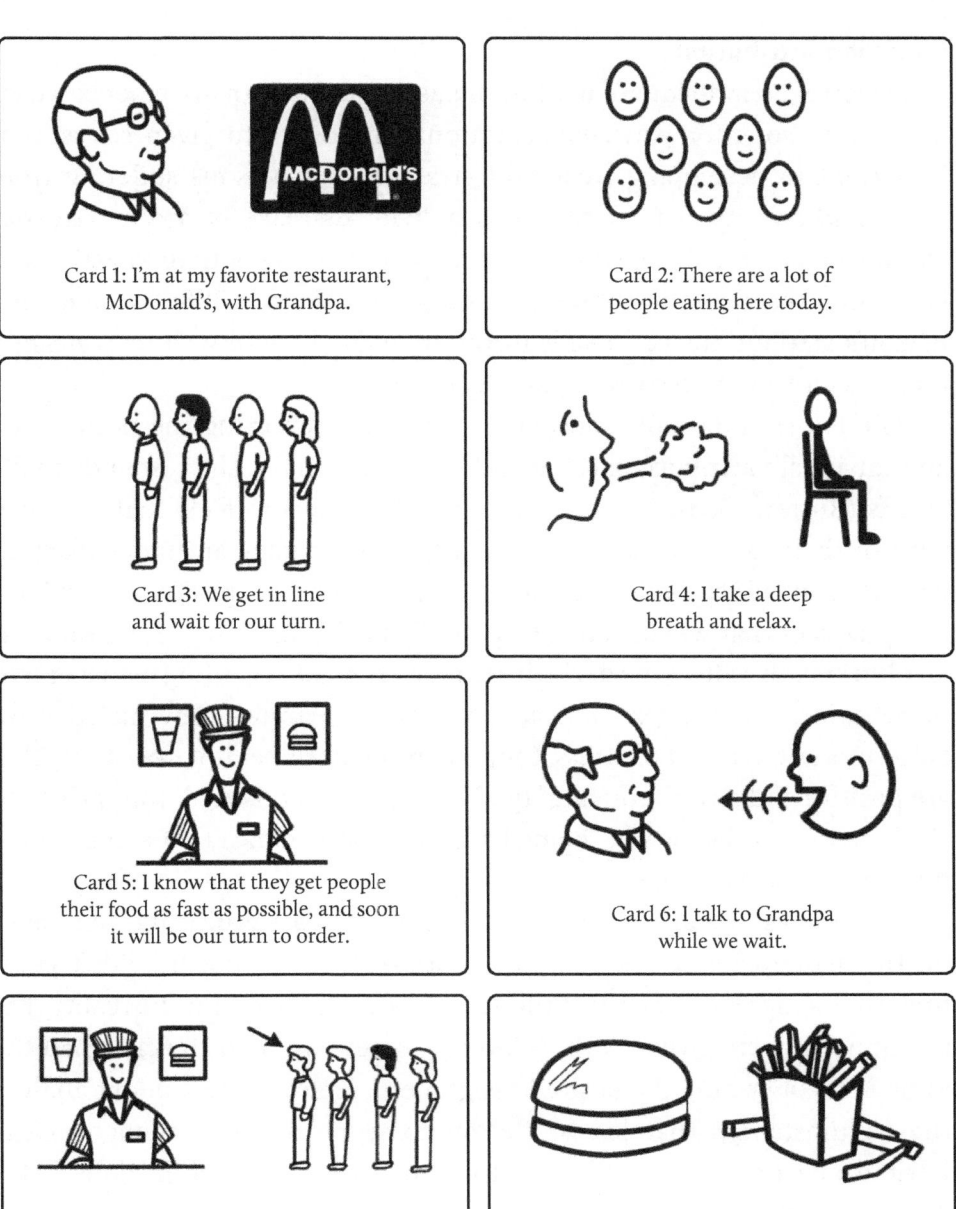

Card 1: I'm at my favorite restaurant, McDonald's, with Grandpa.

Card 2: There are a lot of people eating here today.

Card 3: We get in line and wait for our turn.

Card 4: I take a deep breath and relax.

Card 5: I know that they get people their food as fast as possible, and soon it will be our turn to order.

Card 6: I talk to Grandpa while we wait.

Card 7: Now it is our turn to get our food. That didn't take too long!

Card 8: My hamburger and French fries taste so good. I did a great job waiting!

Figure 9.1 Cognitive Picture Rehearsal Scene that Addresses the Challenge of Waiting in Line at a Restaurant

Source: Reproduced with permission from the Groden Center.

Changing Attributions

Considering an individual's attributions as to the causes of his or her behavior and the reasons for particular emotional responses to given stressors is important in developing treatment strategies for persons suffering from stress and anxiety. The attributions individuals make regarding stressful circumstances have been shown to be good predictors of their affective and behavioral responses in subsequent situations (Weiner, 1986). Changing a person's attributions can result in the individual's ability to respond in a more adaptive way to stressors as they occur.

Groden *et al.* (2006) reported on research supporting the notion that an individual's attributional style influences how he or she responds to life events (Rutter, 1983). The authors write: "If a person feels that they can control their fate and have positive attributions, they are more likely to use self-control, self-reinforcement, positive imagery, positive assertions, and practices that will lead to a brighter future" (p.27). They point out that attributions also affect the decisions caregivers make regarding management of behavioral challenges. "If teachers, staff, or parents view maladaptive behaviors as the result of stress, they will more likely set up procedures that are positive and stress reducing" (p.27). On the other hand, if they attribute the behavior to the person "being bad," there is a chance that some sort of punishment will be imposed.

Sometimes, the attributions individuals make are faulty and not based on the actual causes. For example, a student may think he didn't get a preferred assignment because the teacher doesn't like him. In reality, the assignments were given out by a lottery and everyone in the class had the same odds of getting the desired assignment. Helping the student analyze the circumstances that led to the outcome results in a change in the attribution from "I am not likeable" to "It was just the luck of the draw." This change in thinking can reduce negative feelings and stress. It is important to consider the attributions a person is making in order to develop treatment strategies to address the stress. By identifying stressors and the attributions a person makes about the stressors, it is possible to help the individual change the attribution before the event occurs, thus minimizing or eliminating associated stress.

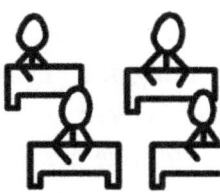

Card 1: I'm in my classroom.

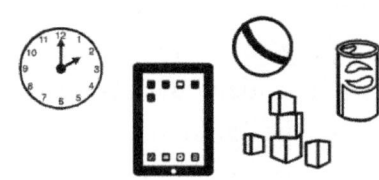

Card 2: It's almost time for me to earn
my reward for having a great day!

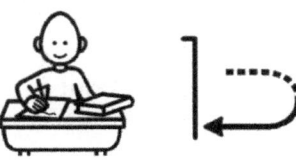

Card 3: I have to wait for my teacher to come
back to the classroom. (Challenging situation)

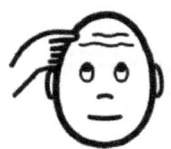

Card 4: I know that my teacher is very busy
and has lots to do. She'll be back soon to give
me my reward. (Changing attribution)

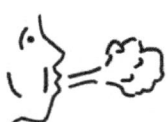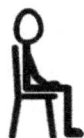

Card 5: I take a deep breath and relax. I
say to myself, "It's only a minute or two.
I can wait." (Self-control strategy)

Card 6: I decide to read a book while
I wait. (Coping strategy)

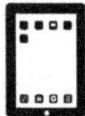

Card 7: I did a great job waiting. I am so proud
of myself. Now I imagine...(*insert something
particularly rewarding for the student such as...*
using my tablet or drinking this soda).

Figure 9.2 Cognitive Picture Rehearsal Scene that Incorporates Changing Attributions

Source: Reproduced with permission from the Groden Center.

An example of how changing attributions can be incorporated into programming for individuals with ASD is shown in Figure 9.2. In this situation, a student with ASD is stressed by waiting for positive events. Previously, the child had said that waiting was related to the teacher forgetting about the student and his reward. A cognitive picture rehearsal scene was created to help the student cope with waiting and change his attribution about it. The scene focuses on the fact that waiting is temporary and not related to the teacher forgetting, and provides the student with stress reduction and self-control activities that can be incorporated to ease the challenge of waiting. The scene ends with the student receiving positive reinforcement for waiting appropriately, and feeling good about his ability to control himself.

Positive Psychology and Stress

To more effectively deal with stress and anxiety in persons with autism and developmental disabilities, we have focused on adapted coping strategies and interventions that foster a person's ability to handle a particular stressor. We also have discussed strategies that can be used on a regular basis, such as relaxation, to reduce general stress and anxiety levels and promote self-control before, during, and after a stressful event. In addition to these options, there are a wide variety of positive psychology traits that can be targeted over time to indirectly assist someone in dealing with stress and anxiety. Examples of these traits include resilience, flow, optimism, self-efficacy, forgiveness, gratitude, empathy, and humor, among others. The development of any one of these traits has the potential to modify a person's response, by affecting how the stressor is initially perceived or encountered. For example, someone who has developed his or her sense of self-efficacy (or the sense that one can handle situations effectively and achieve goals) will encounter a stressor with a more robust sense of confidence in his or her ability to successfully handle that situation. Or someone with a more developed sense of humor can draw on that resource to more effectively see the humorous side of a stressful situation, which can be beneficial indeed.

Another positive psychology trait is resilience, which is a person's ability to "bounce back" from challenges that are encountered in everyday life. In the book *How Everyone on the Autism Spectrum, Young and Old, can...become Resilient, be more Optimistic, enjoy Humor, be Kind, and increase Self-Efficacy*

(Groden *et al.*, 2011), the authors note that Ann Masten defined resilience as "the process of, capacity for, or outcome of successful adaptation despite challenging or threatening circumstances" (Masten *et al.*, 1990). Persons who have a high level of resilience are more able to cope effectively with stress because they not only have the ability to successfully adapt in this manner, but also feel or know that they have this ability to succeed. Such confidence in one's abilities is often half the battle when dealing with challenges, and for persons with autism, the situation is no different. A person with autism has undoubtedly encountered a number of common and less common stressors and problems, and has also likely experienced a significant amount of failure in coping. Knowing or thinking that he or she can get past these failures, re-group and try again (or "bounce back"), and perhaps succeed in the future, is a powerful trait that equips someone with the ability to persevere.

In the book cited above, the authors also reported on the common and more autism-specific stressors that may exist for the person with autism. For example, a person with autism may find the divorce of his or her parents challenging, as anyone would, but additionally situations such as common daily-living activities (entering a public place or riding a bus, for example) may induce unusually high levels of stress. This may be due not only to compromised social skills and increased rigidity, but also to intellectual challenges that may be present. Limited social support resources, frequent failures, and a lack of encouragement from others may also exacerbate the stress levels for persons with autism in areas that typically developing persons might not even consider. Interventions that have promise in promoting resilience are offered by the authors, and include relaxation techniques and targeted cognitive picture rehearsal scenes mentioned previously in this chapter. They also suggest other interventions such as finding areas where a person can realize success. To this end, the authors recommend identifying "islands of competence" where a person's special abilities are highlighted and celebrated, in an effort to acknowledge that person's ability to succeed. For example, a photography program was initiated at the Groden Center to foster these skills and create a sense of accomplishment and competency. This program, entitled My Own World, resulted in photography shows where the students' work was exhibited. The authors also recommend setting reasonable expectations so a person is likely to succeed, encouraging the development of new skills, emphasizing a person's linkage between efforts and success, and celebrating each success no matter how small.

In working with persons with autism who also have intellectual challenges, it is especially important to pursue these goals in a measured and pervasive manner. In other words, it is important to understand that great and immediate gains in traits such as resilience are unlikely, and those working with this population need to be aware of each and every small step made in this direction. Further, efforts such as those noted above need to be throughout the person's environment, and be reflected in teaching materials, statements made by teachers, modeling, attitudes of parents, and all areas of functioning. It is not enough to be a single statement or activity, it must be a goal that penetrates all areas of a person's experience. Knowledge of positive traits and the potential for these traits to better equip a person with autism and intellectual disability to more effectively deal with stress and anxiety must be part of the culture of the organization that works with that person, as well as the home environment. This and other positive psychology traits, when adapted properly, have the potential to give a person tremendous resources in more effectively managing the special challenges encountered in the everyday world.

Integrating New Frontiers in Managing Stress: Mindfulness and Acceptance and Commitment Therapy (ACT)

The adapted coping interventions discussed create both a philosophical and a functional foundation for integrating new trends in the field of psychology. Two current approaches to treatment, mindfulness and Acceptance and Commitment Therapy (ACT), contain strategies that have the potential to greatly enhance services for individuals with autism and other developmental disabilities. Certain elements of these approaches may be applied directly. Others can be woven into established procedures such as cognitive picture rehearsal, and still others will require adaptation for use with this population. In this section, we discuss some of the key elements and the process of adapting them for persons with autism.

Mindfulness

Mindfulness means different things to different people, and has been defined in many ways. One definition is "the awareness that emerges through paying attention on purpose, in the present moment and non-judgmentally to the unfolding of experience moment by moment" (Kabat-Zinn, 2003, p.145). Another definition is "maintaining a moment-by-moment awareness of our thoughts, feelings, bodily sensations, and surrounding environments" (Greater Good Science Center at the University of California at Berkeley, n.d.). The definition of mindfulness can be seen from two perspectives: the Eastern religious tradition in which a state of mindfulness can be achieved through meditation, yoga, and other methods, and a Western scientific perspective as described in *Mindfulness* (Langer, 2014). We will mainly be referring to this Western scientific method, which focuses on paying more attention to the world around us, to context, and the variability within ourselves. However, the two perspectives have a lot in common, in that they both emphasize the importance of awareness, being non-judgmental and being "in the moment." Note that in the relaxation procedure described earlier, becoming aware of muscle groups when they are tense and then learning to relax the tense muscles are essential components of the program. These procedures in and of themselves promote a more mindful state, encouraging the learner to focus on different parts of the body, as well as breathing. Additionally, Langer discusses the key qualities of a mindful state of being: the creation of new categories; openness to new information; and awareness of more than one perspective.

Creating New Categories

Langer (2014) suggests that in creating new categories, we are challenged with thinking of events and situations in new and different ways to better problem-solve or re-frame an event. The purpose is to better identify the core issue by thinking about the situation differently, perhaps breaking it down and making it more tolerable. Given the rigidity and difficulty of seeing things from other perspectives, which is common to persons on the spectrum, making a new category may be very difficult. An individual with autism may get set in a particular speech pattern or sameness of thinking, and find change very difficult. Behaviorally, persons on the spectrum often display stereotypic speech and repeat the same word, idea, or thought over and over, and it is often difficult to break this pattern. However, one way to teach a person with autism to make new categories that assist with coping would be to use small steps. A person with autism, for example, may always give the same answer when asked about gym class, relating an event that causes anxiety. They might consistently and only say, "played in the noisy gym" when asked about activities. Pointed questions could be asked to prompt thinking about this experience in more positive ways such as "What did you do in gym that was fun?" "Exercises" might be a response, and further questioning with some cues might lead to responses like "played with my friends," or "went through the fun tunnel." In this way the person becomes more mindful of the enjoyable aspects of gym rather than the noise, and is less apt to respond in a rote, negative, or automatic manner.

Openness to New Information and Awareness of More than One Perspective

Openness to new information and awareness of different points of view are also important components that can lend themselves to a more mindful state. Exposing students to new experiences and having them reflect on their-own preferences or perceptions, and those of the persons around them, expands awareness and increases focus on the world around them. These abilities, like the creation of new categories, can be fostered by going into new environments, having new experiences in the classroom, and then via sharing in a classroom setting. For example, a class might go on a field trip to the zoo, a restaurant, or the park. After a class has returned from the field trip, students could discuss the trip and make a list of things they saw and what they liked about the trip. Or, photographs could be taken on the field trip, and those with limited speech can point to the pictures of their favorite parts of the outing. Each student could have a turn to present their likes and discuss why they chose those events, giving each one the opportunity to attend to the elements of the experience that he or she found important. Each presentation would generate new information, and these would be from many points of view. The teacher can then discuss how nice it is to hear what each person saw and chose, and then ask the students to describe what they learned from each other. By engaging in this activity, students with autism have the opportunity to receive new information and receive the points of view of their classmates, increasing important elements of mindfulness.

Some of the programs that are designed for persons with autism do have elements of the mindful experience. For example, learning to identify one's own emotions, self-cuing, self-monitoring, and becoming more attuned to the behavior of others all rely on awareness of the self and others. These ideas can be woven into strategies discussed previously, such as CPR. CPR is an excellent way to add mindfulness to scripts that can be personalized. For example, consider Glen, a 20-year-old young man who is functioning in the below average IQ range. He is starting a new job in the supermarket packaging groceries at the checkout counter. He is anxious about beginning his job, and is worried that it will be difficult work and the people he meets may not be nice. A CPR script that incorporates mindful concepts may be of help, such as that given in Figure 9.3.

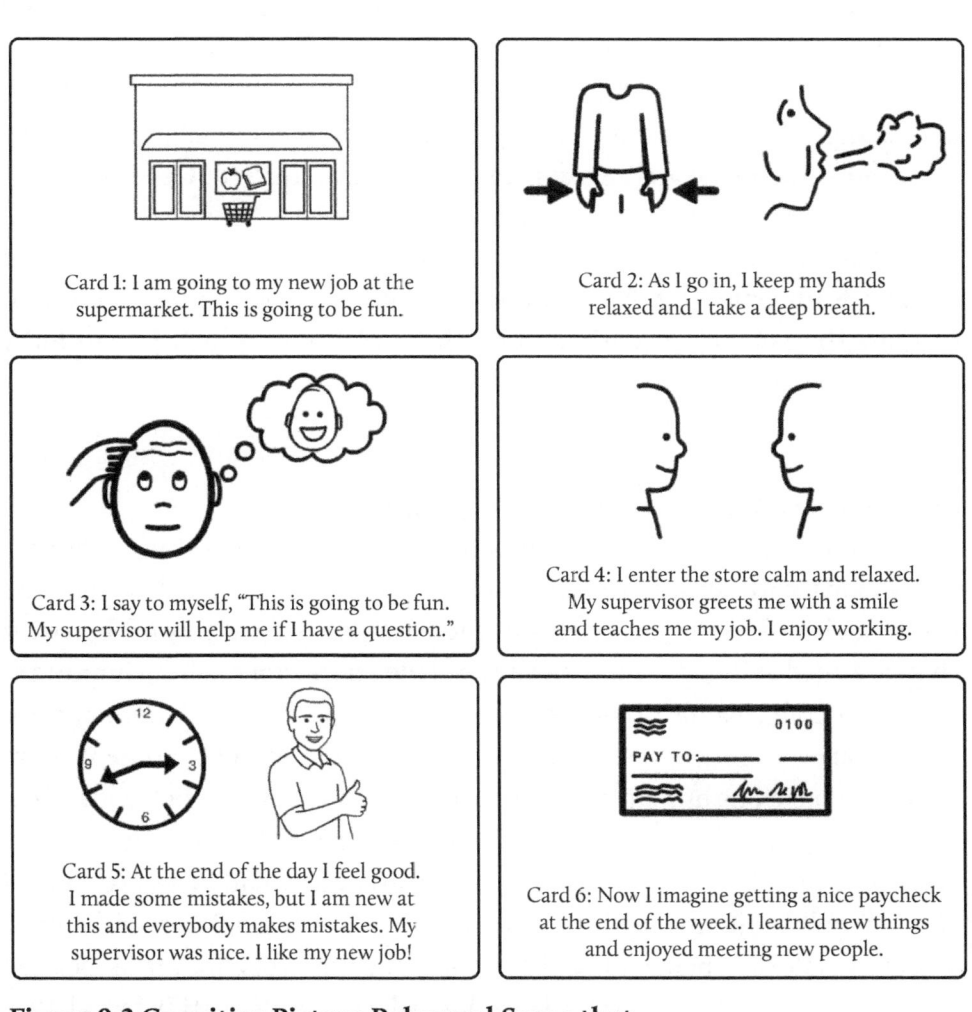

Figure 9.3 Cognitive Picture Rehearsal Scene that Incorporates Elements of Mindfulness

Source: Reproduced with permission from the Groden Center.

In this script, we emphasize that it is important to self-monitor and be aware of fostering a calm and relaxed state. Relaxation is built into the script to cue Glen to be mindful of using relaxation to reduce the stress of starting a new job. We promote new experiences, as well as the points of view of other people. We suggest that work can be fun and the worker can feel good; these may be new categories of ideas for a person who has had less-than-ideal experiences with others. These are all important parts of mindfulness, and can be easily incorporated into CPR scenes. We are also promoting a new attribution: that people can be nice and friendly. Glen would practice this script several times a day for at least two weeks before beginning the job and then it would be changed accordingly once he is on the job.

In this way CPR can incorporate relaxation, components of mindfulness, and changes in attribution. These procedures all blend well and have the same aims—being aware, relaxed, and feeling less stressed. Other ideas for integrating mindfulness might include integrating a "body scan" section in relaxation, developing CPR scenes that are walking meditations in imagery form, or asking, "What are you doing right now?" during relaxation to draw the person's attention to the here and now, which is a primary mindfulness goal.

Acceptance and Commitment Therapy (ACT)

ACT, like mindfulness, has elements that can be integrated into strategies for persons with autism to decrease stress. ACT is designed to increase psychological flexibility, and also to increase persistence toward behavior change aimed at living a more meaningful life and accomplishing important goals. Psychological flexibility is at the core of the ACT model of behavior change, and is defined as the "ability to contact the present moment more fully as a conscious human being and to change or persist in behavior when doing so serves valued ends" (Hayes *et al.*, 2006, p.6). The opposite of this is psychological inflexibility, which focuses on avoidance and excessive control of a person's thoughts, feelings, and emotions. Psychological well-being is reflected in flexible behavior, and behavioral health problems are associated with psychologically inflexible behavior. Gloster *et al.* (2017) found that psychological flexibility moderated a wide variety of stressors in a large Swiss sample, and proposed that increasing psychological flexibility could be a desirable and achievable public health target. Another core component involves encouraging the person to identify the negative effects of avoidance while fostering positive tools to make relevant life changes (Maisel *et al.*, 2019). In an online article describing how ACT works, Ackerman (2017) quotes Dr. Russell Harris's 2011 definition of ACT as a "mindfulness-based therapy that challenges the ground rules of most Western psychology. Its unique goal is to help patients create a rich and meaningful life and develop mindfulness skills alongside the existence of pain and suffering" (paragraph 11). ACT supports people in learning not to overreact to non-desired feeling states, and instead accept these negative feelings and the situations that cause them. People are assisted in making small steps toward what really matters to them, increasing their quality of life and personal meaning. For the purposes of this chapter we will focus on three components of ACT— acceptance, committed action, and cognitive defusion.

Acceptance and Committed Action

Acceptance is an alternative to the instinct to avoid negative (or potentially negative) experiences without trying to change them. In the case of persons with autism, this might mean accepting the diagnosis of autism and understanding the characteristics of the diagnosis, or perhaps accepting some of the challenges and limitations that autism causes. For example, someone with autism may find social interactions or sensory experiences challenging; accepting this and learning ways to cope with these events is more productive than avoiding them or denying them. This entails mustering the courage to face these personal limitations, and the willingness to address problems that hinder the enjoyment of one's life. Another example of this can be seen in the area of difficulty in making changes in employment settings. Working in a job that requires shifting to new assignments or changing day-to-day tasks can be stressful for a person with autism. Accepting this limitation and learning to relax when given a new assignment would be an effective coping skill. The employee might add a cognitive strategy by saying to himself, "I know changing tasks is part of my work and I can handle it. It may be difficult for me, but it is something I need to just accept and deal with. I know I can do it." Deciding to move forward in the face of a challenge and committing to change, and using other coping skills such as learning to ask for help when needed, or focusing on the present and becoming aware of the changes needed for a new task are all examples of positive acceptance. They accept the fact that changing tasks is difficult and they represent a commitment to using strategies that will effect change.

A client came to the Groden Center at age 22 for individual therapy. He had graduated from a good college and had earned a Ph.D. in engineering, but he and his family knew he had many unusual problems that were causing difficulties both at home and at work. Neither he nor his family knew what the cause was, and that he had autism. He had no friends and no social life, and he had difficulty in processing simple information, except for the high-level information at his job and in his earlier coursework. After his assessment was completed and he received a formal diagnosis of autism, he and his family were relieved to finally understand the basis for so many of his problems. Accepting the diagnosis of autism was challenging, but ultimately he met this challenge in a positive way, and was committed to participating in therapies that could assist him in adjusting to the demands of his work and social life. These therapies included social skills training, vocational training (interviewing, dressing for work, using transportation, and other work skills), and behavioral therapy. The behavioral therapy that he did individually included a number of stress-reduction techniques, such as relaxation, cognitive picture rehearsal, practice problem solving, and work on awareness training, changing attributions, and other therapies addressing personal problems. By focusing on accepting the diagnosis of autism and its challenges, and committing to learning positive ways to cope with these challenges, he was able to improve his quality of life; he has since married, holds a good job, and is enjoying many aspects of an enriched and active life.

Cognitive Fusion

Cognitive fusion is a client's belief that his or her negative thoughts are true. This set of beliefs can have automatic and devastating effects on a person's functioning. Negative thoughts are emotionally disturbing, and "cognitive fusion often leads to acting in accordance with such problematic thoughts" (Tyndall *et al.*, 2018, p.4). The authors go on to explain that cognitive fusion is the process in which the content of one's thoughts comes to exert excessive control over an individual, leads to difficulty in tracking experiences outside of the actual content of the specific thoughts, and leaves the person feeling restricted and compelled to act on what the thoughts tell him or her to do. Avoidance behavior is often associated with cognitive fusion, because if something negative is automatically accepted as true, then one's first instinct is to move away from that feeling or event. Avoidance temporarily reduces the stress of negative experiences, but doesn't offer the opportunity for new or better learning to take place. It reduces the chance of experiencing positive reinforcement by dealing with the negative feeling or participating in what could be pleasurable events. This perpetuates the avoidance behavior.

In order to counteract cognitive fusion, we suggest cognitive defusion; it is a dynamic and ongoing process. Rather than seeing the world as organized through one's own negative thoughts, cognitive defusion "aims to reduce the impact of these arbitrarily derived stimulus functions by teaching people to challenge conventions of language in order to relate to their thoughts in less rigid ways" (Maisel *et al.*, 2019, p.35). Cognitive defusion fosters an examination of internal messages and language, and encourages people to reduce the believability of any given negative thought. This concept can be adapted for persons with autism and various levels of cognitive functioning, and can be of value because persons with autism will have many negative life experiences if he or she has not experienced supportive home and school environments, proper teaching methods, appropriate curricula, and caretakers who understand the social, sensory, and other challenges of persons on the spectrum. These repeated experiences can quickly lead to negative thoughts that are automatic, and that begin to govern a person's behavior. In early years, this may lead to a negative self-image, avoidance of socializing and playing with friends, refusal to engage in academic tasks that are difficult, and disruptive, tantrum, or aggressive behavior to avoid further negative experiences. As a person with autism ages, much like persons who are typically developing, these negative thoughts become more and more entrenched, affect all areas of functioning, and become "true."

Bernie is a 14-year-old boy with autism. He is functioning below average, and has problems with tantrum behavior and avoidance whenever he is asked to do something that is new or difficult for him. Math is especially hard, and in the past, not all his teachers have been supportive and encouraging. He has had many assessments to correctly place him on the right level of the academic curriculum, but because of these behaviors, he has difficulty making and keeping friends and avoids social encounters. One can easily imagine how these math challenges have led to further negative experiences, and negative thoughts such as "I'm stupid," "no one likes me," "I will never be able to do math," or "when someone asks me to do math, I will get very angry." Cognitive defusion challenges the person to look at these thoughts and decide whether or not they are true. In this case it would be difficult to address thinking and reflection with Bernie, due to his limited communication skills and cognitive functioning. Instead, the cognitive picture rehearsal script shown in Figure 9.4 has been designed for him and incorporates acceptance, commitment, and challenging of these negative thoughts by positing replacement thinking.

In this CPR scene, we have combined components of acceptance, relaxation, and new ideas that directly challenge established negative thoughts. Bernie practices thinking that he is smart and people like him, and that he can stay calm rather than display problem behaviors. Note that challenging thinking is very similar to changing attributions, and that these interventions begin to overlap and complement each other. Each scene also includes positive reinforcement, because we want the person to immediately see the positive outcome of this line of thinking, and we want this behavior to increase. Bernie is also accepting the fact that math is hard for him, and he is committed to becoming aware of the problems he is working on and trying to solve them. He should practice this scene three times each day with his teacher and repeat it before math class. The more this type of thinking is rehearsed, the better it is for the individual whose behavior is targeted for change. As always, it is important to include parents and caregivers in the behavior change program by providing them with a copy of the scene to practice with the student at home.

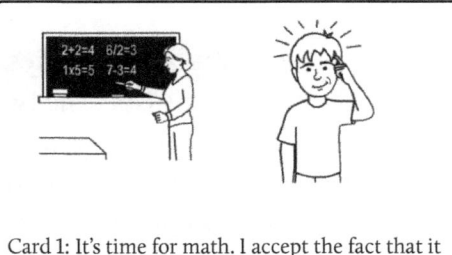

Card 1: It's time for math. I accept the fact that it is difficult for me, but that doesn't bother me.

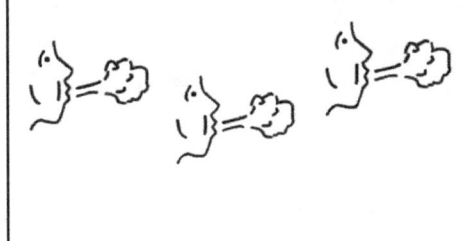

Card 2: I relax and take three deep breaths.

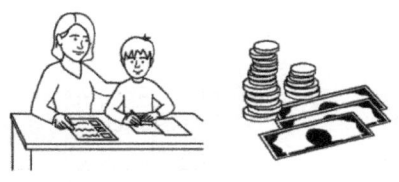

Card 3: My teacher comes to my desk to work with me. I am working on counting money so I can use it when I go shopping.

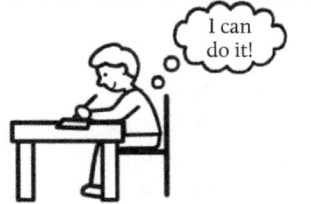

Card 4: I say to myself, "I can do it!" and I can ask for help if I need it.

Card 5: I correct the paper and I feel great that I am learning math and becoming really good at it.

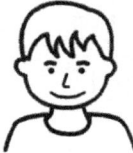

Card 6: I am beginning to like math and am able to stay calm. When I go to the store with my friends, I can buy something. This is fun!

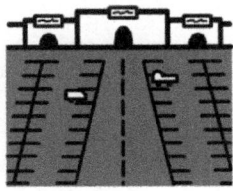

Card 7: Now I think about being at the store, picking out something I like.

Figure 9.4 Cognitive Picture Rehearsal Scene that Incorporates Elements of Acceptance and Commitment Therapy

Source: Reproduced with permission from the Groden Center.

Summary

In this chapter we have addressed the salient issues in the areas of stress, anxiety, and coping with stress within the population with autism. The two figures below summarize our discussion. Figure 9.5, "Challenging Issues in Research and Treatments on Stress and Anxiety in Autism," is a depiction of the problems that we have identified. Figure 9.6, "Recommendations for Research and Treatments on Stress and Anxiety in Autism," lays out our suggestions to strengthen the research and resulting treatments.

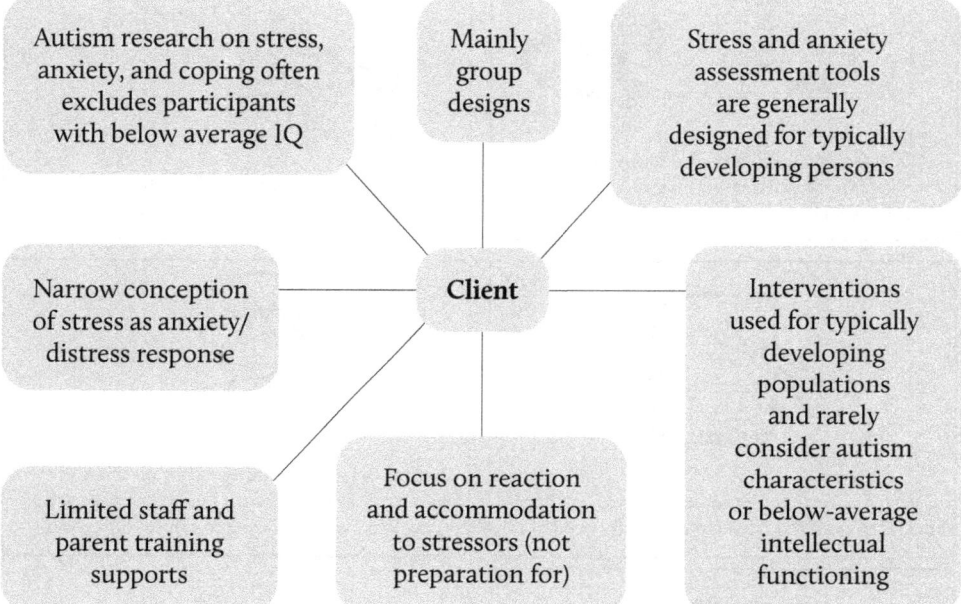

Figure 9.5 Challenging Issues in Research and Treatments on Stress and Anxiety in Autism

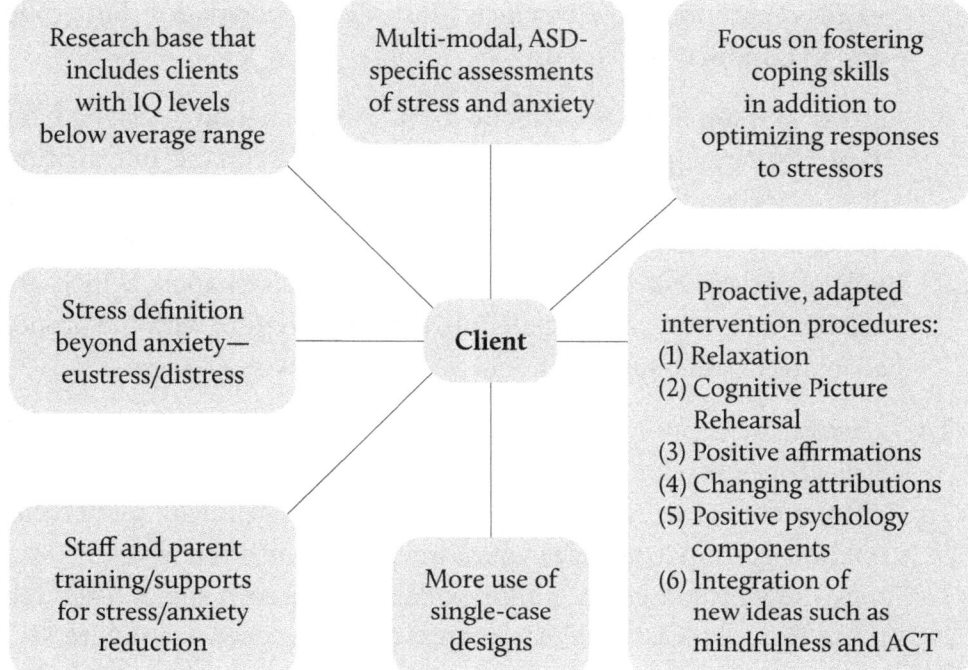

Figure 9.6 Recommendations for Research and Treatments on Stress and Anxiety in Autism

The following is a brief description of the seven major issues outlined in Figure 9.5, and the recommendations offered in Figure 9.6 to address these concerns:

1. Autism Research on Stress, Anxiety, and Coping Often Excludes Participants with Below Average IQ: Participants in recent research on stress and autism are mainly average or above average IQ although two-thirds of the population are below average IQ. Therefore, the results of the research do not necessarily apply to a large percentage of the population.

2. Mainly Group Designs: The autism spectrum is comprised of persons who have a range of IQs, vary widely in behavioral problems, have a variety of speech problems from non-verbal to echolalia, limited comprehension, and difficulty with idioms, and there is much diversity in the ability to speak and understand language. Because of this wide range, single-case design in research (Hersen and Barlow,

1976) is appropriate and beneficial to study this population, but group design is more widely used.

3. Stress and Anxiety Assessment Tools Are Generally Designed for Typically Developing Persons: In order to obtain suitable information during assessments, it is important to use tools that are specifically designed for this population—otherwise appropriate treatments may not be prescribed. Procedures described in this chapter, which are used for a neurotypical population, can be successful with the proper adaptations. Adaptations should be informed by assessments.

4. Narrow Conception of Stress as Anxiety/Distress Response: Eustress as described by Hans Selye is not considered in much of the research or treatment of stress in this population. It can be difficult for persons on the spectrum to engage in pleasant events, and often when they do, they show responses like jumping, flapping, or even anger. Although the events are pleasurable, these stress responses need to be addressed.

5. Limited Staff and Parent Training Supports: This is a problem in many inclusive environments such as schools, nursing homes, and vocational sites where teachers, parents, co-workers, and caregivers are not given training and information relevant to working with people with autism.

6. Focus on Reaction and Accommodation to Stressors (not preparation for): Following a multi-modal stress assessment and the identification of stressors, proactive coping strategies that can be used before the stressor occurs can lead to prevention of maladaptive stress responses. Procedures such as relaxation and CPR can be taught and used for self-control. Although these procedures might take longer to master, in the long run they are more useful than quick reactive strategies such as punishment.

7. Proactive, Adapted Intervention Procedures: The adapted procedures are listed in Figure 9.6 and thoroughly discussed in this chapter. All the treatments work well together and are complementary. There are a number of commonalities among them. They:

   • are personalized—individual needs are considered

- are applicable to all ages, developmental needs, behavioral challenges, and environmental effects

- can be used at home, in school, and in all community environments

- include participation and input from learners

- are based on effective procedures in the literature

- are positive procedures

- are incorporated within a setting that offers high-quality curricula (if in school), team working that includes medical services, other appropriate therapies, and other strong and functionally based programs.

At the Groden Center, we have tried to isolate the components of effective treatment for many of our children and adults, and time after time we have come to the conclusion that it was not a single treatment that contributed to the success of the behavioral treatment, but always a combination. These were different for each person, because they were individualized to meet each person's needs. This provides support for a broad spectrum, rather than relying on single measures.

In closing, it is important to remember that it is not stress that controls us but how we handle stress that impacts our health and wellness.

References

Ackerman, C. (2017). How does Acceptance and Commitment Therapy (ACT) work? Positive Psychology Program. com. Retrieved from www.positivepsychologyprogram.com/act-acceptance-and-committment-therapy.

Baer, D. M., Peterson, R. F., and Sherman, J. A. (1967). The development of imitation by reinforcing behavioral similarity to a model. *Journal of the Experimental Analysis of Behavior, 10*(5), 405–416.

Baron, M. G., Lipsitt, L. P., and Goodwin, M. S. (2006). Scientific foundations for research and practice. In M. G. Baron, J. Groden, G. Groden and L. P. Lipsitt (Eds.), *Stress and Coping in Autism.* New York, NY: Oxford University Press.

Bellini, S. (2004). Social skills deficits and anxiety in high-functioning adolescents with autism spectrum disorders. *Focus on Autism and Other Developmental Disabilities, 19*(2), 78–86.

Benson, H. (1984). *Beyond the Relaxation Response.* New York, NY: Times Books.

Bishop-Fitzpatrick, L., Mazefsky, C. A., Minshew, N. J. and Eack, S. M. (2014). The relationship between stress and social functioning in adults with autism spectrum disorder and without intellectual disability. *Autism Research, 8*(2), 1–18.

Chorpita, B. F., Yim, L., Moffitt, C., Umemoto, L. A., and Francis, S. E. (2000). Assessment of symptoms of DSM-IV anxiety and depression in children: A revised child and anxiety and depression scale. *Behavior Research and Therapy, 38,* 835–855.

Corbett, B. A., Schupp, C. W., Levine, S., and Mendoza, S. (2009). Comparing cortisol, stress and sensory sensitivity in children with autism. *Autism Research, 2*(1), 39–49.

Gillott, A. and Standen, P. J. (2007). Levels of anxiety and sources of stress in adults with autism. *Journal of Intellectual Disabilities, 11*(4), 359–370.

Gloster, A. T., Meyer, A. H., and Lieb, R. (2017). Psychological flexibility as a malleable public health target: Evidence from a representative sample. *Journal of Contextual Behavioural Science, 6*(2), 166–171.

Goldsmith, H. H., Reilly, J., Lemery, K. S., Longley, S., and Prescott, A. (1999). *The Laboratory Temperament Assessment Battery: Preschool Version.* Madison, WI: University of Wisconsin.

Goodwin, M. S., Groden, J., Velicer, W., Lipsett, L., Baron, M. G., Hofmann, S. G., and Groden, G. (2006). Cardiovascular arousal in individuals with autism. *Focus on Autism and Other Developmental Disabilities, 21*(2), 100–123.

Goodwin, M. S., Groden, J., Velicer, W., and Diller, A. (2007). Validating the stress survey schedule for persons with autism and other developmental disabilities. *Focus on Autism and other Developmental Disabilities, 22*(3), 3, 183–189.

Greater Good Science Center at the University of California at Berkeley (n.d.). What is mindfulness? Retrieved from https://greatergood.berkeley.edu/topic/mindfulness/definition.

Groden, G. and Baron, M. G. (Eds.) (1988). *AUTISM, Strategies for Change: A Comprehensive Approach to the Education and Treatment of Children with Autism and Related Disorders.* New York, NY: Gardner Press.

Groden, J., Cautela, J., Prince, S., and Berryman, J. (1994). The impact of stress and anxiety on individuals with autism and developmental disabilities. In E. Schopler and G. E. Mesibov (Eds.), *Behavioral Issues in Autism.* New York, NY: Plenum Press.

Groden, J., and LeVasseur, P. (1995). Cognitive Picture Rehearsal: A system to teach self-control. In K. Quill (Ed.), *Teaching Children with Autism: Strategies to Enhance Learning, Communication and Socialization.* Albany, NY: Delmar Publishing Company.

Groden, G., Stevenson, S., and Groden, J. (1996). *Understanding Challenging Behavior: A Step-by-Step Behavior Analysis Guide.* Worthington, OH: Ids Publishing Corporation.

Groden, J., Diller, A., Bausman, M., Velicer, W., Norman, G., and Cautela, J. (2001). The development of a stress survey schedule for persons with autism and other developmental disabilities. *Journal of Autism and Developmental Disorders, 17*(2), 207–217.

Groden, J., LeVasseur, P., Diller, A. and Cautela, J. (2002). *Coping with Stress through Picture Rehearsal: A How-to Manual for Working with Individuals with Autism and Developmental Disabilities.* Providence, RI: The Groden Center, Inc.

Groden, J., Baron, M. G., and Groden, G. (2006). Assessment and coping strategies. In M. G. Baron, J. Groden, G. Groden, and L. P. Lipsett (Eds.), *Stress and Coping in Autism,* New York, NY: Oxford University Press.

Groden, J., Kantor, A., Woodard, C. R., and Lipsitt, L. (2011). *How Everyone on the Autism Spectrum, Young and Old, can ..become Resilient, be more Optimistic, enjoy Humor, be Kind, and increase Self-Efficacy.* Philadelphia, PA: Jessica Kingsley Publishers.

Groden, J., Weidenman, L., and Diller, A. (2016a). *Relaxation: A Comprehensive Manual for Children and Adults with Autism and Other Developmental Disabilities* (2nd ed.). Champaign, IL: Research Press.

Groden J., Weidenman, L., and Woodard, C. R. (2016b). A stress-reduction approach to addressing self-injurious behavior in individuals with autism. In S. M. Edelson and J. Botsford Johnson (Eds.), *Understanding and Treating Self-Injurious Behavior in Autism.* Philadelphia, PA: Jessica Kingsley Publishers.

Harmony, C., Woodard, C. R., and Groden, J. (2019). A comparison of the Stress Survey Schedule in children with autism and typically developing children: A brief report. Under review.

Hayes, S. C., Luoma, J. B., Bond, F. W., Masuda, A. and Lillis, J. (2006). Acceptance and Commitment Therapy: Models, processes and outcomes. *Behavior Research and Therapy, 44,* 1–25.

Hersen, M. and Barlow, D. H. (1976). *Single Case Experimental Designs.* New York, NY: Pergamon Press.

Hirvikoski, T., and Blomqvist, M. (2015). High self-perceived stress and poor coping in intellectually able adults with autism spectrum disorder. *Autism, 19*(6), 752–757.

Hobfoil, S. E. (2001). The influence of culture, community, and all nested-self in the stress process: Advancing conservation of resources theory. *Applied Psychology: An International Journal, 50,* 337–421.

Hodgdon, L. (1995). *Visual Strategies for Improving Communication.* Troy, MI: Quirk Roberts Publishing.

Hollocks, M. J., Howliln, P., Papadopoulos, A. S., Khondoker, M., and Simonoff, E. (2014). Differences in HPA-axis and heart rate responsiveness to psychosocial stress in children with autism spectrum disorders with and without co-morbid anxiety. *Psychoneuroendocrinology, 46*, 32–45.

Hufnagel, C., Chambres, P., Bertrand, P. R., and Dutheil, F. (2017). The need for objective measures of stress in autism. *Frontiers in Psychology, 8*, 1–4.

Jacobson, E. (1938). *Progressive Relaxation*. Chicago, IL: University of Chicago Press.

Kabat-Zinn, J. (2003). Mindfulness-based interventions in context: Past, present, and future. *Clinical Psychology: Science and Practice, 10*(2), 144–156.

Kerns, C. M., Kendall, P. C., Berry, L., Souders, M. C., Franklin, M. E., Schultz, R. T., Miller, J., and Herrington, J. (2014). Traditional and atypical presentations of anxiety in youth with autism spectrum disorder. *Journal of Autism and Developmental Disorders, 44*(11), 2851–2861.

Langer, E. J. (2014). *Mindfulness: 25th Anniversary Edition*. Philadelphia, PA: Da Capo Press.

Lanni, K. E., Schupp, C. W., Simon, D. and Corbett, B. A. (2012). Verbal ability, social stress, and anxiety in children with autistic disorder. *Autism, 16*(2), 123–138.

Lazarus, R. S. and Folkman, S. (1984). *Stress, Appraisal and Coping*. New York, NY: Springer.

Lovaas, O. I., Koegel, R., Simmons, J. Q., and Long, J. S. (1973). Some generalization and follow-up measures on autistic children in behavior therapy. *Journal of Applied Behavior Analysis, 6*(1), 131–166.

MacNeil, B., Lopes V. A., and Minnes, P. M. (2008). Anxiety in children and adolescents with Autism Spectrum Disorder. *Research in Autism Spectrum Disorders, 3*, 1–21.

Maisel, M., Stephenson, K., Cox, J. and South, M. (2019). Cognitive defusion for reducing distressing thoughts in adults with autism. *Research in Autism Spectrum Disorders, 59*, 34–45.

Masten, A. S., Best, K. M., and Garemezy, N. (1990). Resilience and development: Contributions from the study of children who overcome adversity. *Development and Psychopathology, 2*(4), 425–444.

Panju, S., Brian, J., Dupuis, A., Anagnostou, E., and Kushki, A. (2015). Atypical sympathetic arousal in children with autism spectrum disorder and its association with anxiety symptomatology. *Molecular Autism, 6*(64), 1–19.

Rance, G., Chisari, D., Saunders, K., and Rault, J. (2017). Reducing listening-related stress in school-aged children with autism spectrum disorder. *Journal of Autism and Developmental Disorders, 47*(7), 2010–2022.

Rodgers, J., Wigham, S., McConachie, H., Freeston, M., Honey, E., and Parr, J. R. (2016). Development of the Anxiety Scale for Children with Autism Spectrum Disorder (ASC-ASD). *Autism Research, 9*, 1205–1215.

Romanczyk, R. G., and Gillis, J. M. (2006). Autism and the physiology of stress and anxiety. In M. G. Baron, J. Groden, G. Groden, and L. P. Lipsett (Eds.), *Stress and Coping in Autism*, New York, NY: Oxford University Press.

Rutter, M. (1983). Stress, coping and development: Some issues and some questions. In N. Garmezy and M. Rutter (Eds.), *Stress, Coping, and Development in Children*. New York, NY: McGraw-Hill.

Selye, H. (1956). *The Stress of Life*. New York, NY: McGraw-Hill.

Spratt, E. G., Nicholas, J. S., Brady, K. T., Carpenter, L. A., Hatcher, C. R., Meekins, K. A., Furlanetto, R. W., and Charles, J. A. (2012). Enhanced cortisol response to stress in children in autism. *Journal of Autism and Developmental Disorders, 42*, 75–81.

Thoits, P. A. (1995). Stress, coping, and social support processes: Where are we? What next? *Journal of Health and Social Behavior, 35*, 53–79.

Turner, R. J., and Roszell, P. (1994). Psychosocial resources and the stress process. In W. R. Avison and I. H. Gotlib (Eds.), *Stress and Mental Health: Contemporary Issues and Prospects for the Future*. New York, NY: Plenum Press.

Tyndall, I., Waldeck, D., Pancani, L., Whelan, R., Roche, B., and Pereira, A. (2018). Profiles of psychological flexibility: A latent class analysis of the Acceptance and Commitment Therapy model. *Behavior Modification*, 1–29.

Weiner, B. (1986). *An Attributional Theory of Motivation and Emotion*. New York, NY: Springer.

White, S. W., Oswald, D., Ollendick, T., and Scahill, L. (2009). Anxiety in children and adolescents with autism spectrum disorders. *Clinical Psychology Review, 29*, 216–229.

Wolpe, J. (1958). *Psychotherapy by Reciprocal Inhibition*. Stanford, CA: Stanford University Press.

Zantinge, G., van Rijn, S., Stockmann, L., and Swaab, H. (2017). Physiological arousal and emotion regulation strategies in young children with autism spectrum disorders. *Journal of Autism and Developmental Disorders, 47*(9), 1–15.

CHAPTER 10

Assessing and Treating Anxiety in Individuals with Autism Spectrum Disorder

Lauren J. Moskowitz, Ph.D., Megan Braconnier, M.A., and Melissa Jeffay, M.S., St. John's University, New York

In spite of the fact that anxiety is one of the most common presenting problems for individuals with autism spectrum disorder (ASD) (White *et al.*, 2009), symptoms of anxiety often go unrecognized or overlooked in this population. Although part of that may be due to diagnostic overshadowing, or the belief that symptoms of anxiety are "better explained by the ASD itself" (White *et al.*, 2009), this is also in large part due to the difficulty of assessing anxiety in individuals with ASD. "Anxiety" is a multi-component construct that involves *feelings* or affective states (e.g., subjective fear and panic experienced), *cognitions* (thoughts, beliefs, and images, such as worry and dread), *behavioral* escape or avoidance of the feared situation (and nonverbal behaviors such as crying, whining, and visible muscle tension), and associated *physiological arousal* (Barlow, 2000; Wolpe, 1958). The emotions, cognitions, and physiological arousal are more difficult to assess than overt behaviors in individuals with ASD. In general, anxiety is difficult to assess in this population because of the communication deficits that are inherent in ASD, the presence of co-occurring intellectual disability (ID) in some individuals with ASD, symptom overlap between ASD and anxiety disorders in our current diagnostic classification system, and the fact that symptoms of anxiety can manifest differently in individuals with ASD (see Moskowitz *et al.*, 2017a and the Introduction in this book for more detail). In particular, individuals with ASD are more likely to express fear or anxiety through "problem behaviors" such as aggression, self-injury, and tantrums

(White *et al.*, 2009). Thus, it may be that parents, teachers, or clinicians may not recognize fear or anxiety in individuals with ASD—especially in those who are minimally verbal and/or have ID—and may even attribute their problem behavior to noncompliance, disobedience, oppositionality, or anger/irritability rather than attributing their problem behavior to fear or anxiety. For this reason, and given the functional impairments that are associated with comorbid anxiety in individuals with ASD (see e.g., Kerns *et al.*, 2015), it is important for parents, teachers, and practitioners to learn how to identify and treat anxiety in persons with ASD.

Methods of Assessing Anxiety in ASD
Self-Report Questionnaires
As previously mentioned in the Introduction to this book, the most commonly used method to assess anxiety in typically developing (TD) individuals is self-report, which involves asking the individuals themselves to report on their thoughts, feelings, and behaviors. Although these self-reports were not specifically designed to assess anxiety in ASD, self-report questionnaires such as the Multidimensional Anxiety Scale for Children (MASC-C; March *et al.*, 1997) and the Screen for Child Anxiety Related Emotional Disorders (SCARED-C; Birmaher *et al.*, 1999) are appropriate for screening and measuring treatment outcome in youth with ASD who have greater verbal ability, whereas the Revised Child Anxiety and Depression Scale (RCADS; Chorpita *et al.*, 2000) may be useful for youth with ASD who have less verbal ability. Additionally, the Anxiety Scale for Children—ASD (ASC-ASD; Rodgers *et al.*, 2016) is a self- or parent-report questionnaire that is an adapted version of the RCADS with additional items related to sensory anxiety, uncertainty, and phobias; it is validated with youth with ASD (ages 8–16 years) and is free to download.

There is not as much research on assessing anxiety in adults with ASD, although the Depression Anxiety Stress Scales (DASS-21; Lovibond and Lovibond, 1995) and mini Social Phobia Inventory (mini-SPIN) have been used with adults with ASD as rapid screening devices (Nah *et al.*, 2018) and the Hospital Anxiety and Depression Scale (HADS; Uljarevic *et al.*, 2018) has also been used with adults with ASD. The Spence Children's Anxiety Scale—Parent Version has been modified for use with adults with ASD (Gillott and

Standen, 2007). Finally, Rodgers *et al.* (2016) are in the process of adapting the ASC-ASD for adults.

Although most self-reports require a second- or third-grade reading level and thus may be inappropriate for individuals with ASD who have comorbid ID, some self-reports can be used for individuals with ID and/ or minimal verbal ability if they are modified. Modifications include asking questions both verbally and visually, using simpler language, limiting the number of words, and providing pictures of response options (i.e., a visual scale of facial expressions of fear) (Hartley and MacLean, 2006).

Other-Informant-Report Questionnaires

Many self-report questionnaires, such as the MASC, SCARED, and ASC-ASD, also have versions that can be completed by other informants, such as parents and teachers. However, in our clinical and research experience, some parents of youth with ASD expressed that they felt unable to accurately answer many of the items on parent-report measures (such as "My child worries about other people liking him" on the SCARED) because they were not sure what their children were thinking. As such, the Parent-rated Anxiety Scale for ASD (PRAS-ASD; Scahill *et al.*, 2019) was recently created because, on most anxiety questionnaires, parents of youth with ASD often fail to endorse language-dependent items such as "worries" or "complains," particularly when the child also has ID. The PRAS-ASD was validated with parents of 990 youth with ASD, including those with ID (Scahill *et al.*, 2019). In general, other-informant reports are important to obtain, given that youth with ASD show poor diagnostic agreement with parents and clinical consensus, whereas parents of youth with ASD show better diagnostic agreement with clinical consensus (Storch *et al.*, 2012). Even in clinical samples that include other disorders, youth self-reports were less discriminating than parent reports, whereas combined parent and youth reports were more discriminating, which was replicated across several different measures (Kuhn *et al.*, 2017). Thus, although the combination of parent and self-reports generally does best, when only the parent or the adolescent can be assessed, the findings of Kuhn *et al.* (2017) suggest that parents will generally be the informants of choice.

Interviews

Although questionnaires are less time- and resource-intensive than interviews, diagnoses of anxiety disorders tend to be more accurately made using interviews, which provide more detailed information from the child's and/or parent's verbal reports as well as allow for observations of the child's behavior during the interview. Although most interviews used to assess anxiety in youth with ASD have been designed for TD youth, the Anxiety Disorders Interview Schedule for DSM-IV, Child and Parent Versions (ADIS-IV-C/P; Silverman and Albano, 1996) and the Schedule for Affective Disorders and Schizophrenia in School-Aged Children (K-SADS-PL; Kaufman *et al.*, 1997) have been used with youth with ASD. However, these interviews do not have a systematic approach to differentiate symptoms of anxiety from core features of ASD and may not capture the idiosyncratic manifestations of anxiety in ASD. More recently, Kerns *et al.* (2014b) developed the Autism Spectrum Addendum to the ADIS-P (the ADIS/A), which differentiates DSM anxiety disorders in ASD from the more atypical anxiety (e.g., worries regarding schedule or environmental changes) often present in ASD. Although interviews may be more accurate or detailed than questionnaires, it still may be challenging for individuals with ASD to verbally report their symptoms of anxiety and/or for informants to recognize the symptoms of anxiety in ASD. See Moskowitz *et al.* (2017a) for a more thorough review of self-report questionnaires, other-informant questionnaires, interviews, physiological measures, and direct observation measures to assess anxiety in youth with ASD.

Again, there is less research on adults with ASD, but the Anxiety Disorders Interview Schedule (ADIS-IV; Brown *et al.*, 1994), a semi-structured interview, and the MINI-Plus (Sheehan *et al.*, 1998), a structured diagnostic interview, have been used with adults with ASD. Additionally, the Mini PAS-ADD Clinical Interview, an abbreviated version of the Psychiatric Assessment Schedule for Adults with Developmental Disability (PAS-ADD; Moss *et al.*, 1998), was designed for adults with ID.

Direct Observation

Given that the usefulness of self-report and informant-report is often limited in individuals with ASD due to their aforementioned communication difficulties, anxiety in individuals with ASD must often be inferred from the individual's overt behavior or "fear responses" using direct observation (Moskowitz *et al.*, 2017a; Rosen *et al.*, 2016). Unstructured behavioral observation typically takes place during the initial interview (e.g., the clinician observes the child's body posture, facial expressions, verbalizations, etc.) and can also occur in the child's natural environment (e.g., home, school, community). For a more structured observation, the practitioner can use a Behavioral Approach Test (BAT), also known as a Behavioral Avoidance Test (BAT; Dadds *et al.*, 1994), which involves progressively exposing the person to the feared stimulus or situation along some dimension (e.g., distance, time), while the practitioner assesses the person's avoidance response, subjective level of anxiety, physiological reactions, and/or behavioral responses (Velting *et al.*, 2004). BATs can be used to observe levels of anxiety during assessment as well as during and after intervention to evaluate treatment outcomes. The BAT may be more useful to assess for phobias and obsessive-compulsive disorder (OCD) than for persons with more generalized anxiety, in which it may be more challenging to identify or control stimuli that evoke anxiety (Hagopian and Jennett, 2008).

As such, Hagopian and Jennett (2014) differentiated between "simple avoidance" in which the person with ASD avoids non-preferred stimuli or situations (such as a disliked academic task) versus "anxious avoidance" in which the person exhibits avoidant behavior accompanied by traditional symptoms of anxiety including facial expressions indicative of fear, increased physiological arousal and, if possible, self-reported anxiety. One way to differentiate between simple avoidance versus anxious avoidance is to assess the context in which avoidant behavior and physiological arousal occur, as part of a multi-method assessment.

Multi-Method Assessment of Anxiety in ASD

Given the aforementioned limitations of self-reports, other-informant-reports, interviews, physiological methods, and direct observations in assessing anxiety in ASD, it is important to use multiple methods to assess anxiety in ASD rather than just relying on one single method. For example, Moskowitz *et al.* (2013) developed a multi-method assessment strategy to assess anxiety in children with ASD and ID. We will describe this process in detail.

Behavioral Component of Anxiety

First, we assessed the *behavioral* component of anxiety by identifying the particular idiosyncratic behaviors that indicate anxiety (e.g., crying, pacing, freezing, following parent, reassurance-seeking), unique to each child with ASD. As Rodgers (2018) noted, there may be some behaviors people with ASD exhibit when they are feeling anxious that may not readily be recognized as anxiety. For example, adolescents and adults with ASD reported that, when they are feeling anxious, they may become more repetitive in their actions and more insistent on routines, perhaps as a way of dealing with uncertainty, fear of failure, and sensory input (Joyce *et al.*, 2017; Rodgers, 2018). For those individuals with ASD who cannot self-report what they do when they feel anxious, it is important for parents, teachers, and caretakers to carefully observe and identify behaviors that might indicate anxiety. Although any behavior on its own does not necessarily indicate anxiety (e.g., a child may cry because he is feeling afraid, sad, frustrated, tired, ill, or in pain), multiple sources of converging data may suggest that the behavior is a sign or marker of anxiety. We identified these behaviors from a comprehensive list of behavioral indicators of fear/anxiety (see Appendix A) derived from a variety of sources, such as the Cues for Tension and Anxiety Survey Schedule (CTASS; Cautela, 1977), the Affex Facial Coding System for Negative Facial Expressions (Izard *et al.*, 1989), the Behavioral Relaxation Scale (BRS; Poppen, 1988), behavioral indicators from Lesniak-Karpiak *et al.* (2003), Richards *et al.* (2009), and Sullivan *et al.* (2007), as well as from clinical observations of each child and from interviews with parents and teachers.

Given that it can be difficult to differentiate "anxious behavior" from "problem behavior" (e.g., aggression, tantrums, yelling/screaming) in individuals with ASD (since anxiety is often expressed as problem behavior), it is important to try to define the two behaviors separately, and identify behaviors in disliked situations versus anxiety-provoking situations. For example, in Moskowitz *et al.* (2017a, 2017b), we described how Jon behaved differently in response to situations he simply disliked versus anxiety-provoking situations. He often verbally objected to things he did not like (such as if he were served pasta with tomato sauce instead of plain pasta, he would say, "No!" and push it away) and he yelled or tantrummed when he was denied access to something such as his favorite video, but this was very different from the crying and fearful facial expression that occurred in response to his feared situation (birthday parties). Anxious behaviors for

Jon included clinging onto his mother, crying/tearfulness, freezing (lack of movement except for respiration), cowering (e.g., turning into corner), anxious vocalizations (e.g., whimpering, moaning, or idiosyncratic throat noises), specific perseverative phrases (e.g., "Here we go!"), and a fearful/anxious facial expression consisting of eyes wide open or eyes rapidly darting back and forth, eyebrows sloping down in an inverted V-shape, and frowning (turning down of the mouth). Problem behaviors identified for Jon were yelling or screaming, elopement (running away; leaving the room or attempting to leave the room), pushing another person, and pulling his mother's hair. Although Jon exhibited both anxious behavior and problem behavior in the context of a birthday party (given that his anxious behavior often escalated into problem behavior), he exhibited only problem behaviors such as yelling—not anxious behaviors—in contexts that were merely disliked versus anxiety-provoking.

Physiological Component of Anxiety

Second, we assessed the *physiological* component of anxiety by examining sympathetic activity (heart rate) and parasympathetic activity (respiratory sinus arrhythmia (RSA)) as well as observable indicators of physiological arousal (e.g., flushed face, visible muscle tension). Although there are increasingly affordable, non-intrusive, portable monitors that parents, teachers, or clinicians could use to assess the physiological component of anxiety (e.g., heart activity, breathing, or skin conductance) (Goodwin *et al.*, 2008), physiological devices may not be realistic for parents or teachers to use. However, it is still possible to assess observable symptoms of physiological arousal such as rapid breathing or sweating or trembling or visible muscle tension. Although signs of physiological arousal appear difficult for caretakers to recognize in individuals with ASD and ID, increasing caretakers' awareness can help them to recognize signs such as tenseness and restlessness (Helverschou and Martinsen, 2011).

Cognitive/Affective Component of Anxiety

Third, we assessed the cognitive/affective component of anxiety (i.e., subjective fear or panic experienced) by examining parent-reports on the contexts or situations that elicited anxiety in each individual with ASD and ID. One way to identify anxiety-provoking situations could be to use informant-report questionnaires such as the Stress Survey Schedule (SSS; Groden *et al.*, 2001), but the parents we work with often identify idiosyncratic contexts/situations that are not listed on the SSS. As part of assessing the cognitive/affective component of anxiety, we also had blinded observers rate the child's appearance of fear/anxiety on a 4-point Likert-type scale with 3 being high fear/anxiety and 0 indicating no fear/anxiety (see Appendix B). The rationale for using these contextual measures is that the process of labeling one's state of affective arousal as "anxiety" or any other emotion is highly influenced by the situational context in which the arousal occurs (Bandura, 1988). For example, if one's heart were racing while exercising, the arousal would not likely be interpreted as anxiety, whereas if one's heart were racing while taking an exam, the arousal might be interpreted as anxiety because of the context in which the arousal occurs.

In sum, it is important to conduct a multi-method assessment incorporating multiple informants and direct observation when assessing for the presence of anxiety in individuals with ASD and ID because, although any behavior on its own does not necessarily indicate anxiety, just as physiological arousal on its own does not indicate anxiety, collecting multiple converging pieces of evidence that point towards anxiety may support the presence of anxiety.

Differential Diagnosis of Anxiety Disorders in ASD

In addition to the difficulty distinguishing anxious behavior from problem behavior, it is also difficult to distinguish impairment in functioning due to symptoms of anxiety from impairment due to symptoms of ASD (e.g., a lack of participation in class due to social anxiety rather than due to communication deficits). As such, practitioners should use a multi-step approach, such as that described by Kerns and colleagues (2016b), to differentially diagnose anxiety disorders in anxious individuals with ASD.

Alternatively, Moskowitz *et al.* (2017a) suggest that the practitioner could prioritize a pragmatic approach, and conceptualize and treat patterns of behavior that are 'phobia-like' or 'anxiety-like' as phobias or anxiety, even when it may be suspected that these behaviors might be due to features of ASD such as hyperacusis or sensory over-reactivity or insistence on sameness (e.g., difficulty with transitions or changes in routine). In other words, although from an assessment or diagnostic standpoint it may sometimes be difficult to discriminate if an individual with ASD is running away from a blender while crying and covering his ears because he is anxious or afraid of the blender, versus because he is hypersensitive to auditory stimuli, one could argue that, from a pragmatic treatment standpoint, it may not matter (Moskowitz et al., 2019). Put simply, if it looks like a duck and quacks like a duck, we should probably treat it as a duck. That is, regardless of whether running away from the blender is due to a specific phobia of blenders versus hyperacusis, our intervention goals and procedures would likely be the same: to encourage the individual with ASD to approach rather than avoid the given stimulus (e.g., the blender), and to engage in the formerly avoided activity, or at the very least to calmly tolerate that stimulus or situation without aggression, self-injury, tantrums, or other problem behaviors (Moskowitz *et al.*, 2019). For example, Koegel *et al.* (2004) treated hypersensitivity to auditory stimuli (e.g., sounds from a vacuum cleaner, blender, hand-mixer, toilet flushing) in three children with ASD using the same type of systematic desensitization approach we would use to treat phobias/fears or anxiety: gradual exposure to the feared or avoided stimulus (e.g., Steps 1–2 of the hierarchy for one child involved placing a turned-off vacuum in the child's environment to expose him to seeing the feared stimulus, Steps 3–12 exposed him to an out-of-sight vacuum that became increasingly louder as it was moved closer to the child, and Steps 13–14 exposed the child to both seeing and hearing the vacuum).

Intervention for Anxiety in Individuals with ASD

First, we will describe the intervention components used to treat anxiety in individuals with high-functioning ASD, which are components of cognitive behavioral therapy (CBT), followed by the interventions used to treat anxiety in individuals with low-functioning ASD, which are rooted in applied behavior analysis (ABA) and positive behavior support (PBS). (See Appendix C.) We use the term "high-functioning" to refer to persons who are cognitively able and/or have adequate verbal abilities, whereas we use the term "low-functioning" to refer to persons with ASD who have ID and/or are nonverbal or minimally verbal. Although the terms "high-functioning" and "low-functioning" can be misleading and controversial, because even those individuals with high IQs and verbal abilities can experience substantial impairments in their functioning, and conversely individuals with lower IQs and verbal abilities can still function well in some areas, we will use these terms because they are commonly used in the literature and are an easier shorthand than referring to cognitive abilities and language repeatedly.

Treating Anxiety in Individuals with High-Functioning ASD

CBT is widely considered to be the most effective evidence-based treatment for both neurotypical children and adults with anxiety disorders as well as youth with high-functioning ASD (van Steensel and Bogels, 2015). In fact, a meta-analysis of 14 studies involving 511 youth with high-functioning ASD (HFA) found that the efficacy of CBT for treating anxiety in youth with HFA is fairly robust (Ung et al., 2015). Similarly, CBT has been shown to effectively reduce anxiety in adults with HFA (Lang et al., 2010). The most well-researched CBT programs to treat anxiety for children and adolescents with HFA are Behavioral Interventions for Anxiety in Children with Autism (BIACA; Ehrenreich-May et al., 2014; Storch et al., 2013, 2014; Wise et al., 2019; Wood et al., 2009, 2015), Facing Your Fears (FYF; Reaven et al., 2009, 2011, 2012), Multimodal Anxiety and Social Skills Intervention (MASSI; White et al., 2010, 2013), and a modified version of the Coping Cat (Keehn et al., 2013).

Most CBT programs to address anxiety generally cover the following seven steps. Step 1 typically involves *psychoeducation* about anxiety (explaining the nature of anxiety and the rationale for treatment). Step 2 involves *somatic management* (teaching the individual to identify his/her bodily cues for anxiety, increasing awareness of somatic sensations associated with anxiety). Step 3 involves *cognitive restructuring* (identifying anxious thoughts, teaching the individual to challenge those anxious thoughts, teaching coping-focused thinking). Step 4 involves teaching coping skills such as *relaxation* (belly breathing, progressive muscle relaxation (PMR)) and/or *coping self-talk* (coping statements). Step 5 is developing a *hierarchy* of feared stimuli/situations. Step 6 is developing a *positive reinforcement* system (reward system) for rewarding brave behavior (exposure to those feared situations). Last but not least, Step 7 involves *gradual exposure* to those feared situations, which is arguably the most important component of treatment. These components will be described in more detail below. It is important to note that these components are often not covered in the order or sequence that these seven steps were just listed. Rather, many of the CBT programs used to treat youth with HFA use a flexible, modular approach to therapy in which therapists select treatment modules from the manual based on the individual's anxiety symptoms and most impairing difficulties (e.g., Storch *et al.*, 2013; White *et al.*, 2013). Thus, each of the following interventions we will describe are often individualized to the child with ASD rather than implemented in a set sequence of steps.

Gradual Exposure

The most critical intervention to use when treating anxiety in people with ASD (or in people without ASD, for that matter) is exposure, which means "facing your fears," or exposing people to their feared stimuli or situations. Exposure involves confronting the feared situation, whether that situation is real (in vivo exposure, such as confronting a spider or swimming pool or taking an exam) or imagined (imaginal exposure, such as imagining a loved one dying or being fired from your job). Most researchers would agree that engaging in exposure is necessary for positive treatment outcome when treating anxiety (Kendall *et al.*, 2005). This exposure is typically done in a gradual or hierarchical fashion, also known as "graded exposure" or "graduated exposure" or "systematic desensitization," in which the individual is gradually exposed to increasing proximity, intensity, or amounts of the feared stimulus or situation (i.e., from situations that are rated as less anxiety-provoking to those rated as more anxiety-provoking). In other words, if a person is afraid of a swimming pool, we would not tell him to simply jump in the deep end of the swimming pool; rather, we would encourage him to first dip his toe in the shallow end of the pool, progressing to his whole foot, leg, up to the stomach, up to the chest, etc., gradually progressing to the deep end. The pool might feel very cold at first but, after a while when you get used to it, the water does not feel so cold anymore. This process of "getting used to it" is known as habituation, meaning that if we stay in a feared situation rather than avoiding it, our anxiety will eventually diminish as we habituate or get used to that situation/stimulus. To use an example of one of our clinical cases, Jane was a nine-year-old girl with high-functioning ASD who had a phobia of thunder and lightning (more so thunder than lightning). Prior to coming to see us, her previous therapist had recommended that she wear headphones whenever it thundered outside so that she did not have to hear the thunder. However, avoiding what makes us anxious does not help us learn to cope with it in the long run. Therefore, at our clinic, although Jane was at first allowed to listen to music on her headphones while it thundered, she was encouraged to gradually lower the volume of her music so that she was hearing the thunder more and more, eventually removing her headphones so that she could hear the thunder at full volume with no distractions. Exposures to thunder could involve gradually increasing the volume of thunder or gradually increasing the time spent listening to thunder.

Hierarchy

A fear-and-avoidance hierarchy refers to ranking the feared stimuli/ situations according to how anxiety-provoking they are to the individual with ASD. Although this treatment component of "hierarchy" overlaps with the previous component of "gradual exposure," this component refers to actually creating the steps in the hierarchy, whereas gradual exposure refers to progressively moving the individual with ASD through each step in that hierarchy. For example, in many of the CBT programs that treat anxiety in youth with HFA (e.g., IQ above 70 or 80), at least one session or module of the program focuses on creating a hierarchy, in which the individual with ASD is helped to rank-order his/her fears in preparation for the gradual exposures (e.g., Reaven et al., 2009). See Appendix D for an example of a hierarchy (called a "fear ladder" or "fear staircase" or something to denote different levels) we created for Jane who, as just described, had a phobia of thunder. Higher-functioning individuals with ASD may be able to rank-order these situations from least to most anxiety-provoking on their own, as Jane did, or may need assistance from parents or teachers. In most studies and in clinical practice, progression to the next step of the hierarchy is typically contingent on a certain number of successfully completed trials of the previous step. For example, once Jane was able to listen to thunder *inside* while rating a low level of fear/anxiety (e.g., down from a 6 to a 0, 1, or 2), we moved on to tackling the exposure of listening to thunder *outside*. Given that Jane could not always accurately report her level of anxiety (e.g., sometimes she would still continue to rate a situation as a 5 or 6 even though she was no longer crying or covering her ears or giving any indication of anxiety, or conversely rate a situation as 0 or 1 even though she appeared to be very anxious), we often encouraged her to reconsider her rating and move on to the next exposure if she was no longer exhibiting the appearance of anxiety. Jane's difficulty rating her anxiety is consistent with data suggesting that even high-functioning youth with ASD tend to underreport their anxiety (Storch *et al.*, 2012). Regardless, even if Jane's self-reported anxiety was not actually decreasing from an 8 to a 1, some newer research (e.g., Craske *et al.*, 2014) suggests that whether a person's anxiety decreases during the exposure (i.e., habituation) may not matter as much as the learning that occurs during the exposure. New learning occurs during the exposure that contradicts or counteracts the fear-based association, meaning we learn through repeated exposures that the spider has not killed us, or that the elevator did not crash, or that all of the people in the audience did not laugh at us.

Psychoeducation

Psychoeducation refers to educating the individual with ASD (and often his/her caretakers) about the nature of anxiety, providing corrective information about fear and anxiety, and explaining the rationale for treatment (e.g., expose yourself to the feared situation until you habituate or get used to it). This often includes explaining the difference between a real danger (e.g., smoke alarm going off because there is a fire) versus a false alarm (e.g., smoke alarm going off because there is burnt toast) and how the individual with an anxiety disorder may have an overly sensitive smoke alarm. Psychoeducation for Jane, who was afraid of thunder, involved educating her about thunderstorms, such as how they are formed, how they are often important for bringing rain to nourish grass and plants, and how they very rarely result in harm or danger.

Cognitive Restructuring

Cognitive restructuring refers to identifying anxious thoughts or "self-talk"; challenging or disputing the accuracy, likelihood, or usefulness of those anxious thoughts; and replacing anxious self-talk with more accurate, probable, or productive thoughts that promote coping with anxiety-provoking situations rather than avoiding them (i.e., teaching coping self-talk). Most CBT protocols devote several sessions to helping the individual come up with a toolkit to fight anxiety, including generating helpful thoughts/coping self-talk, other cognitive restructuring strategies, and relaxation, before moving on to conducting exposures. Perhaps the main goal of psychoeducation and cognitive restructuring is to help the individual with anxiety to learn that, as Mark Twain said, "Courage is resistance to fear, mastery of fear—not absence of fear." In other words, we aim to teach the individual who is suffering from anxiety that being brave is not about eliminating fear or anxiety, but rather confronting the things that make you anxious and coping with them.

The first step in cognitive restructuring is typically to help the individual with ASD to identify his/her anxious thoughts (known as cognitive distortions or "thinking traps"). To illustrate with a specific example of cognitive restructuring for Lily, after we helped her to identify her anxious thoughts surrounding performing in her school musical (e.g., "What if I mess up? What if I sing out of tune? What if people don't like it?"), we helped her to challenge these anxious thoughts by asking herself questions such as "What is the evidence that will happen? What is the evidence that won't happen? What else might happen? If that happens, can I handle it? Have I coped with this before?" Ultimately, Lily was able to generate coping thoughts such as "There is no evidence that I would mess up or sing off tune...it's never happened before," "Even if I did mess up, there will be a lot of people singing over me, so no one will probably notice," and "Even if people *did* notice, they might think it's part of the show or they might forget about it, or they might not care... I wouldn't care if someone else messed up." She wrote these thoughts down on Coping Cards and was able to read herself these coping thoughts before she went on stage to encourage herself to confront her fears.

Modifications to Cognitive Restructuring for ASD

Given that it is often challenging for youth with ASD to understand and recognize the thoughts and feelings of others and within themselves, CBT protocols have been modified for youth with HFA (Ung *et al.*, 2015). Some of these modifications include longer sessions to allow for more opportunities for repetition and practice; adding extra modules to cover ASD-specific difficulties (e.g., social skills, independence) that may contribute to anxiety symptoms; emphasis on a reward system; incorporating the child's perseverative interests into treatment; increasing the amount of separate parent training sessions; involving parents in all treatment sessions; adding a school consultation component; and using more concrete, visual strategies such as visual schedules, written instead of verbal examples, Social Stories to explain others' thoughts and feelings and teach cognitive restructuring and problem-solving, use of video modeling and role-play to teach coping strategies, and worksheets with multiple choice lists instead of open-ended questions (e.g., Moree and Davis, 2010; Reaven *et al.*, 2012; Storch *et al.*, 2013; Walters *et al.*, 2016; Wise *et al.*, 2019; Wood *et al.*, 2009). Walters *et al.* (2016) also noted that in CBT programs that were modified for youth with HFA, cognitive restructuring was often delivered through the use of acronyms such as KICK—Knowing I'm nervous, Icky thoughts, Calming thoughts, Keep practicing (Wood *et al.*, 2015)—and "through the use of lists of unhelpful and helpful thoughts from which alternative thinking strategies could be chosen rather than generated" (Walters *et al.*, 2016, p.146). Similarly, to address anxiety in cognitively able adults with ASD, adaptations to CBT can include working as a team with other providers, increasing structure and routine, making abstract concepts into concrete activities, normalizing symptoms, using simple coping thoughts, and teaching problem-solving strategies (Kerns *et al.*, 2016a).

One important modification for individuals with ASD who present with more generalized anxiety (rather than more circumscribed fears, as in specific phobias) might be the need to address uncertainty and unpredictability, since many if not most interventions for individuals with ASD involve increasing predictability. Although it is important to reduce uncertainty and unpredictability by ensuring (when possible) that people with ASD know what to expect, we must keep in mind that this is often a strategy to prevent challenging behavior in the short term rather than help individuals to cope with inevitable uncertainty and unpredictability in the long term. Thus, it is also important to gradually expose individuals with ASD to uncertain situations (Rodgers, 2018) and slowly build in changes to routine and unpredictable situations over time. One approach to CBT is based on the intolerance of uncertainty (IU) model. Rodgers *et al.* (2017) recently developed a parent group-based manualized treatment program for young people with ASD (without ID) which focuses on IU. IU is a risk factor for anxiety even in neurotypical populations but may be a particular issue for those with ASD, given the insistence on sameness, inflexible adherence to routines, and difficulty tolerating change that are characteristic of ASD. Rather than treating the cognitive *content* of the person's anxiety, the program by Rodgers *et al.* (2017) targets the cognitive *process* of anxiety in that it aims to increase individuals' tolerance of uncertainty. Preliminary data suggests this program has promise as a treatment of anxiety in ASD (Rodgers *et al.*, 2017).

Relaxation Training

Relaxation typically involves deep breathing and/or progressive muscle relaxation (PMR; Jacobson, 1938). Although there are no studies that examine the effect of relaxation on its own for individuals with ASD, relaxation is typically part of a wider CBT program for individuals with HFA. In a systematic review of effective modifications to CBT for young people with ASD, Walters *et al.* (2016) noted that the majority of studies reduce the cognitive component of CBT while increasing the use of behavioral strategies such as exposure and relaxation. They also noted that relaxation activities were delivered in a more directive way for individuals with ASD than would be expected in CBT with TD individuals (Walters *et al.*, 2016). Although relaxation is always taught in some CBT programs, in other modular programs, a relaxation module is only taught if needed; for example, in an open trial of modular CBT for late adolescents and young adults with HFA (adapted from the BIACA protocol), the relaxation skills of deep breathing and PMR were sometimes used with more physiologically reactive individuals (Wise *et al.*, 2019).

Mindfulness and Acceptance-Based Interventions

"Third wave" CBT includes mindfulness and acceptance-based interventions such as acceptance and commitment therapy (ACT), dialectical behavior therapy (DBT), and mindfulness-based cognitive therapy (MBCT). These approaches retain elements of traditional CBT (i.e., emphasizing the connection between thoughts, feelings, and behavior) but focus less on challenging/changing thoughts and more on radical acceptance of those thoughts and oneself.

DBT incorporates skills training (mindfulness, interpersonal effectiveness, emotion regulation, distress tolerance), contingency management, exposure, and cognitive restructuring (Linehan, 2014). Although there has been some consideration of how to adapt DBT for individuals with ASD, Mazefsky and

White (2014) noted there had been no randomized controlled trials (RCTs) or published outcome research on DBT with individuals with ASD.

Mindfulness interventions such as MBCT often combine elements of cognitive therapy with breathing meditations and yoga exercises to help increase the individual's awareness of the present moment and bodily sensations without attempting to get rid of those sensations. Mindfulness relies less on verbal exchange than traditional CBT, which could make it a good fit for individuals with ASD (particularly those with ID). A recent systematic review found that mindfulness training reduced anxiety in children with ASD in one study and reduced anxiety in adults with ASD in two studies, though there is not enough evidence to determine whether mindfulness reduces anxiety in adolescents with ASD (Cachia *et al.*, 2016). However, as the literature in this area is scarce, this systematic review was based on few studies with various methodological concerns. Although the Soles of Feet mindfulness program (which involves directing attention to a neutral part of the body—i.e., the soles of the feet—when aggression-triggering emotions or thoughts occur) has been shown to reduce aggressive behavior in adolescents with ASD (Singh *et al.*, 2011a, 2011b), it is unclear whether this approach would similarly reduce anxiety, or whether the reduction in aggression may be attributed to a decrease in anxiety, given that anxiety has not been assessed. Thus, further research is needed to determine the effectiveness of mindfulness and acceptance-based programs for treating anxiety in individuals with ASD.

Treating Anxiety in Individuals with Lower-Functioning ASD

Although the efficacy of CBT for treating anxiety in youth with HFA is fairly strong, there is limited research on CBT to treat anxiety in individuals with lower-functioning ASD (LFA). In fact, RCTs that examine the effectiveness of CBT in youth with ASD exclude children or adolescents with an IQ below 70 (e.g., Storch *et al.*, 2013; White *et al.*, 2009; Wood *et al.*, 2009) or IQ below 80 (e.g., Reaven *et al.*, 2011, 2012) or in some cases IQ below 85 (e.g., Ehrenreich-May *et al.*, 2014; Wood *et al.*, 2015). For the two studies that used CBT to treat anxiety in children with borderline IQ (Neil *et al.*, 2017) or ID (Moskowitz *et al.*, 2017b), modifications to CBT included increased structure and emphasis on visuals, presenting concepts more concretely, more practice opportunities to use concepts and skills, increased parental involvement, incorporation of the child's special interests and, in some cases, a reduced focus on thoughts.

When individuals have a cognitive impairment or are minimally verbal, the cognitive components of CBT (i.e., cognitive restructuring, psychoeducation) are often de-emphasized, simplified, modified, adapted to the individual's level, or most commonly excluded altogether so that the intervention is more "behavioral" rather than "*cognitive*-behavioral" (Moskowitz *et al.*, 2019). Rosen *et al.* (2016) reviewed the literature on behavioral interventions for treating anxiety in individuals with LFA and found that systematic desensitization (essentially the same thing as gradual exposure) and positive reinforcement were *efficacious* treatments for anxiety; prompting, modeling, and anti-anxiety stimuli were *possibly efficacious* in treating anxiety in individuals with LFA; and blocking and safety signals were *undetermined* (not enough studies). We will review these intervention components below and several other possible interventions for this population. We will describe the intervention components mentioned in the reviews by Rosen *et al.* (2016) and Jennett and Hagopian (2008) from ABA that have been used to treat fear or "phobic avoidance" or "anxiety-like" behaviors in individuals with ID. In addition, we will describe the interventions that have been used to treat "problem behavior" or "challenging behavior" (e.g., aggression, self-injury, tantrums) in the PBS literature, but not fear or anxiety per se, although these interventions have been used in our research to treat anxiety in children with ASD and ID (Moskowitz *et al.*, 2017b) as well as in our clinical experience treating fear or anxiety in this population.

Gradual Exposure/Systematic Desensitization

To illustrate gradual exposure, in Moskowitz *et al.* (2017b), Jon, a child with ASD and ID, was exposed to people singing "Happy Birthday," progressing from a cake with the candles unlit to a cake with the candles lit, and gradually increasing his proximity to the cake, little by little, until he was eventually sitting in a chair right next to the birthday cake and even attempting to blow out the candles. Similarly, for Sam, who had a fear of left/right turns while riding in the car, he first engaged in activities that we predicted would provoke relatively low levels of anxiety: listening to audio-recordings of the sound of blinkers and then watching internet videos of cars making left and right turns. He then engaged in an activity that we predicted might evoke moderate levels of anxiety: Sam and his parents practiced listening to the real blinker in their car when the car was stationary (parked in their driveway), first with the car door open and then with the door closed. Finally, Sam engaged in activities that we predicted would evoke high levels of anxiety because they all involved riding in the car. We moved up the exposure hierarchy from right and left turns that were thought to be less anxiety-provoking (e.g., a small intersection on a side street with a stop sign) to more anxiety-provoking (e.g., major intersections with traffic lights).

Hierarchy/Shaping

Even for those lower-functioning individuals who cannot rank-order their fears as some higher-functioning individuals can do (see above), creating a fear-and-avoidance hierarchy still involves breaking down the task of approaching or engaging with the feared stimulus or situation into baby steps, with gradual increases in response requirements or successive approximations towards the final goal/step (known as "shaping" in the ABA/PBS literature). Steps can be broken down sequentially into a task analysis, such as sitting in the dental chair, leaning back in the dental chair, opening mouth for the dentist's mirror, etc. (Luscre and Center, 1996). Alternatively, steps can include time exposed to the stimulus, amount of the stimulus, size of the stimulus (e.g., increasingly larger dogs), intensity of the stimulus (e.g., increasing volume of audio-recordings of fire alarms), or distance to the stimulus (e.g., exposing a boy with ASD and ID to gradually greater distances from his house; Love *et al.*, 1990).

Positive Reinforcement

This refers to providing the person with ASD with some type of positive reinforcement for "brave behavior," such as social reinforcement (e.g., praise, high-fives) and/or tangible reinforcement (e.g., favorite toy, tokens/points to be exchanged for desired item), contingent upon the person approaching the feared stimulus or engaging in a feared activity/task, or contingent on the person remaining in a feared situation without resisting or engaging in problem behavior. Most of the intervention studies that target fear or anxiety in individuals with ASD (both individuals with HFA and LFA) involved some type of reinforcement for approach or completing an exposure. For example, in Moskowitz *et al.* (2017b), after a certain number of trials in which Jon was reinforced non-contingently, we switched to contingent reinforcement in that, if Jon approached the birthday cake and attempted to blow out the candle, he immediately received his favorite *Sesame Street* pop-up toy, along with enthusiastic praise. That is, he received the pop-up toy and praise *contingent upon* attempting to blow out the candle.

Although the parent, teacher, or therapist may often provide reinforcement to the individual with ASD, if the individual is more cognitively able, then he or she is typically taught to deliver self-reinforcement (e.g., Keehn *et al.*, 2013; Reaven *et al.*, 2009).

Of note, positive reinforcement includes both *differential reinforcement of alternative behavior* (DRA), in which approach behavior or compliance is reinforced (e.g., moving closer to a dog, petting the dog, sitting still during blood draw); and *differential reinforcement of other behavior* (DRO), in which the absence of escape/avoidance behavior is reinforced (e.g., *not* running out of the room, *not* asking mother reassurance-seeking questions, *not* washing hands if you fear they are germy). Although DRA is usually preferable because our goal is to teach skills (alternative behaviors), DRO can also be useful. For example, Ed's mother awarded him a sticker for every ten minutes, then every 20 minutes, and then every 30 minutes that he engaged in "brave behavior" (i.e., doing anything *other* than asking his mother questions about his health, such as "Mom, am I sick?"). The stickers counted towards larger prizes from his Reward Menu. The DRO system helped to prevent him from ritualizing (i.e., asking his mother reassurance-seeking questions). Regardless of the specific approach used, it is important for individuals with ASD to be rewarded as they attempt increasingly anxiety-provoking activities.

Prompting

Prompting is the presentation of any antecedent stimulus—such as physical guidance or verbal directions or an auditory cue—to help get a behavior started. Hagopian and Jennett (2008) suggested including prompting as a way to help individuals with ASD and ID to comply with the steps of the exposure hierarchy, which may be especially important when the individual is displaying highly intense anxiety behaviors or not approximating the approach response. Many if not most intervention studies that target fear or anxiety in individuals with ASD involved assisting the individual to approach or engage with the feared stimulus using verbal prompts (e.g., mother verbally prompting her child to speak to a stranger) or physical prompts (e.g., physically guiding a child to enter a feared setting at school, as Schmidt et al. (2013) did with an adolescent with autism).

One note of caution is that prompting should be used to *teach* or encourage approach responses rather than *force* them, as this can lead to negative emotions and problem behavior (Hagopian et al., 2017). To illustrate, in Moskowitz et al. (2017b), the third time we exposed Jon to the birthday cake with the candles lit, he was cowering in the corner approximately 4 meters away from the birthday cake; we prompted an "approach response" (i.e., prompted him to approach the cake) by gently physically guiding Jon to sit in a chair that was approximately 2 meters away from the cake. When Jon made a distress vocalization in response to being physically prompted, we realized we were moving too fast and instead switched to using a verbal prompt (e.g., "Jon, first blow out the candle, then you get the *Sesame Street* pop-up toy!") to encourage Jon to approach the birthday cake, which was very successful.

Modeling

Modeling involves the person with ASD observing another person confront the feared situation or interact with the feared stimulus. With modeling, a therapist, parent, or peer demonstrates engaging in the anxiety-provoking situation or engaging with the feared stimulus appropriately while the individual with ASD observes. This can include the model demonstrating a step in the hierarchy and/or receiving reinforcement for brave behavior. Many studies that treat fear or anxiety in individuals with ASD involve modeling. For example, in a study that treated phobias of children with ASD and ID, the child observed his parent as she modeled approach steps such as turning on the shower (Love et al., 1990). While modeling, the parent verbalized to her child her actions and lack of fear (Love et al., 1990).

Whereas some studies use "in-vivo" or live modeling in person (as in Love et al., 1990), other studies use video modeling. For example, in Luscre and Center's (1996) study treating dental fear in children with autism and ID, four TD children acted as the peer models in a video of a dental exam conducted in the dentist's office. As another example of video modeling, in Moskowitz *et al.* (2017b), a child with ASD and ID who was afraid of "Happy Birthday" viewed several internet videos of his favorite *Sesame Street* characters singing "Happy Birthday" and blowing out candles on a birthday cake. Even CBT programs for youth with high-functioning ASD often use a great deal of modeling. For example, MASSI uses modeling by the therapist in individual CBT and by peer tutors in the group CBT (e.g., "even though I feel nervous about how she will respond, I will smile and say 'hello' because that is how I should greet someone"; White *et al.*, 2010).

Non-Contingent Reinforcement/Counterconditioning/Anti-Anxiety Stimuli

This intervention involves providing the person with ASD with non-contingent access to preferred or "anti-anxiety" stimuli before or during exposure to the feared stimulus/situation in order to override or compete with a fear response. To illustrate, for Sam, who was afraid of his parents making left/right turns on car rides, upon entering the car, Sam immediately was provided non-contingent access to his most highly preferred items: the Dr. Seuss book *The Sneetches*, along with listening to an audio-recording of *The Sneetches* (Moskowitz *et al.*, 2017b). As another example, when we first started treating Jon's phobia of "Happy Birthday," upon presentation of the birthday cake accompanied by the "Happy Birthday" song, Jon was immediately given his most highly preferred item, a *Sesame Street* pop-up toy, non-contingently (meaning without him having to do any behavior to receive the toy) (Moskowitz *et al.*, 2017b). This antecedent-based strategy of pairing anxiety-producing stimuli with positive stimuli non-contingently *before* or *during* the exposure stands in contrast to the consequence-based strategy mentioned above of positive reinforcement contingent upon the person displaying a certain behavior or *after* completing a certain task (e.g., reinforcing Jon only after he attempts to blow out the candles).

This strategy of non-contingent reinforcement can also be conceptualized as counterconditioning, in which the feared stimulus is repeatedly paired with an "anti-anxiety" stimulus. For example, Luscre and Center (1996) paired anti-anxiety stimuli (individualized to each child; e.g., hand-held mirror, Play-Doh, the song "Achy Breaky Heart") with the presentation of dental procedures for children with autism in order to help counter a fear response to dental examinations. Although counterconditioning has not been shown to be more effective than standard exposure (repeated presentation of the feared stimulus) in the treatment of fear/anxiety for individuals with ASD (or without ASD), it should be noted that, in Moskowitz *et al.* (2017b), the anxious behaviors of the children with ASD did *not* decrease throughout the repeated exposures of the baseline (pre-treatment) sessions. That is why we decided to pair the anxiety-provoking situation with a highly preferred and otherwise inaccessible positive reinforcer (e.g., pairing birthday cake/song with *Sesame Street* toy), rather than just exposing the children to the anxiety-provoking situation without any accompanying positive stimuli. Anecdotally, our clinical observations suggest that pairing the anxiety-provoking stimulus with an equally potent or even more powerful "perseverative" stimulus (e.g., *The Sneetches*) served to counteract the individual's fearful/anxious responses in a way that exposure to the feared stimulus alone (without pairing it with anti-anxiety stimuli) may not have been able to accomplish, or at least may not have been able to accomplish as quickly. Thus, clinically, we often tend to use counterconditioning rather than standard exposure for those individuals who are cognitively impaired and/or display severe problem behavior (e.g., self-injurious behavior, aggression), because waiting for them to "get used to" (i.e., habituate to) the feared stimulus through exposure alone may be too dangerous when there is serious problem behavior. In contrast, for a child such as Jane who had a high IQ and was verbal and did not display any problem behavior (beyond yelling/screaming and crying when confronted with thunder), we used standard gradual exposure to thunder without pairing the thunder with anti-anxiety stimuli.

It is important to note that, although using anti-anxiety stimuli would be considered distraction or "safety signals" in the CBT literature and would thus be contraindicated for neurotypical individuals with anxiety, it is possible this may not be as true for those with ASD, who often lack the cognitive capacity to understand that their anxiety will eventually decrease (i.e., they will habituate) if they simply remain in the situation for long enough, without having to do anything at all (Moskowitz and Ritter, 2016; Moskowitz *et al.*, 2017b).

Extinction/Blocking

Escape extinction means that an individual's anxious behaviors (e.g., crying, running away) or problem behaviors (e.g., aggression, self-injury, tantrums) no longer produce reinforcement in the form of escape. Put another way, escape extinction refers to not allowing the person with ASD to escape the anxiety-provoking situation or stop performing the given step in the hierarchy in response to problem behaviors or anxious/avoidance behaviors. This generally involves physically guiding the individual with ASD to engage in a step in the hierarchy (preventing him from escaping) or, in some cases, even blocking the individual from escaping. For example, in Rapp *et al.* (2005), who treated "swimming pool avoidance" in an adolescent with ASD and ID (Amy, who most likely had a phobia of swimming although those words "fear" or "phobia" were not used), two therapists blocked or prevented Amy's attempts to run away from the swimming pool or flop to the ground by prompting her to sit in a rolling chair. A third therapist stood in front of Amy with a food item and verbally prompted her to move toward the pool. If Amy did not comply with the verbal prompt (e.g., "Amy, come over here") after approximately 15 seconds, the two therapists pushed the chair until Amy reached the item.

Similar to response blocking, "response prevention" or "ritual prevention" involves preventing individuals with OCD from engaging in rituals because these rituals serve to reduce (and therefore avoid) their anxiety. The goal of treatment is for individuals to face their fears and expose themselves to anxiety rather than do anything to reduce or avoid anxiety. For example, for Ed, a boy with ASD, OCD, and mild ID who engaged in the ritual of repeatedly asking his mother if he was sick or healthy, ritual prevention involved encouraging Ed *not* to ask his mother questions related to being sick or healthy (these questions were listed) as well as instructing his mother *not* to answer these questions if Ed did ask them. Rather, his mother was encouraged to respond with, "I can't tell you if you're sick. That's just your OCD talking, and we have to fight your OCD!"

In other research studies and in our clinical experience, extinction does not involve response blocking or ritual prevention, but simply involves continuing with the anxiety-provoking situation regardless of the child's problem behavior or anxious behavior. To illustrate, in Moskowitz *et al.* (2017b), for Ben, a child who was afraid of his parents leaving him home with someone other than them (his grandparents or uncle or a babysitter), this meant that, during intervention, his parents had to leave the house regardless of whatever behaviors Ben displayed. Similarly, when Sam was riding in the car with his parents prior to receiving intervention in Moskowitz *et al.* (2017b), his parents often altered their driving route in response to his anxious behavior (e.g., crying "no left!" or "drive straight!") to avoid his feared stimulus of left/right turns, thus reinforcing his anxious behavior. That is, Sam learned that crying or yelling "no left!" would sometimes results in his parents driving straight rather than making a left or right turn. Thus, one component of intervention involved extinction, in which Sam's anxious behavior was no longer reinforced by escape through terminating the task (driving back home) or altering the driving route to accommodate Sam's anxiety (i.e., driving straight instead of turning right left).

Incorporating the Individual's Perseverative Interests

Given the level of anxiety that the targeted contexts appeared to provoke in three children with ASD and ID, Moskowitz *et al.* (2017b) paired the anxiety-provoking situation with stimuli/activities that were not simply reinforcing, but took it one step further by incorporating perseverative items or activities that were *the most* highly salient/preferred in an attempt to override or counteract the aversiveness of the anxiety-provoking contexts. "Perseverative interest" (also called "circumscribed interest" or "special interest" or "obsessive interest") refers to an object, activity, or topic with which the individual is intensely preoccupied. To illustrate, in Moskowitz *et al.* (2017b), for Sam, the boy mentioned above who was afraid of left/right turns while driving in the car, his parents paired Sam's riding in the car with his main perseverative interest (Dr. Seuss). Although Sam's favorite book, *The Sneetches* by Dr. Seuss, was an item he owned before intervention and could access at home, audio-recordings of *The Sneetches* and other Dr. Seuss books were created at the start of intervention; Sam was only allowed to listen to these Dr. Seuss recordings during car rides. It is important to emphasize that, by incorporating perseverative interests, we are not only referring to using the perseverative interest as a reinforcer, but also incorporating the perseverative interest into the exposure itself. For example, Jon had a perseverative interest in *Sesame Street*; in addition to providing Jon with the *Sesame Street* pop-up toy at first non-contingently when presented with the birthday cake, and later contingent upon approaching the birthday cake, we also incorporated *Sesame Street* into the exposure by using *Sesame Street* characters singing "Happy Birthday" in video modeling, by using *Sesame Street* candles in the birthday cake, etc. Perseverative interests also include referring to favorite cartoons or stories or characters, such as the person in the video model saying, "I'm going to be brave like Harry Potter" and coaching the individual with anxiety to use that same self-talk to motivate himself to face his fears. Of note, although incorporating children's "special interests" is a part of CBT treatment protocols to treat anxiety in youth with ASD (e.g., Reaven *et al.*, 2012; Wood *et al.*, 2009), with the exception of Moskowitz *et al.* (2017b) and Neil *et al.* (2017), these treatments have only included youth with HFA. It should also be noted that, in the treatment protocol to address anxiety in ASD by Wood *et al.* (2009), although the children's special interests are initially incorporated into treatment to build rapport and increase attention and motivation, later in treatment, a "suppression" approach is used in which the children are encouraged to refrain from discussing or engaging in the special interests for increasing amounts of time per day, since these special interests can get in the way of friendships.

Cognitive Restructuring

As noted above, the cognitive components of CBT (i.e., cognitive restructuring, psychoeducation) are often de-emphasized, simplified, modified, adapted to the individual's level, or excluded altogether. To illustrate, Moskowitz *et al.* (2017b) used video priming or video modeling to provide a simplified psychoeducation for Jon and Sam, and used Social Stories as a way to provide psychoeducation (e.g., normalizing anxiety, explaining that anxiety has a function or purpose, explaining habituation) and a simplified form of cognitive restructuring for Ben and Sam in a visual modality that could be more easily comprehended (see 'Social Stories' below). Although Moskowitz *et al.* (2017b) did not address identifying or disputing anxious thoughts, which would have been too cognitively and verbally challenging, for Ben, cognitive restructuring took the form of prompting coping self-talk through the use of a Social Story.

Coping self-talk is often used before exposures to help reduce anti-cipatory anxiety and/or during exposures to encourage brave/calm behavior rather than avoidance/anxious behavior. For example, Neil *et al.* (2017) taught a boy with ASD and ID to use coping statements (e.g., "I can do it, I'm not going to let OCD beat me!") to help himself refrain from ritualizing by ripping and sniffing. Similarly, in Moskowitz *et al.* (2017b), Ben's Social

Story provided him with coping statements that he could tell himself when he was feeling anxious, such as "I am going to fight my anxiety and I will win!," that appeared to help calm him when his parents left. However, it is unclear what role—if any—these simplified cognitive elements played in the reduction of anxiety in these multi-component treatments, and whether the same results would have been achieved with the behavioral components (e.g., counterconditioning) alone.

Relaxation Training

Although Bouvet and Coulet (2016) conducted an RCT comparing adults with mild to moderate ID who received PMR with those in a waitlist control group and found that relaxation significantly reduced state anxiety, there are no similar studies that examine the effect of relaxation on its own to treat anxiety for individuals with ASD and ID (or ASD in general). However, Mullins and Christian (2001) taught an abbreviated version of PMR (e.g., "Make your right arm tight, relax your right arm; make your left arm tight, relax your left arm") to a 12-year-old boy with ASD and mild ID. Although Mullins and Christians (2001) did not assess anxiety, they found that overt relaxed behaviors increased following training in PMR and the duration of disruptive behaviors decreased when PMR preceded leisure activity sessions. It is unclear if this decrease in disruptive behaviors is due to a reduction in anxiety, although it is possible. However, the authors cautioned against "concluding that a behavior is caused by stress or anxiety simply because it decreases when relaxation training is implemented" (Mullins and Christian, 2001, p.451).

PBS Prevention Strategies

Positive behavior support (PBS) involves conducting a functional behavior assessment (FBA) to identify the antecedents that precede problem behavior, the consequences that follow problem behavior, and the setting events that make problem behavior more likely to occur, and then designing an intervention plan informed by the FBA that includes "Prevention Strategies" to address the setting events and antecedents that precede problem behavior; "Replacement Strategies" or "Teaching Strategies" to teach desired replacement skills; and "Consequence Strategies" or "Management

Strategies" to reinforce positive behavior rather than problem behavior (see Durand and Hieneman, 2008 and Prevent-Teach-Reinforce; Dunlap *et al.*, 2017). Although the PBS framework was designed to address problem behavior, the same approach and strategies can also apply to addressing anxiety or anxious behavior. For example, Prevention Strategies can include providing choices to increase a child's motivation to face his fears, Replacement Strategies can involve prompting a child and modeling for that child how to face his fears, engage in coping self-talk, or belly breathing, and Consequence Strategies can involve reinforcing approximations of approaching the feared stimulus/situation.

The goal of Prevention Strategies is to prevent anxiety from developing in response to its typical triggers, or at least to prevent the anxiety from escalating into problem behavior. Typically, Prevention Strategies involve altering the antecedents that precede problem behavior. For our purposes, Prevention Strategies involve altering the antecedents that precede anxiety.

Increasing Predictability

Although there is no research showing that predictability decreases anxiety in individuals with ASD, research has shown that problem behavior (e.g., aggression, self-injury, tantrums) is lower when situations are more predictable. Although Flannery and Horner (1994) did not conceptualize the reduction in problem behavior as being due to a reduction in "anxiety," we do conceptualize it as such. After all, startle studies suggest that the ability to predict aversive events attenuates anxious responses (Grillon, 2008). Thus, one PBS prevention strategy entails providing information proactively to reduce anxiety (Lucyshyn *et al.*, 2007). It is important to acknowledge that increasing predictability may often be a temporary PBS prevention strategy, in that things cannot always be predictable in life, so unpredictability has to be introduced into the individual's life systematically in baby steps so that the individual can eventually learn to cope with changes in routine.

Visual Schedules

There are many different ways that a therapist, parent, teacher, or staff member can increase predictability for individuals with ASD. A visual schedule is one way to reduce the unpredictability associated with transitions by informing individuals with ASD about the upcoming sequence of events (Dettmer *et al.*, 2000). For example, to ensure the predictability of Sam's transition, pictures were created to represent the most common locations to which Sam's parents drove, and those pictures were used to construct a visual schedule (Moskowitz *et al.*, 2017b). Before entering the car, Sam was presented with a portable board that contained pictures and words representing the locations he would be traveling to in the community as well as anchor pictures of his home on each end of the schedule (Moskowitz *et al.*, 2017b). As another example, in our clinical experience, for one boy with ASD (Mike) who had anxiety surrounding transitioning from one class to another at school, we created a visual schedule for him. Even though there was a visual schedule in Mike's classroom that was posted for the entire class, given Mike's extreme anxiety that occurred at almost every transition, we decided it could help for Mike to have his own, individualized, personal schedule—a portable visual schedule that was velcroed to his desk and that he could carry around with him from one classroom to another.

Social Stories

Social Stories (Gray and Garand, 1993) are individualized narratives that visually depict the sequence of events involved in a routine or situation and describe appropriate behavior relevant to the situation, which may decrease unpredictability and provide a model for socially acceptable behavior (in this case, non-anxious behavior or "coping behavior"). Gut and Safran (2002) proposed that, since some people with disabilities exhibit anxiety when routines are changed, providing advance information about this type of situation can reduce anxiety and provide alternative coping strategies to deal with such a situation. In illustration, to increase predictability for Sam and provide guidance on how he could understand the situation, a Social Story was created about riding in the car with his parents which included information about what would happen in the car ride, how he should behave, what positive activities he would engage in while riding in the car, and why his parents needed to make left/right turns to get to where they needed to go (Moskowitz *et al.*, 2017b). In addition, to capitalize on Sam's special interest in Dr. Seuss books, a second Social Story was created about making left turns and right turns while driving, which was written in the format of Dr. Seuss' *The Foot Book*.

Although Social Stories have been shown to decrease levels of problem behavior in individuals with ASD and ID (Kokina and Kern, 2010), with the exception of Moskowitz *et al.* (2017b), no other Social Stories studies have targeted or mentioned fear or anxiety specifically. A recent meta-analysis of Social Stories for students with ASD reported that Social Stories are more effective when addressing inappropriate behaviors than when teaching social skills and when participants had lower cognitive ability rather than high or average intelligence (Kokina and Kern, 2010), which suggests that Social Stories could be helpful in treating anxiety or anxiety-related behaviors in individuals with ASD and ID (particularly anxiety that is related to unpredictability), although more research is needed to support this.

For individuals with ASD, especially those with co-occurring ID, we often convey psychoeducation in a visual format or modality, such as using a Social Story. For example, for a boy with ASD and ID who exhibited separation anxiety in Moskowitz *et al.* (2017b), Ben's Social Story:

1. normalized anxiety (e.g., "Everyone feels worried or afraid or anxious sometimes")

2. explained that anxiety has a function or purpose (e.g., "If a lion is chasing you, it is okay to feel afraid, because your fear will make you run from the lion")

3. described the specific nature of Ben's anxiety (e.g., "I am very, very afraid when Mommy or Daddy leave the house and go out without me")

4. explained the concept of habituation (e.g., "After a while longer, I won't be scared anymore; I will see that my anxiety goes down after a while, even when Mommy and Daddy are not home")

5. provided Ben with replacement behaviors that he could do instead of crying, screaming, and trying to run after them (i.e., coping self-statements such as "This is just my anxiety talking," relaxation techniques such as deep breathing, and activities such as playing, watching a movie, and playing video games).

See Appendix D for the full text of Ben's Social Story. (Pictures were also included in the actual Social Story, though are not included here in this chapter because some pictures include identifying information and other pictures are copyrighted.)

As another example, for Ed, who engaged in the ritual of repeatedly asking his mother if he was sick or healthy, his Social Story (given in Appendix E) also explained the concept of ritual prevention (i.e., "To fight my anxiety, I will try not to ask Mom these questions and Mom will try not to answer my questions").

Priming

Another way to increase predictability is through priming, in which a person previews future events so that they become more predictable. For example, we rehearsed Mike's transitions from one classroom to another with him one-on-one, under relaxed conditions, when school was not in session. As another example, for Justin, a child with ASD and ID we worked with who was afraid of giving his items to the cashier on the checkout line at grocery stores, we rehearsed the checkout line at home with a pretend cash register and pretend scanner over and over again until the child appeared to be comfortable giving his items to the pretend cashier to be scanned and returned to him. In addition to live priming, the use of video also allows us to use priming with individuals who are non-verbal or limited in their ability to comprehend verbal descriptions. Similar to advanced warnings, visual schedules, and Social Stories, the research on priming (Wilde *et al.*, 1992) and video priming (Schreibman *et al.*, 2000) has shown that it decreases problem behavior associated with transitions or an upcoming unpredictable situation, but no studies except for Moskowitz *et al.* (2017b) have mentioned treating fear or anxiety using priming or video priming.

To illustrate video priming, Sam, who had a fear of left/right turns while riding in the car, watched videos of cars making left and right turns on YouTube before we conducted exposures to left/right turns while actually riding in the car (Moskowitz *et al.*, 2017b). Watching videos can also be conceptualized as a low-level exposure (see gradual exposure above). As another example, in our clinical experience, Mike's teachers carried a video camera throughout the school to show the school as Mike would see it when progressing through the transition (as was done in Schreibman *et al.*, 2000). This method of video priming is different from video modeling because no model appears in the video; rather, the video was taken as a bird's eye view from Mike's point of view so that, when he watched the video, he would feel as if he was walking through the halls at school. For example, one of the videos can begin exiting the homeroom, show the walk through the halls and up the stairs, show entering the lunchroom, show sitting at the lunch table, and end with showing a reinforcer that Mike will receive upon completing the transition successfully. Video modeling (in which Mike could watch a video of his father, mother, favorite teacher, or preferred peer transitioning from the homeroom to the lunchroom) also might have been successful. As an example of video modeling, Jon, who was afraid of "Happy Birthday," viewed multiple internet videos of his favorite characters (e.g., Ernie and Bert) singing "Happy Birthday" and blowing out candles on a birthday cake (Moskowitz et al., 2017b).

Advanced Warning

Another way to increase predictability is to provide an "advanced warning" to signal upcoming transitions or changes in routine or aversive events, which can provide the individual with time to prepare for the upcoming anxiety-provoking situation (making the transition gradual rather than abrupt), or can signal how much time is left until the anxiety-provoking activity will be over. These advanced warnings can be verbal and/or visual, including countdowns (e.g., "You have ten seconds left until the blood test is finished... 10, 9, 8, 7, 6, 5, 4, 3, 2, 1, it's finished"), picture prompts (Mace et al., 1998), and visual representations of time such as a Time Timer (displaying a section of red indicating the given amount of time, with the red disappearing as the time runs out) (Dettmer et al., 2000). The concept is similar to how most New York City subway stations now have "countdown clocks" that visually display how much time is left until the next train arrives; the purpose of installing these clocks was to reduce the anxiety that comes from not knowing when the next train will arrive. Although almost all of these studies that used advanced warnings with individuals with ASD did not mention fear or anxiety and only mentioned "aversive" events such as transitions, researchers are increasingly recognizing transition/change-related anxiety as being anxiety in individuals with ASD (e.g., Kerns et al., 2014a, 2016b). To illustrate the use of advanced warnings to treat a traditional anxiety disorder (needle phobia) in an adult with autism and ID, after three unsuccessful trials of attempting to treat the phobia with stimulus fading plus DRA, Wolff and Symons (2013) added a timer to visually convey that the trial was of a finite duration and show when the trial would end. Adding the timer corresponded with a change in the adult's behavior (increased compliance, reduced agitation) (Wolff and Symons, 2013). Further, even after the safety signal was later removed, the adult with ASD and ID continued to keep his arm on the table for the duration of the needle exposure, suggesting he may have learned that all trials, with or without the timer, were of a limited duration and would be over soon. Similarly, in our clinical experience, a Time Timer was helpful for Mike because he could see the time visually passing, showing how much time he had left before he had to transition to another classroom or activity.

Providing Choices/Control

Allowing individuals with ASD and other developmental disabilities to choose activities and reinforcers has been shown to increase task engagement and reduce escape-motivated problem behaviors (Shogren *et al.*, 2004). One reason this could be is because providing people with opportunities to make choices increases their sense of control over their environments. Too often, individuals with ASD and other disabilities are not given any choice or control over their lives, which can be extremely anxiety-provoking. Indeed, research has shown that fear is conditioned at a much higher level in animals that are exposed to uncontrollable shock (Mineka *et al.*, 1984) than in those that are able to control the shock. Although the existing research on providing choices/control to individuals with ASD only mentions escape-motivated problem behaviors such as aggression and tantrums and (with the exception of Moskowitz *et al.*, 2017b and Cale *et al.*, 2009) does not mention fear or anxiety, many researchers in the field of anxiety disorders have suggested that a sense of unpredictability and uncontrollability is at the heart of anxiety, and that developing coping responses can provide the individual with a sense of control that can buffer anxiety (Barlow, 2000). For example, Cale *et al.* (2009) presented the children with ASD with a choice between the feared stimulus and an alternative stimulus that was matched with the feared stimulus relative to generic content category, such as a choice between a book without onomatopoeic sounds and a book with them, or a choice between math worksheets without sea creatures versus worksheets with sea creatures. This allowed the children to avoid the feared stimulus without compromising the instructional goal.

However, in many other cases, it may not be possible or desirable/ beneficial for the individual with ASD to choose to avoid the anxiety-provoking activity or situation (even if a comparable activity is available), which is where exposure to the anxiety-provoking situation comes in. Thus, rather than allowing the individual to choose *whether* to complete a disliked or anxiety-provoking activity (e.g., doing homework versus not doing homework), we generally advise parents and teachers and therapists to provide the person with choices over *how* or when or where to complete a disliked or anxiety-provoking activity (e.g., doing spelling or math homework first, using monkey pencil or panda pen to complete homework, doing homework at living room table or kitchen table) or choosing which rewards they want to receive for completing or engaging in the anxiety-provoking activity. For example, in Moskowitz *et al.* (2017b), Sam, who was afraid of left/right turns while riding in the car, was given the opportunity to choose several preferred items (e.g., balls, books) to pack in a "Car Bag" that he could bring with him while riding in the car. In addition, whenever possible, Sam's parents attempted to provide him with a choice of the location to which they would drive. In this way, Sam became an active participant in the process of constructing his schedule and selecting preferred items with which to engage himself on the car ride.

Teaching Replacement Skills

Although the aforementioned PBS "Prevention Strategies" (increasing predictability, providing choices, incorporating perseverative interests) reduce problem behavior that may be related to anxiety by eliminating or minimizing or altering the antecedents that lead to problem behavior, it may not always be possible or desirable to eliminate/alter antecedents. Overreliance on Prevention Strategies in the absence of teaching skills often results in parents, teachers, and providers *avoiding* anxiety-provoking or difficult situations rather than teaching the individual with ASD how to *cope* with those situations (Moskowitz and Ritter, 2016). Thus, it is important to teach "replacement behaviors" or skills for coping with anxiety-provoking situations so that they can be used in any environment, independent of trained staff or caretakers.

Functional Communication Skills

One example of teaching replacement behaviors is functional communication training (FCT; Carr and Durand, 1985), which involves assessing the function(s) of an individual's problem behavior and then teaching him or her a functionally equivalent communicative response(s) that serves the same function or purpose. Although FCT is an evidence-based intervention for reducing problem behavior, there has not been research on using FCT to reduce fear or anxiety per se. However, we have used FCT clinically to reduce anxiety in youth with ASD, in combination with gradual exposure. For example, Wesley, a nine-year-old boy with ASD and ID, became anxious whenever two of his female classmates cried, and he responded by hitting or scratching them. This resulted in his teachers bringing him out of the classroom to a break room. Using FCT, we taught Wesley to ask for a break from class by handing a "Break Card" to the teachers. In this way, Wesley could escape the anxiety-provoking situation by using communication rather than escape the classroom/crying by resorting to aggression, as he had in the past. In other words, the communication replaced the aggression, since both served the same function of escape. Specifically, we gradually exposed Wesley to the sounds and sights of crying, progressing from audio-recordings to video-recordings of children crying, to real-life adults crying, to children in the clinic and siblings crying, and ultimately to the real-life girls in his class crying (Moskowitz and Ritter, 2016). While listening to and watching the audios/videos, Wesley was taught to ask for a break by handing us the Break Card while saying, "I want a break." It is important to note that we used FCT in combination with gradual exposure so that Wesley was not endlessly avoiding the anxiety-provoking stimulus (crying) by using Break Cards, but was increasingly exposed to the crying by gradually reducing the number of Break Cards over time. The rationale for this is that if a person was allowed to constantly ask for a break from anxiety-provoking situations, they would never learn to habituate to those situations or cope with those situations.

Coping Skills

In addition to replacing the problem behavior with a form of communication, we can also replace problem behavior that functions to reduce anxiety with relaxation skills (e.g., deep breathing, PMR) and/or coping self-talk that serves the same function. Coping statements such as "I've handled this before and I will handle it again," or simpler statements such as "I can be brave!" are often used before exposures to help reduce anticipatory anxiety and/or during exposures to help reduce anxiety (Moskowitz and Ritter, 2016).

PBS Consequence Strategies

This section does not represent a separate intervention, as the interventions that comprise Consequence Strategies are all described above, though we wanted to add this section just to represent the PBS framework of Prevention Strategies, Replacement Strategies, and Consequence Strategies. Consequence Strategies include making sure that the anxious behavior or problem behavior is not effective, meaning that we do not reinforce the person's anxious behavior or problem behavior, and that we reinforce alternative skills or "positive" behaviors (e.g., approach behavior) instead. Essentially, the rewards for positive behavior should exceed (or at least be equal to) the rewards for engaging in anxious behavior or problem behavior. Consequences strategies include *positive reinforcement* (delivering reinforcement contingent upon approaching the anxiety-producing stimulus or remaining in a feared situation), *differential reinforcement* (differentially reinforcing non-anxious behavior over anxious behavior, meaning heavily reinforcing brave/non-anxious behaviors while withholding or delaying reinforcement for anxious behaviors), and *extinction* (withholding reinforcement following anxious behavior), all of which were discussed above.

Conclusion

The purpose of this chapter was to serve as a guide for clinicians working with individuals with ASD and comorbid anxiety. We discussed multi-method assessment and evidence-based interventions for anxiety in individuals with ASD. In conclusion, we want to emphasize three points that researchers and practitioners should consider and focus on in the future: (1) the dearth of literature on assessment and treatment of anxiety in *adults* with ASD; (2) the lack of treatment research on individuals with ASD (of all ages) who have *comorbid ID*; and (3) the importance of *individualizing* assessment and treatment. Regarding the third point, Wood *et al.* (2009) noted that the structured, linear format of group therapy (and manualized CBT) may limit the ability to match intervention techniques to the individual characteristics of a child with ASD. They further state that, given the heterogeneity of phenotypes in ASD (and, most likely, the related heterogeneity in underlying pathology), individualized interventions tailored to a child's specific characteristics may be particularly effective.

Moreover, given the heterogeneity of setting events and antecedents of fearful/anxious behavior and the different functions of such behavior, as well as given the idiosyncratic fears that individuals with ASD possess and the idiosyncratic ways in which they express their fear and anxiety, individualized treatments tailored to each specific person with ASD will likely be the most helpful.

In sum, recognizing anxiety in individuals with ASD can help parents, teachers, practitioners, and researchers to view or perceive problem behavior as stemming from anxiety rather than oppositionality, non-compliance, disobedience, or defiance. More important, as noted by Moskowitz *et al.* (2017b), identifying anxiety in individuals with ASD can help to inform treatment in terms of preventing problem behavior before it occurs, and reducing anxiety or teaching the person to cope with anxiety when it does occur.

References

Bandura, A. (1988). Self-efficacy conception of anxiety. *Anxiety, Stress, and Coping, 1,* 77–98.

Barlow, D. H. (2000). Unraveling the mysteries of anxiety and its disorders from the perspective of emotion theory. *American Psychologist, 55,* 1247–1263.

Birmaher, B., Brent, D. A., Chiappetta, L., Bridge, J., Monga, S., and Baugher, M. (1999). Psychometric properties of the Screen for Child Anxiety Related Emotional Disorders Scale (SCARED): A replication study. *Journal of the American Academy of Child and Adolescent Psychiatry, 38,* 1230–1236.

Bouvet, C., and Coulet, A. (2016). Relaxation therapy and anxiety, self-esteem, and emotional regulation among adults with intellectual disabilities: A randomized controlled trial. *Journal of Intellectual Disabilities, 20,* 228–240.

Brown, T. A., Di Nardo, P. A., and Barlow, D. H. (1994). *Anxiety Disorders Interview Schedule for DSM-IV (ADIS-IV)*. San Antonio, TX: Psychological Corporation.

Cachia, R. L., Anderson, A., and Moore, D. W. (2016). Mindfulness in individuals with autism spectrum disorder: A systematic review and narrative analysis. *Review Journal of Autism and Developmental Disorders, 3,* 165–178.

Cale, S. I., Carr, E. G., Blakeley-Smith, A., and Owen-DeSchryver, J. S. (2009). Context-based assessment and intervention for problem behavior in children with autism spectrum disorder. *Behavior Modification, 33,* 707–742.

Carr, E. G., and Durand, V. M. (1985). Reducing behavior problems through functional communication training. *Journal of Applied Behavior Analysis, 18,* 111–126.

Cautela, J. (1977). *Behavior Analysis Forms for Clinical Intervention*. Champaign, IL: Research Press Co.

Chorpita, B. F., Yim, L., Moffitt, C., Umemoto, L. A., and Francis, S. E. (2000). Assessment of symptoms of DSM-IV anxiety and depression in children: A revised child anxiety and depression scale. *Behaviour Research and Therapy, 38,* 835–855.

Craske, M. G., Treanor, M., Conway, C. C., Zbozinek, T., and Vervliet, B. (2014). Maximizing exposure therapy: An inhibitory learning approach. *Behaviour Research and Therapy, 58,* 10–23.

Dadds, M. R., Rapee, R. M., and Barrett, P. M. (1994) Behavioral observation. In T. H. Ollendick, N. J. King, and W. Yule (Eds.), *International Handbook of Phobic and Anxiety Disorders in Children and Adolescents. Issues in Clinical Child Psychology*. Boston, MA: Springer.

Dettmer, S., Simpson, R. L., Myles, B. S., and Ganz, J. B. (2000). The use of visual supports to facilitate transitions of students with autism. *Focus on Autism and Other Developmental Disabilities, 15,* 163–169.

Dunlap, G., Strain, P. S., Lee, J. K., Joseph, J. D., Vatland, C., and Fox, L. (2017). *Prevent, Teach, Reinforce for Families: A Model of Individualized Positive Behavior Support for Home and Community.* Baltimore, MD: Paul H. Brookes Publishing Co.

Durand, V. M., and Hieneman, M. (2008). *Helping Parents with Challenging Children: Positive Family Intervention Parent Workbook.* New York, NY: Oxford University Press.

Ehrenreich-May, J., Storch, E. A., Queens, A. H., Rodriguez, J. H., Ghilain, C. S., Alessandri, M., ... Wood, J. J. (2014). An open trial of cognitive-behavioral therapy for anxiety disorders in adolescents with autism spectrum disorders. *Focus on Autism and Other Developmental Disabilities, 29,* 145–155.

Flannery, B., and Horner, R. H. (1994). The relationship between predictability and problem behavior for students with severe disabilities. *Journal of Behavioral Education, 4,* 157–176.

Florez, I. A., and Bethay, J. S. (2017). Using adapted dialectical behavioral therapy to treat challenging behaviors, emotional dysregulation, and generalized anxiety disorder in an individual with mild intellectual disability. *Clinical Case Studies, 16*(3), 200–215. https://doi.org/10.1177/1534650116687073.

Gillott, A., and Standen, P. J. (2007). Levels of anxiety and sources of stress in adults with autism. *Journal of Intellectual Disabilities, 11,* 359–370.

Goodwin, M. S., Velicer, W. F., and Intille, S. S. (2008). Telemetric monitoring in the behavior sciences. *Behavior Research Methods, 40,* 328–341.

Gray, C. A., and Garand, J. D. (1993). Social stories: Improving responses of student with autism with accurate social information. *Focus on Autistic Behavior, 8,* 1–10.

Grillon, C. (2008). Models and mechanisms of anxiety: Evidence from startle studies. *Psychopharmacology, 199,* 421–437.

Groden, J., Diller, A., Bausman, M., Velicer, W., Norman, G., and Cautela, J. (2001). The development of a stress survey schedule for persons with autism and other developmental disabilities. *Journal of Autism and Developmental Disorders, 31,* 207–217.

Gut, D. M., and Safran, S. P. (2002). Cooperative learning and social stories: Effective social skills strategies for reading teachers. *Reading and Writing Quarterly, 18,* 87–91.

Hagopian, L. P., and Jennett, H. K. (2008). Behavioral assessment and treatment of anxiety in individuals with intellectual disabilities. *Journal of Developmental and Physical Disabilities, 20,* 467–483.

Hagopian, L. P., and Jennett, H. K. (2014). Behavioral assessment and treatment for anxiety for those with autism spectrum disorder. In T. Davis, S. White, and T. Ollendick (Eds.), *Handbook of Autism and Anxiety.* Cham: Springer.

Hagopian, L. P., Lilly, M., and Davis, T. E. (2017). Behavioral treatments for anxiety in minimally verbal children with ASD. In C. M. Kerns, P. Renno, E. A. Storch, P. C. Kendall, and J. J. Wood (Eds.), *Anxiety in Children and Adolescents with Autism Spectrum Disorder: Evidence-Based Assessment and Treatment.* Amsterdam: Elsevier.

Hartley, S. L., and MacLean, W. E. (2006). A review of the reliability and validity of Likert-type scales for people with intellectual disability. *Journal of Intellectual Disability Research, 50,* 813–826.

Helverschou, S. B., and Martinsen, H. (2011). Anxiety in people diagnosed with autism and intellectual disability: Recognition and phenomenology. *Research in Autism Spectrum Disorders, 5,* 377–387.

Idusohan-Moizer, S., Sawicka, A., Dendle, J., and Albany, M. (2015). Mindfulness-based cognitive therapy for adults with intellectual disabilities: An evaluation of the effectiveness of mindfulness in reducing symptoms of depression and anxiety. *Journal of Intellectual Disability Research, 59*(2), 93–104.

Izard, C. E., Dougherty, L. M., and Hembree, E. A. (1989). *A System for Identifying Affect Expressions by Holistic Judgements (Affex).* Newark, DE: University of Delaware.

Jacobson, E. (1938). *Progressive Relaxation.* Chicago, IL: University of Chicago Press.

Jennett, H., and Hagopian, L. P. (2008). Identifying empirically supported treatments for phobic avoidance in individuals with intellectual disabilities. *Behavior Therapy, 39,* 151–161.

Joyce, C., Honey, E., Leekam, S. R., Barrett, S. L., and Rodgers, J. (2017). Anxiety, intolerance of uncertainty and restricted and repetitive behaviour: Insights directly from young people with ASD. *Journal of Autism and Developmental Disorders, 47,* 3789–3802.

Kaufman, J., Birmaher, B., Brent, D. A., Rao, U., Flynn, C., Moreci, P., ... Ryan, N. (1997). Schedule for affective disorders and schizophrenia for school-age children-present and lifetime version (K-SADS-PL): Initial reliability and validity data. *Journal of the American Academy of Child and Adolescent Psychiatry, 36*, 980–988.

Keehn, R. H. M., Lincoln, A. J., Brown, M. Z., and Chavira, D. A. (2013). The Coping Cat Program for children with anxiety and autism spectrum disorder: A pilot randomized controlled trial. *Journal of Autism and Developmental Disorders, 43*, 57–67.

Kendall, P. C., Robin, J. A., Hedtke, K. A., Suveg, C., Flannery-Schroeder, E., and Gosch, E. (2005). Considering CBT with anxious youth? Think exposures. *Cognitive and Behavioral Practice, 12*, 136–150.

Kerns, C. M., Kendall, P. C., Berry, L., Souders, M. C., Franklin, M. E., Schultz, R. T., ... Herrington, J. (2014a). Traditional and atypical presentations of anxiety in youth with autism spectrum disorder. *Journal of Autism and Developmental Disorders, 44*, 2851.

Kerns, C. M., Renno, P., Kendall, P. C., Wood, J. J., and Storch, E. A. (2014b). Anxiety disorders interview schedule – autism addendum: Reliability and validity in children with autism spectrum disorder. *Journal of Clinical Child and Adolescent Psychology, 46*, 88–100.

Kerns, C. M., Kendall, P. C., Zickgraf, H., Franklin, M. E., Miller, J., and Herrington, J. (2015). Not to be overshadowed or overlooked: Functional impairments associated with comorbid anxiety disorders in youth with ASD. *Behavior Therapy, 46*, 29–39.

Kerns, C. M., Roux, A. M., Connell, J. E., and Shattuck, P. T. (2016a). Adapting cognitive behavioral techniques to address anxiety and depression in cognitively able emerging adults on the autism spectrum. *Cognitive and Behavioral Practice, 23*, 329–340.

Kerns, C. M., Rump, K., Worley, J., Kratz, H., McVey, A., Herrington, J., and Miller, J. (2016b). The differential diagnosis of anxiety disorders in cognitively-able youth with autism. *Cognitive and Behavioral Practice, 23*, 530–547.

Kiep, M., Spek, A. A., and Hoeben, L. (2015). Mindfulness-based therapy in adults with autism spectrum disorder: Do treatment effects last? *Mindfulness, 6*, 637–644.

Koegel, R. L., Openden, D., and Koegel, L. K. (2004). A systematic desensitization paradigm to treat hypersensitivity to auditory stimuli in children with autism in family contexts. *Research and Practice for Persons with Severe Disabilities, 29*, 122–134.

Kokina, A., and Kern, L. (2010). Social story interventions for students with autism spectrum disorders: A meta-analysis. *Journal of Autism and Developmental Disabilities, 40*, 812–826.

Kuhn, C., Aebi, M., Jakobsen, H., Banaschewski, T., Poustka, L., Grimmer, Y., ... Steinhausen, H. (2017). Effective mental health screening in adolescents: Should we collect data from youth, parents, or both? *Child Psychiatry and Human Development, 48*, 385–392.

Lang, R., Regester, A., Lauderdale, S., Ashbaugh, K., and Haring, A. (2010). Treatment of anxiety in autism spectrum disorders using cognitive behaviour therapy: A systematic review. *Developmental Neurorehabilitation, 13*, 53–63.

Lesniak-Karpiak, K., Mazzocco, M. M., and Ross, J. L. (2003). Behavioral assessment of social anxiety in females with Turner or Fragile X Syndrome. *Journal of Autism and Developmental Disorders, 33*, 55–67.

Linehan, M. M. (2014). *DBT Skills Training Manual* (2nd ed.). New York, NY: Guilford Press.

Love, S. R., Matson, J. L., and West, D. (1990). Mothers as effective therapists for autistic children's phobias. *Journal of Applied Behavior Analysis, 23*, 379–385.

Lovibond, P. F., and Lovibond, S. H. (1995). The structure of negative emotional states: Comparison of the depression anxiety stress scales (DASS) with the Beck depression and anxiety inventories. *Behaviour Research and Therapy, 33*, 335–343.

Lucyshyn, J. M., Albin, R. W., Horner, R. H., Mann, J. C., and Wadsworth, G. (2007). Family implementation of positive behavior support for a child with autism: Longitudinal, single-case, experimental, and descriptive replication and extension. *Journal of Positive Behavior Interventions, 9*, 131–150.

Luscre, D. M., and Center, D. B. (1996). Procedures for reducing dental fear in children with autism. *Journal of Autism and Developmental Disorders, 26*, 547–556.

Mace, A. B., Shapiro, E. S., and Mace, F. C. (1998). Effects of warning stimuli for reinforcer withdrawal and task onset on self-injury. *Journal of Applied Behavior Analysis, 31*, 679.

March, J. S., Parker, J. D. A., Sullivan, K., Stallings, P., and Conners, K. (1997). The multidimensional anxiety scale for children (MASC): Factor structure, reliability, and validity. *Journal of the American Academy of Child and Adolescent Psychiatry, 36*, 554–565.

Maskey, M., Rodgers, J., Ingham, B., Freeston, M., Evans, G., Labus, M., and Parr, J. R. (2019). Using virtual reality environments to augment cognitive behavioral therapy for fears and phobias in autistic adults. *Autism in Adulthood, 1*, 134–145.

Mazefsky, C. A., and White, S. W. (2014). Emotion regulation: Concepts and practice in autism spectrum disorder. *Child Adolescent Psychiatric Clinics of North America, 23*, 15–24.

McVey, A. J., Dolan, B. K., Willar, K. S., Pleiss, S., Karst, J. S., *et al.* (2016). A replication and extension of PEERS for young adults social skills intervention: Examining effects on social skills and social anxiety in young adults with autism spectrum disorder. *Journal of Autism and Developmental Disorders, 46*(12), 3739–3754.

Mineka, S., Cook, M., and Miller, S. (1984). Fear conditioned with escapable and inescapable shock: Effects of a feedback stimulus. *Journal of Experimental Psychology: Animal Behavior Processes, 10*, 307–323.

Moree, B. N., and Davis, T. E. (2010). Cognitive-behavioral therapy for anxiety in children diagnosed with autism spectrum disorders: Modification trends. *Research in Autism Spectrum Disorders, 4*, 346–354.

Moskowitz, L. J., Mulder, E., Walsh, C., McLaughlin, D. M., Zarcone, J., Hajcak, G., and Carr, E. G. (2013). A multimethod assessment of anxiety and problem behavior in children with autism spectrum disorders and intellectual disability. *American Journal on Intellectual and Developmental Disabilities, 118*, 419–434.

Moskowitz, L. J., and Ritter, A. B. (2016). Assessment and intervention for self-injurious behavior related to anxiety. In S. M. Edelson and J. Johnson (Eds.), *Understanding and Treating Self-Injurious Behavior in Autism: A Multidisciplinary Perspective.* London: Jessica Kingsley Publishers.

Moskowitz, L. J., Rosen, T., Lerner, M. D., and Levine, K. (2017a). Assessment of anxiety in youth with autism spectrum disorder. In C. Kerns, E. Storch, P. Kendall, J. J. Wood, and P. Renno (Eds.), *Evidence Based Assessment and Treatment of Anxiety in Children and Adolescents with Autism Spectrum Disorder.* London: Academic Press.

Moskowitz, L. J., Walsh, C. E., Mulder, E., Magito McLaughlin, D., Hajcak, G., Carr, E. G., and Zarcone, J. R. (2017b). Intervention for anxiety and problem behavior in children with autism spectrum disorder and intellectual disability. *Journal of Autism and Developmental Disorders, 47*, 3930–3948.

Moskowitz, L. J., Braconnier, M. L., and Jeffay, M. (2019). Anxiety and phobias in individuals with intellectual disabilities. In J. L. Matson (Ed.), *Handbook of Intellectual Disabilities: Integrating Theory, Research, and Practice.* Cham: Springer International Publishing.

Moss, S., Prosser, H., Costello, H., Simpson, N., Patel, P., Rowe, S., … Hatton, C. (1998). Reliability and validity of the PAS-ADD Checklist for detecting psychiatric disorders in adults with intellectual disability. *Journal of Intellectual Disability Research, 42*, 173–183.

Mullins, J. L., and Christian, L. (2001). The effects of progressive relaxation training on the disruptive behavior of a boy with autism. *Research in Developmental Disabilities, 22*, 449–462.

Nah, Y., Brewer, N., Young, R. L., and Flower, R. (2018). Brief report: Screening adults with autism spectrum disorder for anxiety and depression. *Journal of Autism and Developmental Disorders, 48*, 1841–1846.

Neil, N., Vause, T., Jaksic, H., and Feldman, M. (2017). Effects of group functional behavior based cognitive-behavioral therapy for obsessive-compulsive behavior in a youth with autism spectrum disorder. *Child and Family Behavior Therapy, 39*, 179–190.

Poppen, R. (1988). *Behavioral Relaxation Training and Assessment.* Elmford, NY: Pergamon.

Rapp, J. T., Vollmer, T. R., and Hovanetz, A. (2005). Evaluation and treatment of swimming pool avoidance exhibited by an adolescent girl with autism. *Behavior Therapy, 36*, 101–105.

Reaven, J. A., Blakeley-Smith, A., Nichols, S., Dasari, S., Flanigan, E., and Hepburn, S. (2009). Cognitive-behavioral group treatment for anxiety symptoms in children with high-functioning autism spectrum disorders: A pilot study. *Focus on Autism and Other Developmental Disabilities, 24*, 27–37.

Reaven, J. A., Blakeley-Smith, A., Nichols, S., and Hepburn, S. (2011). *Facing Your Fears: Group Therapy for Managing Anxiety in Children with High-Functioning Autism Spectrum Disorders.* Baltimore, MD: Paul H. Brookes Publishing Co.

Reaven, J., Blakeley-Smith, A., Culhane-Shelburne, K., and Hepburn, S. (2012). Group cognitive behavior therapy for children with high-functioning autism spectrum disorders and anxiety: A randomized trial. *Journal of Child Psychology and Psychiatry, 53*, 410–419.

Richards, C., Moss, J., O'Farrell, L., Kaur, G., and Oliver, C. (2009). Social anxiety in Cornelia de Lange Syndrome. *Journal of Autism and Developmental Disorders, 39*, 1155–1162.

Rodgers, J. (2018, February 22). Anxiety in autistic people. Retrieved from https://network.autism.org.uk/good-practice/evidence-base/anxiety-autistic-people.

Rodgers, J., Wigham, S., McConachie, H., Freeston, M., Honey, E., and Parr, J. R. (2016). Development of the anxiety scale for children with autism spectrum disorder (ASC-ASD). *Autism Research, 9*, 1205–1215.

Rodgers, J., Hodgson, A., Shields, K., Wright, C., Honey, E., and Freeston, M. (2017). Towards a treatment for intolerance of uncertainty in people with autism spectrum disorder: Development of the coping with uncertainty in everyday situations programme. *Journal of Autism and Developmental Disorders, 47*, 3959–3966.

Rosen, T. E., Connell, J. E., and Kerns, C. M. (2016). A review of behavioral interventions for anxiety-related behaviors in lower-functioning individuals with autism. *Behavioral Interventions, 31*, 120–143.

Scahill, L., Lecavalier, L., Schultz, R. T., Evans, A. N., Maddox, B., Pritchett, J., … Edwards, M. C. (2019). Development of the parent-rated anxiety scale for youth with autism spectrum disorder. *Journal of the American Academy of Child and Adolescent Psychiatry, 58*, 887–896.

Schmidt, J. D., Luiselli, J. K., Rue, H., and Whalley, K. (2013). Graduated exposure and positive reinforcement to overcome setting and activity avoidance in an adolescent with autism. *Behavior Modification, 37*, 128–142.

Schreibman, L., Whalen, C., and Stahmer, A. C. (2000). The use of video priming to reduce disruptive transition behavior in children with autism. *Journal of Positive Behavior Interventions, 2*, 3–11.

Sheehan, D. V., Lecrubier, Y., Sheehan, K. H., Amorim, P., Janavs, J., Weiller, E., … Dunbar, G. C. (1998). The Mini-International Neuropsychiatric Interview (M.I.N.I): The development and validation of a structured diagnostic psychiatric interview for DSM-IV and ICD-10. *The Journal of Clinical Psychiatry, 59*, 22–33.

Shogren, K. A., Faggella-Luby, M. N., Jik Bae, S., and Wehmeyer, M. L. (2004). The effect of choice-making as an intervention for problem behavior: A meta-analysis. *Journal of Positive Behavior Interventions, 6*, 228–237.

Silverman, W. K., and Albano, A. M. (1996). *The Anxiety Disorders Interview Schedule for DSM-IV: Child and Parent Versions*. San Antonio, TX: Psychological Corporation.

Singh, N. N., Lancioni, G. E., Manikam, R., Winton, A. S. W., Singh, A. N. A., Singh, J., and Singh, A. D. A. (2011a). A mindfulness-based strategy for self-management of aggressive behavior in adolescents with autism. *Research in Autism Spectrum Disorders, 5*, 1153–1158.

Singh, N. N., Lancioni, G. E., Singh, A. D. A., Winton, A. S. W., Singh, A. N. A., and Singh, J. (2011b). Adolescents with Asperger syndrome can use mindfulness-based strategy to control their aggressive behavior. *Research in Autism Spectrum Disorders, 5*, 1103–1109.

Sizoo, B. B. and Kuiper, E. (2017). Cognitive behavioural therapy and mindfulness based stress reduction may be equally effective in reducing anxiety and depression in adults with autism spectrum disorders. *Research in Developmental Disabilities, 64*, 47–55. https://doi:10.1016/j.ridd.2017.03.004.

Spek, A., van Ham, N., and Nyklicke, I. (2013) Mindfulness-based therapy in adults with an autism spectrum disorder: A randomized controlled trial. *Research in Developmental Disabilities, 34*, 246–253.

Storch, E. A., Arnold, E. B., Lewin, A. B., Nadeau, J. M., Jones, A. M., De Nadai, A. S., … Murphy, T. K. (2013). The effect of cognitive-behavioral therapy versus treatment as usual for anxiety in children with autism spectrum disorders: A randomized, controlled trial. *Journal of the American Academy of Child and Adolescent Psychiatry, 52*, 132–142.

Storch, E. A., Wood, J. J., Ehrenreich-May, J., Jones, A. M., Park, J. M., Lewin, A. B., and Murphy, T. K. (2012). Convergent and discriminant validity and reliability of the pediatric anxiety rating scale in youth with autism spectrum disorders. *Journal of Autism and Developmental Disorders, 42*, 2374–2382.

Storch, E. A., Lewin, A. B., Collier, A. B., Arnold, E., De Nadi, A. S., Dane, B. F., … Murphy, T. K. (2014). A randomized controlled trial of cognitive-behavioral therapy versus treatment as usual for adolescents with autism spectrum disorders and comorbid anxiety. *Depression and Anxiety, 32*, 174–181.

Sullivan, K., Hooper, S., and Hatton, D. (2007). Behavioural equivalents of anxiety in children with fragile X syndrome: parent and teacher report. *Journal of Intellectual Disability Research, 51*, 54–64.

Uljarevic, M., Richdale, A. L., McConachie, H., Hedley, D., Cai, R. Y., Merrick, H., ... Le Couteur, A. (2018). The hospital anxiety and depression scale: Factor structure and psychometric properties in older adolescents and young adults with autism spectrum disorder. *Autism Research, 11*, 258–269.

Ung, D., Selles, R., Small, B. J., and Storch, E. A. (2015). A systematic review and meta-analysis of cognitive-behavioral therapy for anxiety in youth with high-functioning autism spectrum disorders. *Child Psychiatry and Human Development, 46*, 533–547.

van Steensel, F. J. A., and Bogels, S. M. (2015). CBT for anxiety disorders in children with and without autism spectrum disorders. *Journal of Consulting and Clinical Psychology, 83*, 512–523.

Velting, O. N., Setzer, N. J., and Albano, A. M. (2004). Update on and advances in assessment and cognitive-behavioral treatment of anxiety disorders in children and adolescents. *Professional Psychology: Research and Practice, 35*, 42–54.

Walters, S., Loades, M., and Russell, A. (2016). A systematic review of effective modifications to cognitive behavioural therapy for young people with autism spectrum disorders. *Review Journal of Autism and Developmental Disorders, 3*, 137–153.

White, S. W., Oswald, D., Ollendick, T., and Scahill, L. (2009). Anxiety in children and adolescents with autism spectrum disorders. *Clinical Psychology Review, 29*, 216–229.

White, S. W., Albano, A. M., Johnson, C. R., Kasari, C., Ollendick, T., Klin, A., ... Scahill, L. (2010). Development of a cognitive-behavioral intervention program to treat anxiety and social deficits in teens with high-functioning autism. *Clinical Child and Family Psychology Review, 13*, 77–90.

White, S. W., Ollendick, T., Albano, A. M., Oswald, D., Johnson, C., Southam-Gerow, M., Kim, I., and Scahill, L. (2013). Randomized controlled trial: Multimodal Anxiety and Social Skill Intervention for Adolescents with Autism Spectrum Disorder. *Journal of Autism and Developmental Disorders, 43*, 382–294.

Wilde, L. D., Koegel, L. K., and Koegel, R. L. (1992). *Increasing Success in School through Priming: A Training Manual.* Santa Barbara, CA: University of California.

Wise, J. M., Cepeda, S. L., Ordaz, D. L., McBride, N., Cavitt, M. A., Howie, F. R., ... Storch, E. A. (2019). Open trial of modular cognitive-behavioral therapy in the treatment of anxiety among late adolescents with autism spectrum disorder. *Child Psychiatry and Human Development, 50*, 27–34.

Wolff, J. J., and Symons, F. J. (2013). An evaluation of multi-component exposure treatment of needle phobia in an adult with autism and intellectual disability. *Journal of Applied Research in Intellectual Disabilities, 26*, 344–348.

Wolpe, J. (1958). *Psychotherapy by Reciprocal Inhibition.* Stanford, CA: Stanford University Press.

Wood, J. J., Drahota, A., Sze, K., Har, K., Chiu, A., and Langer, D. A. (2009). Cognitive behavioral therapy for anxiety in children with autism spectrum disorders: A randomized, controlled trial. *The Journal of Child Psychology and Psychiatry, 50*, 224–234.

Wood, J. J., Ehrenreich-May, J., Alessandri, M., Fujii, C., Renno, P., Laugeson, E., ... Storch, E. A. (2015). Cognitive behavioral therapy for early adolescents with autism spectrum disorders and clinical anxiety: A randomized, controlled trial. *Behavior Therapy, 46*, 7.

COMPREHENSIVE LIST OF BEHAVIORAL INDICATORS OF ANXIETY

Physical/Physiological Symptoms Associated with Anxiety	Present	Absent
Rigidity or tenseness (visible muscle tension or stiffness)		
Hyperventilating, heavy breathing, rapid breathing, gasping		
Sweating or perspiration		
Flushed face or neck		
Trembling or shaking		
Lips clenched		
Lips quivering		
Behaviors associated with anxiety	Present	Absent
Withdrawal/avoidance		
Cowering		
Pacing		
Freezing		
Fidgeting		
Twitching or jerky/jumpy movements		
Frowning (turning down of mouth)		
Eyebrows raised in inverted V shape		
Tears		
Rapid clenching and unclenching of fists		
Avoiding eye contact		
Difficulty maintaining eye contact (e.g., eyes rapidly darting back and forth)		
Unusual movements (e.g., eye blinking, twitching, lip licking, head jerking)		

Behaviors associated with anxiety	Present	Absent
Unusual vocal sounds (e.g., coughing, throat clearing, sniffling, grunting)		
Picking or scratching (e.g., picks nose, skin, or other parts of body)		
Hand-wringing		
Teeth-grinding		
Compulsions (i.e., repeats certain acts, words, phrases, sentences, or movements over and over)		
Talking, singing, or vocalizing excessively (more than usual)		
Talking, singing, or vocalizing too loudly (more than usual) or for longer than usual		
Escalation (movements or vocalizations increase in volume, speed, or intensity)		
Stuttering or dysfluent speech, such as repetitions, interjections, pauses/blocks, or revisions		
Reassurance-seeking		

ANXIETY RATING SCALE

Please rate this child's anxiety by choosing the number that best described his state of anxiety in the activity you just observed.

0 No anxiety (i.e., comfortable)	1 Mild anxiety	2 Moderate anxiety	3 High anxiety
Absence of any apparent anxiety relating to the stimulus or situation.	The child displayed symptoms of anxiety—such as rigidity or tenseness (visible muscle tension), heavy or rapid breathing, freezing, flushed face, and trembling—to a **mild** degree, but these symptoms did not significantly interfere with the activity.	The child displayed symptoms of anxiety—such as pulling/pushing away from the stimulus, cling to parent, cowering, rigidity or tenseness (visible muscle tension), heavy or rapid breathing, freezing, flushed face, trembling or shaking, tearfulness (eyes tearing or watering)—to a **moderate** degree, to the extent that he could *rarely* participate, play, or interact appropriately.	The child exhibited symptoms of anxiety—such as crying, sobbing, or screaming, running away from the stimulus or situation, pulling/pushing away from the stimulus, clinging to parent, cowering, trembling or shaking, freezing, rigidity or tenseness (visible muscle tension), heavy or rapid breathing, and flushed face—to a **high** degree, to the extent that he could *not* participate, play, or interact appropriately.

0 No anxiety (i.e., comfortable)	1 Mild anxiety	2 Moderate anxiety	3 High anxiety
The child appeared to be relaxed, engaged happily in typical play and interactions, and unaffected by the presence of the stimulus or situation.	The child *occasionally* displayed an anxious or fearful facial expression (e.g., lips stretched back, tensing of lower eyelid, furrowing of brow and eye areas, eyebrows brought together somewhat) or mild apprehension expression (e.g., eyebrow somewhat raised and pulled together in an inverted V shape)	The child *frequently* displayed an anxious or fearful facial expression (e.g., eyebrows raised and drawn together in an inverted V shape, wide open eyes, stretched lips).	The child *constantly* displayed an anxious or fearful facial expression (e.g., eyebrows raised and drawn together in an inverted V shape, wide open eyes, stretched lips).

TABLE OF EVIDENCE-BASED INTERVENTIONS

Evidence-based Intervention	Description	Treatment Study Examples	
		Children	Adults
In vivo/ Imaginal exposure	Confronting the feared stimulus or situation, either real (in vivo exposure) or imagined (imaginal exposure)		Maskey *et al.* (2019)
Hierarchy	Breaking down the task of approaching or engaging with the feared stimulus or situation into small steps with gradual increases in response requirements		
Contingent reinforcement	Providing the individual with some type of positive reinforcement contingent upon approaching the feared stimulus, engaging in a feared activity, or remaining in a feared situation without engaging in a problem behavior		
Prompting	Presenting an antecedent stimulus (physical, verbal, or sensory) to initiate a response		
Modeling	Observing another person confronting the feared situation or interacting successfully with the feared stimulus		McVey *et al.* (2016)
Extinction/ Blocking	Preventing the person from escaping the anxiety-provoking situation		

Evidence-based Intervention	Description	Treatment Study Examples	
		Children	Adults
Increasing predictability	Increasing predictability in anxiety-provoking situations using advanced warnings, individualized narratives, and priming		
Providing choices	Allowing individuals to choose activities and reinforcers		
Perseverative interests	Pairing the anxiety-provoking situation with stimuli/activities that incorporate the person's perseverative interests or obsessions		
Cognitive behavioral therapy	Providing therapy that focuses on the connection between thoughts, feelings and behaviors, usually involving graduated exposure, psychoeducation, cognitive restructuring, somatic management, and relapse prevention	Wise *et al.* (2019)	Sizoo and Kuiper (2017)
Relaxation	Instructing the person on techniques to reduce anxiety, including deep breathing and progressive muscle relaxation		
Acceptance-based therapy/ Mindfulness-based therapy/ Dialectical behavioral therapy	Providing therapy that focuses on radical acceptance of one's thoughts and oneself		Idusohan-Moizer *et al.* (2015); Florez and Bethay (2017); Sizoo and Kuiper (2017); Spek *et al.* (2013); Kiep *et al.* (2015)

JANE'S FEAR STAIRCASE FOR THUNDER AND LIGHTNING

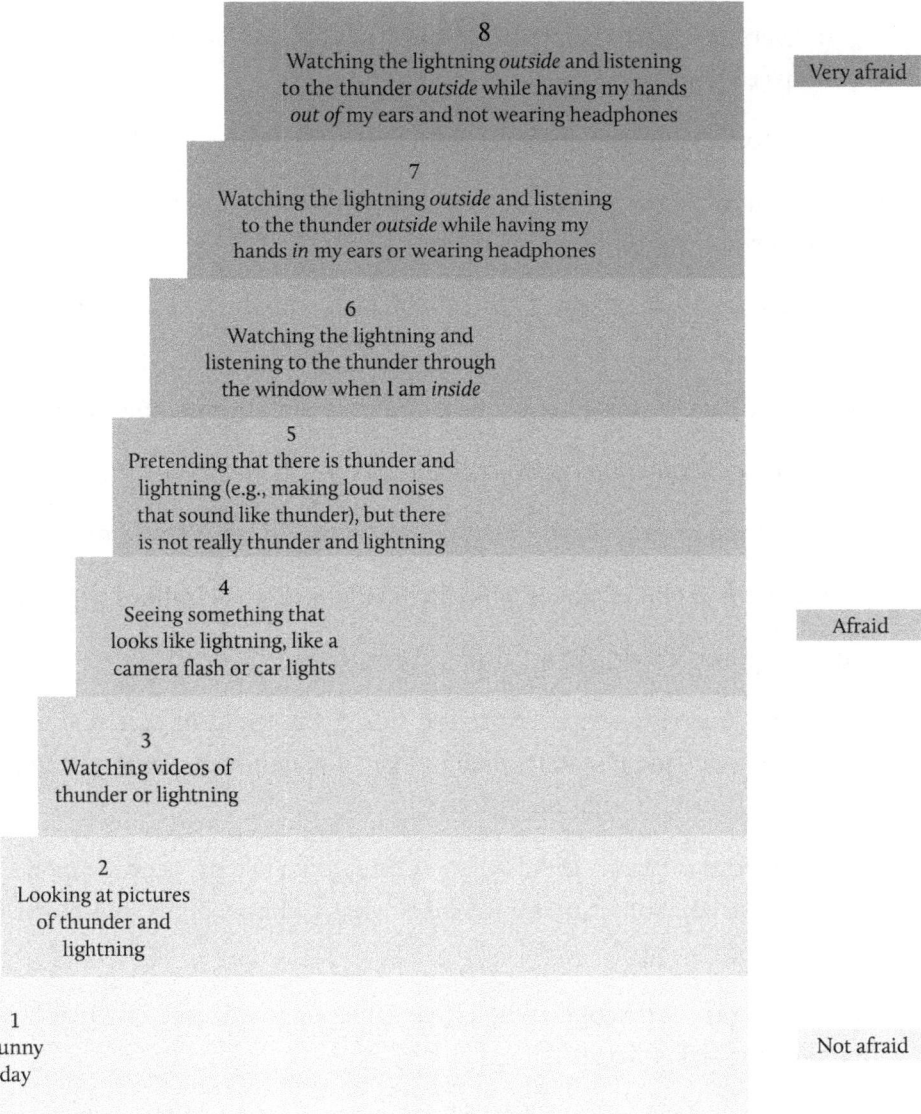

8
Watching the lightning *outside* and listening to the thunder *outside* while having my hands *out of* my ears and not wearing headphones

Very afraid

7
Watching the lightning *outside* and listening to the thunder *outside* while having my hands *in* my ears or wearing headphones

6
Watching the lightning and listening to the thunder through the window when I am *inside*

5
Pretending that there is thunder and lightning (e.g., making loud noises that sound like thunder), but there is not really thunder and lightning

4
Seeing something that looks like lightning, like a camera flash or car lights

Afraid

3
Watching videos of thunder or lightning

2
Looking at pictures of thunder and lightning

1
Sunny day

Not afraid

SOCIAL STORIES

Ed's Social Story

- Pg. 1: Everyone feels worried or afraid or anxious sometimes—kids and grownups too. (pictures)

- It is okay to feel worried or afraid or anxious sometimes.

- Pg. 2: If a lion is chasing you, it is okay to feel afraid, because your fear will make you run from the lion! (picture)

- Pg. 3: There are some things I'm afraid of and some things I am not afraid of. (picture)

- Some other kids are afraid of thunderstorms and lightning. (picture)

- Some kids are afraid of dogs. (picture)

- I am not afraid of thunderstorms and lightning. I am not afraid of dogs.

- Pg. 4: I am a little bit afraid of going up a ladder or a tall building. (pictures)

- I am very afraid of flying in an airplane. (picture)

- Pg. 5: I am very, very afraid of getting sick. I am afraid of catching a virus, throwing up, getting a sore throat, and getting asthma. I am afraid that if I breathe really fast, I might die. (picture)

- Pg. 6: Sometimes I want to know something, like if I am healthy, or if I am going to get sick. Sometimes I REALLY want to know. This makes me feel bad. (picture)

- Pg. 7: This worry can happen when I see someone who is sick or when I think about getting sick. (picture)

- Pg. 8: When I feel bad and anxious, I want to go find Mom and ask her a question. I might ask, "Mom, am I going to get sick?" or "Mom, is the medicine going to work?" (picture with word bubble) These thoughts are just my anxiety talking. These thoughts are not real.

- Pg. 9: So, to fight my anxiety, I will try not to ask Mom these questions. (picture with word bubble crossed out)

- Pg. 10: And to help me fight my anxiety, Mom will try NOT to answer my questions by saying, "Yes, you're healthy" or "No, you're not going to get sick." (picture with word bubble crossed out) Instead, mom will say, "That's just your anxiety talking. I can't tell you if you're going to get sick." (picture with word bubble)

- Pg. 11: Then, Mom and I can do other things together, like play or read or cook. (pictures)

- Pg. 12: So, from now on, Mom is not going to tell me that I'm not going to get sick. She is not going to tell me that because we want to fight my anxiety and beat my anxiety. (picture with word bubble crossed out)

- Pg. 13: At first, when Mom says, "I don't know" or "I can't tell you," I will feel scared. But, after a while, I will be less scared. Then, after a while longer, I won't be scared anymore. I will see that my anxiety goes down after a while, even if mom doesn't answer me.

- Pg. 14: My anxiety will go away. I will see that I'm okay, even if Mom doesn't tell me that I'm okay. (picture with word bubble)

- Pg. 15: Sometimes I need help coping with this bad feeling. So here are some things I can do when I feel anxious. When I feel worried or anxious, I can tell myself, "This is just my anxiety talking. I am not really sick." (picture)

- Pg. 16: When I feel anxiety, I can tell myself, "I may get sick, but that is okay. Even if I get sick, I will get better." (picture)

- Pg. 17: When I feel anxiety, I can distract myself and go do something else, like play Tech Deck Skateboarding or watch wrestling or play a video game. Or I can think of something funny. (pictures)

- Pg. 18: When I feel anxiety, I can breathe nice and slow while I count to ten. (picture)

- Pg. 19: This will help me feel calm. I am going to fight my anxiety and I will win!

Text of Ben's Social Story (for Separation) from Moskowitz *et al.* (2017b)

- Everyone feels worried or afraid or anxious sometimes—kids and grownups too.

- It is okay to feel worried or afraid or anxious sometimes. If a lion is chasing you, it is okay to feel afraid, because your fear will make you run from the lion!

- There are some things I'm afraid of and some things I am not afraid of. Some other kids are afraid of thunderstorms and lightning. Some kids are afraid of dogs. I am not afraid of thunder and lightning. I am not afraid of dogs.

- I am a little bit afraid of fireworks. I am very afraid of walking over railroad tracks. I am very afraid of bees.

- I am very, very afraid when Mom or Dad leave the house and go out without me.

- I am afraid because I really want to go with them. I really want Mommy and Daddy.

- But I don't have to be afraid when Mommy or Daddy leaves the house and I stay with Uncle or Grandma or Grandpa. I don't have to be afraid because Mommy and Daddy will always come back. (picture of Mommy and Daddy walking through the front door and hugging Ben)

- At first, when Mommy and Daddy leave, I will feel scared. Then, after a while longer, I will feel less scared. Then, after a while longer, I won't be scared anymore. I will see that my anxiety goes down after a while, even when Mommy and Daddy are not home.

- I don't have to be afraid. My anxiety will go away. I will see that I am okay, even if Mommy and Daddy are not home.

- When Mommy and Daddy are not home, here are some things I can do when I feel afraid.

- When I feel worried or anxious, I can tell myself, "This is just my anxiety talking. I don't have to be afraid. I am okay. I can beat my anxiety."

- When Mommy and Daddy are gone, I can tell myself, "Mommy and Daddy always come home. So I won't be afraid."

- When Mommy and Daddy are gone, I will go do something fun, like play Leapster or Math Desk, or watch a movie, like the Muppet movie.

- When Mommy and Daddy are gone and I feel afraid, I can breathe nice and slow while I count to ten. This will help me feel calm.

- So, from now on, when Mommy and Daddy go out, I am going to be brave because I want to fight my anxiety and beat my anxiety.

- I am going to fight my anxiety and I will win. (picture of Kai-Lan saying, "We can do it!")

- When Mommy and Daddy come home, they will bring me a special prize for being so brave. Mommy and Daddy will be so proud of me for being brave and staying with Uncle or Grandma or Grandpa.

Conclusion

Stephen M. Edelson, Ph.D., Autism Research Institute, California

Anxiety is a complex, largely "invisible" condition, affecting a large proportion of individuals with ASD, across all ages and across the entire spectrum. As this book demonstrates, anxiety involves numerous interacting biological systems as well as internal sensations and behavioral responses. Providing the best treatment for people on the spectrum who suffer from anxiety requires a multi-disciplinary approach that effectively addresses all of these elements.

Survey Questions

Results from a recent Autism Research Institute survey of 2328 individuals were analyzed with respect to aspects of anxiety. The responses to specific questions related to topics mentioned in this book are reported below. A Bonferroni Correction (a multiple-comparison correction used when several dependent or independent statistical tests are being performed at the same time) for multiple comparisons was calculated into the analyses.

These results should be interpreted with respect to the question raised, rather than whether or not the person experiences anxiety or nervousness. For example, the second part of Table 1 shows responses to the question, "What is the average amount of time your child sleeps in a 24-hour period?" This table shows that among those who sleep less than eight hours, 69 percent are anxious. These results should not be interpreted to mean that 69 percent of anxious individuals sleep less than eight hours.

A synopsis of the significant findings is presented following the table.

Table 1. Analyses of ASD Individuals Who Were Described as "Often Anxious or Nervous" Versus Those Who Were Not

Child's sex (N = 2150)*

Source	Often anxious or nervous		Not descriptive	
	n	%	n	%
Boy	995	55.31	804	44.69
Girl	225	64.10	126	35.90

* χ^2 = 9.25, p<.05

What is the average amount of time your child sleeps in a 24-hour period? (N = 2129)*

Source	Often anxious or nervous		Not descriptive	
	n	%	n	%
About 8 hours	480	56.47	370	43.43
Less than 8 hours	286	69.42	126	30.58
More than 8 hours	437	50.40	430	49.60

* χ^2 = 41.08, p<.05

Does your son/daughter seem depressed or sad? (N = 2105)*

Source	Often anxious or nervous		Not descriptive	
	n	%	n	%
Yes, most of the time	110	86.61	17	13.39
Yes, some of the time	562	78.71	152	21.29
No	519	41.06	745	58.94

* χ^2 = 312.91, p<.05

Sensory Processing

Covers ears at many sounds (N = 2139)*

Source	Often anxious or nervous		Not descriptive	
	n	%	n	%
Very true	446	68.20	208	31.80
True	371	58.80	260	41.20
False	395	46.25	459	53.75

* χ^2 = 62.72, p<.05

Only certain sounds seem painful to him (N = 2138)*

Source	Often anxious or nervous		Not descriptive	
	n	%	n	%
Very true	382	65.64	200	34.36
True	563	58.10	406	41.90
False	268	45.66	319	54.34

* χ^2 = 40.46, p<.05

Fails to blink at bright lights (N = 2119)*

Source	Often anxious or nervous		Not descriptive	
	n	%	n	%
Very true	93	72.66	35	27.34
True	250	59.22	170	40.48
False	857	54.55	714	45.45

* χ^2 = 17.58, p<.05

Intensely aware of odors (N = 2129)*

Source	Often anxious or nervous		Not descriptive	
	n	%	n	%
Very true	293	78.13	82	21.87
True	329	62.19	200	37.81
False	584	47.69	641	52.32

* χ^2 = 94.58, p<.05

Seems not to feel pain (N = 2136)*

Source	Often anxious or nervous		Not descriptive	
	n	%	n	%
Very true	264	63.31	153	36.70
True	433	55.30	350	44.70
False	511	54.59	425	45.41

* χ^2 = 2.61, n.s.

Gastrointestinal Distress

Constipation: Commonly experienced by your child (N = 2159)*

Source	Often anxious or nervous		Not descriptive	
	n	%	n	%
True	647	62.33	350	37.67
False	578	51.56	425	48.44

* χ^2 = 6.78, n.s.

Diarrhea: Commonly experienced by your child (N = 2159)*

Source	Often anxious or nervous		Not descriptive	
	n	%	n	%
True	418	59.54	284	40.46
False	807	55.39	350	44.61

* χ^2 = 3.33, n.s.

Challenging Behavior

How does child usually react to being interrupted at what he is doing? (N = 2127)*

Source	Often anxious or nervous		Not descriptive	
	n	%	n	%
Rarely or never gets upset	97	39.75	147	60.25
Sometimes gets mildly upset; rarely very upset	482	50.58	471	49.42
Typically gets very upset	633	68.06	297	31.94

* χ^2 = 92.09, p<.05

Does the child get very upset if certain things he is used to are changed? (N = 2129)*

Source	Often anxious or nervous		Not descriptive	
	n	%	n	%
No	325	43.05	430	56.95
Yes, definitely	500	72.78	187	27.22
Slightly true	387	56.33	300	43.67

* χ^2 = 129.84, p<.05

Is the child destructive? (N = 2129)*

Source	Often anxious or nervous		Not descriptive	
	n	%	n	%
No	275	67.73	131	32.27
Yes, this is definitely true	415	57.24	310	42.76
Not especially destructive	525	52.61	473	47.39

* χ^2 = 26.97. p<.05

Is there a problem in that the child hits, pinches, bites or otherwise injures himself or others? (N = 2131)*

Source	Often anxious or nervous		Not descriptive	
	n	%	n	%
Yes, self only	159	69.43	70	30.57
Yes, others only	198	56.73	151	43.27
Yes, self and others	287	68.33	133	31.67
No (not a problem)	569	50.22	564	49.78

* χ^2 = 57.68, p<.05

In summary, these results indicate that anxiety/nervousness occurs more often in those who:

- are female

- sleep less than eight hours

- are depressed or sad

- cover their ears at many sounds

- experience pain in response to certain sounds

- do not blink at bright lights

- are intensely aware of odors

- react unusually when interrupted

- are upset when certain things are changed

- are destructive

- injure themselves.

Interestingly, there was no significant association between anxiety/nervousness and frequent constipation or diarrhea. It is possible that many of those who completed the survey were not aware of the status of the individual's bowel movements, or that these two gastrointestinal problems were simply not common in this sample.

Commentary

Up to this point, progress in understanding and treating anxiety in individuals on the autism spectrum has been slow. To some degree, this is a result of "tunnel vision" on the part of professionals in the autism field.

Clinicians who treat individuals on the spectrum typically do not evaluate them for autonomic nervous system dysregulation, gastrointestinal problems, or sensory processing issues. Often, the treatments prescribed by clinicians or therapists depend on their background or training. Such interventions are not necessarily optimal for a specific individual. Furthermore, there is no empirical evidence indicating that a single approach or discipline is the most effective in treating anxiety for all individuals on the autism spectrum. Instead, they should understand that anxiety is a complicated issue and work in collaboration with specialists in other fields when developing an effective treatment plan.

Like their clinical peers, researchers studying anxiety in individuals with ASD rarely look outside of their own area of expertise. As a result, much of the research on the biology of autism has focused on one or at most two components of anxiety. However, as this book shows, several systems involved in anxiety are interrelated, and some of these relationships are bi-directional. The combination of these factors could be additive (i.e., sum of the parts), synergistic (i.e., greater than the sum), or even antagonistic (i.e., less than the sum). Understanding such uni- and bi-directional interactions, especially in cases where multiple biological processes are dysregulated, will provide much-needed insight into the causes of the anxiety suffered by so many individuals with ASD.

A multi-disciplinary approach to studying anxiety in ASD should include biological, cognitive, and behavioral assessments. As several authors have noted, a number of well-accepted standardized assessments tools have been adapted to evaluate individuals with ASD. Although studies that involve administering a wide range of such assessments may appear costly, these studies will provide us with a wealth of information not available from the hundreds of studies focusing on only one or two components of anxiety.

Analysis of the data obtained from numerous multi-disciplinary assessment measures could help elucidate the role of each system as well as their interactions. Besides examining various biological processes in general, statistical algorithms (or formulas) could also account for individual differences. Sensory function and observable behaviors could also be integrated into these formulas, resulting in a more in-depth understanding of anxiety in autism. This could be taken a step further by adding the prescribed treatments into the algorithms. Eventually, these analyses could be used to predict, based on likelihood, optimal treatment strategies for each individual.

This book is the second in a series on understanding and treating autism by taking a multi-disciplinary perspective. The first book, *Understanding and Treating Self-Injurious Behavior in Autism*, complements this book well, as both books approach challenging symptoms in multiple ways. Obviously, other symptoms and behaviors of concern can and should be approached using a similar multi-disciplinary perspective. These include aggression, eating problems, severe tantrums, sleeping problems, and toileting issues, as well as conditions such as depression, obsessions/compulsions, and suicidal ideation.

The multi-disciplinary approach, which is still in its infancy, may seem "eclectic"—a term used by some critics who view it merely as a miscellaneous assortment of treatments. However, continued research within each discipline, as well as collaborative research among disciplines, will eventually refine and optimize multi-disciplinary treatments for ASD and validate their effectiveness.

Currently, research on understanding and treating anxiety in individuals with ASD is not well coordinated across disciplines. Even within each discipline, the degree of collaboration is far from optimal. A network of researchers in the autism community, as well as researchers studying anxiety in other populations (for example, the general population, or individuals with depression or schizophrenia), is needed to expedite the relatively slow progress in identifying effective interventions. Establishing such a network will involve recognizing the important contributions of each discipline, organizing an efficient way to communicate within and among disciplines, and encouraging collegial collaboration. Most importantly, it will require researchers, clinicians, and therapists in the autism field to understand that *we are all in it together.*

SUBJECT INDEX

AUTHOR INDEX